BEYOND
THERAPY

For sale by the Superintendent of Documents, U.S. Government Printing Office
Internet: bookstore.gpo.gov Phone: toll free (866) 512-1800; DC area (202) 512-1800
Fax: (202) 512-2250 Mail: Stop SSOP, Washington, DC 20402-0001

ISBN 0-16-073099-6

BEYOND THERAPY

BIOTECHNOLOGY AND THE PURSUIT OF HAPPINESS

A Report by the President's Council on Bioethics

CONTENTS

MEMBERS OF
THE PRESIDENT'S COUNCIL
ON BIOETHICS

Leon R. Kass, M.D., Ph.D., Chairman
Addie Clark Harding Professor, The College and the Committee on
Social Thought, University of Chicago. Hertog Fellow, American
Enterprise Institute.

Elizabeth H. Blackburn, Ph.D.
Professor, Department of Biochemistry and Biophysics, University of
California, San Francisco.

Rebecca S. Dresser, J.D., M.S.
Daniel Noyes Kirby Professor of Law and Professor of Ethics in Medicine,
Washington University, St. Louis.

Daniel W. Foster, M.D.
Donald W. Seldin Distinguished Chair in Internal Medicine, Chairman
of the Department of Internal Medicine, University of Texas
Southwestern Medical School.

Francis Fukuyama, Ph.D.
Dean of the Faculty, Bernard L. Schwartz Professor of International
Political Economy, Paul H. Nitze School of Advanced International
Studies, Johns Hopkins University.

Michael S. Gazzaniga, Ph.D.
Dean of the Faculty, David T. McLaughlin Distinguished Professor, Professor of Psychological and Brain Sciences, Dartmouth College.

Robert P. George, J.D., D.Phil.
McCormick Professor of Jurisprudence, Director of the James Madison Program in American Ideals and Institutions, Princeton University.

Mary Ann Glendon, J.D., M.Comp.L.
Learned Hand Professor of Law, Harvard University.

Alfonso Gómez-Lobo, Dr. phil.
Ryan Family Professor of Metaphysics and Moral Philosophy, Georgetown University.

William B. Hurlbut, M.D.
Consulting Professor in Human Biology, Stanford University.

Charles Krauthammer, M.D.
Syndicated Columnist.

William F. May, Ph.D.
Fellow, Institute for Practical Ethics and Public Life. Visiting Professor, Department of Religious Studies, University of Virginia.

Paul McHugh, M.D.
University Distinguished Service Professor of Psychiatry, Johns Hopkins School of Medicine. Professor, Department of Mental Health, Bloomberg School of Public Health, Johns Hopkins University.

Gilbert C. Meilaender, Ph.D.
Phyllis & Richard Duesenberg Professor of Christian Ethics, Valparaiso University.

Janet D. Rowley, M.D.
Blum-Riese Distinguished Service Professor of Medicine, Molecular Genetics and Cell Biology, and Human Genetics, Pritzker School of Medicine, University of Chicago.

Michael J. Sandel, D.Phil.
Anne T. and Robert M. Bass Professor of Government,
Harvard University.

James Q. Wilson, Ph.D.
James A. Collins Professor of Management and Public Policy Emeritus, University of California-Los Angeles. Reagan Professor of Public Policy, Pepperdine University.

LETTER OF TRANSMITTAL
TO THE PRESIDENT

The President's Council on Bioethics
October 15, 2003

The President
The White House
Washington, D.C.

Dear Mr. President:

I am pleased to present to you Beyond Therapy: Biotechnology and the Pursuit of Happiness, a report of the President's Council on Bioethics.

The product of more than sixteen months of research, reflection, and deliberation, we hope this report will prove a worthy contribution to public understanding of the important questions it considers. In it, we have sought to live up to the charge you gave us when you created this Council, namely, "to undertake fundamental inquiry into the human and moral significance of developments in biomedical and behavioral science and technology" and "to facilitate a greater under-standing of bioethical issues."

Biotechnology offers exciting and promising prospects for healing the sick and relieving the suffering. But exactly because of their impressive powers to alter the workings of body and mind, the "dual uses" of the same technologies make them attractive also to people who are not sick but who would use them to look younger, perform better, feel happier, or become more "perfect." These applications of biotechnology are already presenting us with some unfamiliar and very difficult challenges. In this report, we consider such possible "beyond therapy" uses, and explore both their scientific basis and the ethical and social issues they are likely to raise.

We have structured our inquiry around the desires and goals of human beings, rather than around the technologies they employ, the better to keep the important ethical questions before us. In a quartet of four central chapters, we consider how pursuing the goals of better children, superior performance, ageless bodies, or happy souls might be aided or hindered, elevated or degraded, by seeking them through a wide variety of technological means.

Among the biotechnical powers considered are techniques for screening genes and testing embryos, choosing sex of children, modifying the behavior of children, augmenting muscle size and strength, enhancing athletic performance, slowing senescence, blunting painful memories, brightening mood, and altering basic temperaments. In a concluding chapter, we consider together the several "beyond therapy" uses of these technologies, in order to ask what kinds of human beings and what sort of society we might be creating in the coming age of biotechnology.

On the optimistic view, the emerging picture is one of unmitigated progress and improvement. It envisions a society in which more and more people are able to realize the American dream of liberty, prosperity, and justice for all. It is a nation whose citizens are longer-lived, more competent, better accomplished, more productive, and happier than human beings have ever been before. It is a world in which many more human beings—biologically better-equipped, aided by performance-enhancers, liberated from the constraints of nature and fortune—can live lives of achievement, contentment, and high self-esteem, come what may.

But there are reasons to wonder whether life will really be better if we turn to biotechnology to fulfill our deepest human desires. There is an old expression: to a man armed with a hammer, everything looks like a nail. To a society armed with biotechnology, the activities of human life may seem more amenable to improvement than they really are. Or we may imagine ourselves wiser than we really are. Or we may get more easily what we asked for only to realize it is much less than what we really wanted.

We want better children—but not by turning procreation into manufacture or by altering their brains to gain them an edge over their peers. We want to perform better in the activities of life—but not by becoming mere creatures of our chemists or by turning ourselves into tools designed to win or achieve in inhuman ways. We want longer lives—but not at the cost of living carelessly or shallowly with diminished aspiration for living well, and not by becoming people so obsessed with our own longevity that we care little about the next generations. We want to be happy—but not because of a drug that gives us happy feelings without the real loves, attachments, and achievements that are essential for true human flourishing.

I believe the report breaks new ground in public bioethics, by dealing with a topic not treated by previous national bioethics commissions. And it approaches the topics not on a piecemeal basis, but as elements of one large picture: life in the age of biotechnology. Beginning to paint that picture is the aim of this report. We hope, through this document, to advance the nation's awareness and understanding of a critical set of bioethical issues and to bring them beyond the narrow circle of bioethics professionals into the larger public arena, where matters of such moment rightly belong.

In enjoying the benefits of biotechnology, we will need to hold fast to an account of the human being, seen not in material or mechanistic or medical terms but in psychic and moral and spiritual ones. As we note in the Conclusion, we need to see the human person in more than therapeutic terms:

> as a creature "in-between," neither god nor beast, neither dumb body nor disembodied soul, but as a puzzling, upward-pointing unity of psyche and soma whose precise limitations are the source of its—our—loftiest aspirations, whose weaknesses are the source of its—our—keenest attachments, and whose natural gifts may be, if we do not squander or destroy them, exactly what we need to flourish and perfect ourselves—as human beings.

We close the inquiry with a lingering sense that tremendous new biotechnical powers may blind us to the larger meaning of our own

American ideals and may narrow our sense of what it is, after all, to live, to be free, and to pursue happiness.

But we are also hopeful that, by informing and moderating our desires, and by grasping the limits of our new powers, we can keep in mind the true meaning of our founding ideals—and thus find the means to savor the fruits of the age of biotechnology, without succumbing to its most dangerous temptations.

Mr. President, allow me to join my Council colleagues and our fine staff in thanking you for this opportunity to set down on paper, for your consideration and that of the American public, some (we hope useful) thoughts and reflections on these important subjects.

Sincerely,
Leon R. Kass, M.D.
Chairman

PREFACE

B*eyond Therapy: Biotechnology and the Pursuit of Happiness* is a report
by the President's Council on Bioethics, which was created by President
George W. Bush on November 28, 2001, by means of Executive Order
13237.

The Council's purpose is to advise the President on bioethical issues
related to advances in biomedical science and technology. In connection with
its advisory role, the mission of the Council includes the following functions:

- To undertake fundamental inquiry into the human and moral
  significance of developments in biomedical and behavioral science and technology.

- To explore specific ethical and policy questions related to these
  developments.

- To provide a forum for a national discussion of bioethical issues.

- To facilitate a greater understanding of bioethical issues.

President Bush left the Council free to establish its own priorities
among the many issues encompassed within its charter, and to determine
its own modes of proceeding.

In keeping with our mission, we have undertaken an inquiry into the
potential implications of using biotechnology "beyond therapy," in order
to try to satisfy deep and familiar human desires: for better children, superior performance, ageless bodies, and happy souls. Such uses of biotechnology, some of which are now possible and some of which may become

possible in the future, are likely to present us with profound and highly consequential ethical challenges and choices. They may play a crucial role in shaping human experience in the fast-approaching age of biotechnology.

We believe that the promises and perils of this prospect merit the attention of the nation. They are a worthy target for fundamental inquiry, an appropriate arena for exploring specific ethical questions, an important subject for ongoing national discussion, and (through such discussion) perhaps also a means of facilitating greater understanding of bioethical issues. Our intention in this report is to clarify the relevant scientific possibilities and, especially, to explore the ethical and social implications of using biotechnical powers for purposes beyond therapy.

The Council has been attentive to this subject from its very earliest days, beginning with a discussion at its first meeting, in January of 2002, of the purposes and motivations underlying biomedical science. The Council has also devoted time expressly to this particular project at nine of its meetings in the past two years (in April, July, September, October, and December of 2002, and in January, March, June, and July of 2003), taking testimony from experts in the relevant scientific, ethical, and social arenas, receiving public comment, and engaging in serious deliberation among the Members. All told, twenty-two sessions, of ninety minutes each, were devoted to the subject at public meetings. Complete transcripts of all these sessions are available to the public on the Council's website at www.bioethics.gov.

This report draws directly upon those sessions and discussions, as well as on written material prepared by some Council members and staff during the process. Given that context, it is crucial to understand the precise nature of this document: The final document is not a research report, but an ethical inquiry. It makes no pretense of comprehensiveness; it does not report exhaustively on the literature, scientific or ethical. Rather, it aspires to thoughtful reflection and represents mainly a (partial) distillation of the Council's own thinking. Not every Member shares every concern here expressed, or every scientific speculation or ethical assessment offered, and a few disagreements on particular points are noted in the text. Different Members care more about different topics, and all of us are aware that there are issues not addressed, and scientific opinions and ethical viewpoints not reflected. Yet, as a Council, we offer the entire document as a guide to further thinking on this very important subject.

We hope, through this report, to advance the nation's awareness and understanding of a critical set of bioethical issues and to bring them beyond the narrow circle of bioethics professionals into the larger public arena, where questions of such consequence rightly belong.

In creating this Council, President Bush expressed his desire to see us

> consider all of the medical and ethical ramifications of biomedical innovation. . . . This council will keep us apprised of new developments and give our nation a forum to continue to discuss and evaluate these important issues. As we go forward, I hope we will always be guided by both intellect and heart, by both our capabilities and our conscience.

It has been our goal in the present report, as in all of our work, to live up to these high hopes and noble aspirations.

—LEON R. KASS, M.D.
Chairman

1

Biotechnology and the Pursuit of Happiness: An Introduction

What is biotechnology for? Why is it developed, used, and esteemed? Toward what ends is it taking us? To raise such questions will very likely strike the reader as strange, for the answers seem so obvious: to feed the hungry, to cure the sick, to relieve the suffering—in a word, to improve the lot of humankind, or, in the memorable words of Francis Bacon, "to relieve man's estate." Stated in such general terms, the obvious answers are of course correct. But they do not tell the whole story, and, when carefully considered, they give rise to some challenging questions, questions that compel us to ask in earnest not only, "What is biotechnology for?" but also, "What should it be for?"

Before reaching these questions, we had better specify what we mean by "biotechnology," for it is a new word for our new age. Though others have given it both narrow and broad definitions,* our purpose—for reasons that

---

* These range from "engineering and biological study of relationships between human beings and machines" (*Webster's II New Riverside University Dictionary*, 1988), to "biological science when applied especially in genetic engineering and recombinant DNA technology" (*Merriam-Webster OnLine Dictionary*, 2003), to "the use of biological processes to solve problems or make useful products" (Glossary provided by BIO, the Biotechnology Industry Organization, www.bio.org, 2003). In the broader sense of the term that we will follow here, older biotechnologies would include fermentation (used to bake bread and brew beer) and plant and animal hybridization. Newer biotechnologies would include, among others, processes to produce genetically engineered crops, to repair genetic defects using genomic knowledge, to develop new drugs based on knowledge of biochemistry or molecular biology, and to improve biological capacities using nanotechnology. They include also the products obtained by these processes: nucleic acids and proteins, drugs, genetically modified cells, tissues derived from stem cells, biomechanical devices, etc.—in short, any industrially developed, useful agent that can alter the workings of the body or mind.

will become clear—recommends that we work with a very broad meaning: the processes and products (usually of industrial scale) offering the potential to alter and, to a degree, to control the phenomena of life—in plants, in (non-human) animals, and, increasingly, in human beings (the last, our exclusive focus here). Overarching the processes and products it brings forth, biotechnology is also a *conceptual and ethical outlook*, informed by progressive aspirations. In this sense, it appears as a most recent and vibrant expression of the technological spirit, a desire and disposition rationally to understand, order, predict, and (ultimately) control the events and workings of nature, all pursued for the sake of human benefit.

Thus understood, biotechnology is bigger than its processes and products; it is a form of human empowerment. By means of its techniques (for example, recombining genes), instruments (for example, DNA sequencers), and products (for example, new drugs or vaccines), biotechnology empowers us human beings to assume greater control over our lives, diminishing our subjection to disease and misfortune, chance and necessity. The techniques, instruments, and products of biotechnology— like similar technological fruit produced in other technological areas— augment our capacities to act or perform effectively, for many different purposes. Just as the automobile is an instrument that confers enhanced powers of "auto-mobility" (of moving *oneself*), which powers can then be used for innumerable purposes not defined by the machine itself, so DNA sequencing is a technique that confers powers for genetic screening that can be used for various purposes not determined by the technique; and synthetic growth hormone is a product that confers powers to try to increase height in the short or to augment muscle strength in the old. If we are to understand what biotechnology is for, we shall need to keep our eye more on the new abilities it provides than on the technical instruments and products that make the abilities available to us.*

---

* The importance, for assessing biomedical technologies, of the distinction between (1) the techniques and (2) the powers they make available was first developed nearly thirty years ago in a report from the National Research Council/National Academy of Sciences, *Assessing Biomedical Technologies: An Inquiry into the Nature of the Process* (Committee on Life Sciences and Social Policy, National Academy of Sciences, Washington, D.C., 1975). The report recommended (and illustrated by example) that assessment of biomedical technologies concern itself with implications of both the techniques and the perfected powers they provide. (See pages 1 and 9, and the

This terminological discussion exposes the first complication regarding the purposes of biotechnology: the fact that means and ends are readily detached from one another. As with all techniques and the powers they place in human hands, the techniques and powers of biotechnology enjoy considerable independence from ties to narrow or specific goals. Biotechnology, like any other technology, is not for anything in particular. Like any other technology, the goals it serves are supplied neither by the techniques themselves nor by the powers they make available, but by their human users. Like any other means, a given biotechnology once developed to serve one purpose is frequently available to serve multiple purposes, including some that were not imagined or even imaginable by those who brought the means into being.

Second, there are several questions regarding the overall goal of biotechnology: improving the lot of humankind. What exactly is it about the lot of humankind that needs or invites improvement? Should we think only of specific, as-yet-untreatable diseases that compromise our well-being, such ailments as juvenile diabetes, cancer, or Alzheimer disease? Should we not also include mental illnesses and infirmities, from retardation to major depression, from memory loss to melancholy, from sexual incontinence to self-contempt? And should we consider in addition those more deep-rooted limitations built into our nature, whether of body or mind, including the harsh facts of decline, decay, and death? What exactly is it about "man's estate" that most calls for relief? Just sickness and suffering, or also such things as nastiness, folly, and despair? Must "improvement" be limited to eliminating these and other evils, or should it also encompass augmenting our share of positive goods—beauty, strength, memory, intelligence, longevity, or happiness itself?

Third, even assuming that we could agree on which aspects of the human condition call for improvement, we would still face difficulties deciding how to judge whether our attempts at improving them really made things better—both for the individuals and for the society. Some of

structure of the analysis in each chapter.) We generally prefer the more energetic word "power," with its implication of efficacy, to the more prosaic "capacity" or "ability," but we mean by it nothing ominous or sinister. As we use it, "power" is to be understood as neutral or better, certainly when compared to its opposite, "impotence." At the same time, however, this term invites us to think about power's misuse or abuse; such reminders do not shadow the more quiescent near-synonyms, "capacity" or "ability."

the goals we seek might conflict with each other: longer life might come at the price of less energy; superior performance for some might diminish self-esteem for others. Efforts to moderate human aggression might wind up sapping ambition; interventions aimed at quieting discontent might flatten aspiration. And, unintended consequences aside, it is not easy to say just how much less aggression or discontent would be good for us. Once we go beyond the treatment of disease and the pursuit of health, there seem to be no ready-made or reliable standards of better and worse available to guide our choices.

As this report will demonstrate, these are not idle or merely academic concerns. Indeed, some are already upon us. We now have techniques to test early human embryos for the presence or absence of many genes: shall we use these techniques only to prevent disease or also to try to get us "better" children? We are acquiring techniques for boosting muscle strength and performance: shall we use them only to treat muscular dystrophy and the weak muscles of the elderly or also to enable athletes to attain superior performance? We are gradually learning how to control the biological processes of aging: should we seek only to diminish the bodily and mental infirmities of old age or also to engineer large increases in the maximum human lifespan? We are gaining new techniques for altering mental life, including memory and mood: should we use them only to prevent or treat mental illness or also to blunt painful memories of shameful behavior, transform a melancholic temperament, or ease the sorrows of mourning? Increasingly, these are exactly the kinds of questions that we shall be forced to face as a consequence of new biotechnical powers now and soon to be at our disposal. Increasingly we must ask, "What is biotechnology for?" "What should it be for?"

I. THE GOLDEN AGE: ENTHUSIASM AND CONCERN

By all accounts, we have entered upon a golden age for biology, medicine, and biotechnology. With the completion of (the DNA sequencing phase of) the Human Genome Project and the emergence of stem cell research, we can look forward to major insights into human development, normal and abnormal, as well as novel and more precisely selected treatments for human diseases. Advances in neuroscience hold out the promise of powerful new understandings of mental processes and behavior, as well as remedies for devastating mental illnesses. Ingenious nanotechnological devices, implantable into the human body and brain, raise hopes for overcoming blindness and deafness, and, more generally, of enhancing native human capacities of awareness and action. Research on the biology of aging and senescence suggests the possibility of slowing down age-related declines in bodies and minds, and perhaps even expanding the maximum human lifespan. In myriad ways, the discoveries of biologists and the inventions of biotechnologists are steadily increasing our power ever more precisely to intervene into the workings of our bodies and minds and to alter them by rational design.

For the most part, there is great excitement over and enthusiasm for these developments. Even before coming to the practical benefits, we look forward to greatly enriched knowledge of how our minds and bodies work. But it is the promised medical benefits that especially excite our admiration. Vast numbers of people and their families ardently await cures for many devastating diseases and eagerly anticipate relief from much human misery. We will surely welcome, as we have in the past, new technological measures that can bring us healthier bodies, decreased pain and suffering, peace of mind, and longer life.

At the same time, however, the advent of new biotechnical powers is for many people a cause for concern. First, the scientific findings themselves raise challenges to human self-understanding: people wonder, for example, what new knowledge of brain function and behavior will do to our notions of free will and personal moral responsibility, formed before the advent of such knowledge. Second, the prospect of genetic engineering, though welcomed for treatment of inherited genetic diseases, raises for some people fears of eugenics or worries about "designer babies." Psychotropic drugs, though welcomed for treatment of depression or schizophrenia, raise fears of behavior control and worries about diminished autonomy or confused personal identity. Precisely because the new knowledge and the new powers impinge directly upon the human person, and in ways that may affect our very humanity, a certain vague disquiet hovers over the entire enterprise. Notwithstanding the fact that almost everyone, on balance, is on the side of further progress, the new age of biotechnology will bring with it novel, and very likely momentous, challenges.

While its leading benefits and blessings are readily identified, the ethical and social concerns raised by the march of biotechnology are not easily articulated. They go beyond the familiar issues of bioethics, such as informed consent for human subjects of research, equitable access to the fruits of medical research, or, as with embryo research, the morality of the means used to pursue worthy ends. Indeed, they seem to be more directly connected to the ends themselves, to the uses to which biotechnological powers will be put. Generally speaking, these broader concerns attach especially to those uses of biotechnology that go "beyond therapy," beyond the usual domain of medicine and the goals of healing, uses that range from the advantageous to the frivolous to the pernicious. Biotechnologies are already available as instruments of bioterrorism (for example, genetically engineered super-pathogens or drugs that can destroy the immune system or erase memory), as agents of social control (for example, tranquilizers for the unruly or fertility-blockers for the impoverished), and as means to improve or perfect our bodies and minds and those of our children (steroids for body-building or stimulants for taking exams). In the first two cases, there are concerns about what others might do to us, or what some people, including governments, might do to other people. In the last case, there are concerns about what we might voluntarily do to ourselves or to our society. People worry both that our society might be harmed and that we ourselves might be diminished in ways that could undermine the highest and richest possibilities for human life.

Truth to tell, not everyone who has considered these prospects is worried. On the contrary, some celebrate the perfection-seeking direction in which biotechnology may be taking us. Indeed, some scientists and biotechnologists have not been shy about prophesying a better-than-currently-human world to come, available with the aid of genetic engineering, nanotechnologies, and psychotropic drugs. "At this unique moment in the history of technical achievement," declares a recent report of the National Science Foundation, "improvement of human performance becomes possible," and such improvement, if pursued with vigor, "could achieve a golden age that would be a turning point for human productivity and quality of life."[1] "Future humans—whoever or whatever they may be—will look back on our era as a challenging, difficult, traumatic moment," writes a scientist observing present trends. "They will likely see it as a strange and primitive time when people lived only seventy or eighty years, died of awful diseases, and conceived their children outside a laboratory by a random, unpredictable meeting of sperm and egg."[2] James Watson, co-discoverer of the structure of DNA, put the matter as a simple question: "If we could make better human beings by knowing how to add genes, why shouldn't we?"[3]

Yet the very insouciance of some of these predictions and the confidence that the changes they endorse will make for a better world actually serve to increase public unease. Not everyone cheers a summons to a "post-human" future. Not everyone likes the idea of "remaking Eden" or of "man playing God." Not everyone agrees that this prophesied new world will be better than our own. Some suspect it could rather resemble the humanly diminished world portrayed in Aldous Huxley's novel *Brave New World*, whose technologically enhanced inhabitants live cheerfully, without disappointment or regret, "enjoying" flat, empty lives devoid of love and longing, filled with only trivial pursuits and shallow attachments.

II. THE CASE FOR PUBLIC ATTENTION

Despite the disquiet it arouses, the subject of using biomedical technologies for purposes "beyond therapy" has received remarkably little public attention. Given its potential importance, it is arguably the most neglected topic in public bioethics. No previous national bioethics commission has considered the subject, and for understandable reasons. The realm of biotechnology "beyond therapy" is hard to define, a gray zone where judgment is, to say the least, difficult. Compared with more immediate topics in bioethics, the questions raised by efforts to "improve on human nature" seem abstract, remote, and overly philosophical, unfit for public policy; indeed, many bioethicists and intellectuals believe either that there is no such thing as "human nature" or that altering it is not ethically problematic. The concerns raised are complicated and inchoate, hard to formulate in general terms, especially because the differing technologically based powers raise different ethical and social questions: enhancing athletic performance with steroids and genetic selection of embryos for reproduction give rise to different concerns. Analysis often requires distinguishing the primary and immediate uses of a technology (say, mood-elevating drugs to treat depression or memory-blunting drugs to prevent post-traumatic stress disorder) from derivative and longer-term uses and implications (the same drugs used as general mood-brighteners or to sanitize memories of shameful or guilty conduct). Speculation about those possible implications, never to be confused with accurate prediction, is further complicated by the fact that the meaning of any future uses of biotechnology "beyond therapy" will be determined at least as much by the goals and practices of an ever-changing society as by the technologies themselves. Finally, taking up these semi-futuristic prospects may seem a waste of public attention, especially given the more immediate ethical issues that clamor for attention. Some may take us to task for worrying about the excesses and abuses of biotechnology and the dangers of a "brave *new* world" when, in the present misery-ridden world, millions are dying of AIDS, malaria, and malnutrition, in part owing to the *lack* of already available biomedical technologies.

Yet despite these genuine difficulties and objections, we believe that it is important to open up this subject for public discussion. For it raises some of the weightiest questions in bioethics. It touches on the ends and goals to be served by the acquisition of biotechnical power, not just on the safety, efficacy, or morality of the means. It bears on the nature and meaning of human freedom and human flourishing. It faces squarely the alleged threat of dehumanization as well as the alleged promise of "super-humanization." It compels attention to what it means to *be* a human being and to be *active as* a human being. And it is far from being simply futuristic: current trends make clear how the push "beyond therapy" and "toward perfection and happiness" is already upon us—witness the growing and increasingly acceptable uses of cosmetic surgery, performance-enhancing drugs, and mood- or attention-altering agents.* Given the bur-

---

* The already widely accepted "beyond therapy" uses of biomedical technologies include: pills for sleep and wakefulness, weight loss, hair growth, and birth control; surgery to remove fat and wrin-

geoning research in neuroscience and the ever-expanding biological approaches to psychiatric disorders and to all mental states, it seems clear that the expected new discoveries about the workings of the psyche and the biological basis of behavior will surely increase both our ability and our desire to alter and improve them. Decisions we are making today—for instance, what to do about sex selection or genetic selection of embryos, or whether to prescribe behavior-modifying drugs to preschoolers, or how vigorously to try to reverse the processes of senescence—will set the path "beyond therapy" for coming generations. And fair or not, the decisions and choices of the privileged or *avant-garde* often will pave the way that others later follow, in the process sometimes changing what counts as "normal," often irreversibly.

Taking up this topic is, in fact, responsive to the charge President Bush gave to this Council, formed by executive order "to advise the President on bioethical issues that may emerge as a consequence of advances in biomedical science and technology." Among the specific functions set forth in connection with our mission, the Council was instructed in the first place "to undertake fundamental inquiry into the human and moral significance of developments in biomedical and behavioral science and technology," and then "to explore specific ethical and policy questions related to these developments." Anticipating, as we do, the arrival of technological powers that are likely to affect profoundly the nature, shape, and content of human experience, human character, and human society, we believe that it is highly desirable that we try to articulate as best we can their likely "human and moral significance."

The Council has not only the mandate but also the opportunity to take a more long-range view of these matters. Unlike legislators caught up in the demands of pressing business, we have the luxury of being able carefully and disinterestedly to consider matters before they become hotly contested items for public policy. Unless a national bioethics council takes up this topic, it is unlikely that anyone else in public life will do so. And if

---

kles, to shrink thighs, and to enlarge breasts; and procedures to straighten teeth and select the sex of offspring. These practices are already big business. In 2002 Americans spent roughly one billion dollars on drugs used to treat baldness, about ten times the amount spent on scientific research to find a cure for malaria, a disease that afflicts hundreds of millions of people worldwide.

we do not prepare ourselves in advance to think about these matters, we shall be ill prepared to meet the challenges as they arrive and to make wisely the policy decisions they may require.

III. DEFINING THE TOPIC

Having offered our reasons for taking up the topic, we need next to define it more carefully and to indicate how we mean to approach it. As already suggested, the "beyond therapy" uses of biotechnology on human beings are manifold. We shall not here consider biotechnologies as instruments of bioterrorism or of mass population control. The former topic is highly specialized and tied up with matters of national security, an area beyond our charge and competence. Also, although the practical and political difficulties they raise are enormous, the ethical and social issues are relatively uncomplicated. The main question about bioterrorism is not what to think about it but how to prevent it. And the use of tranquilizing aerosols for crowd control or contraceptive additions to the drinking water, unlikely prospects in liberal democratic societies like our own, raise few issues beyond the familiar one of freedom and coercion.

Much more ethically challenging are those "beyond therapy" uses of biotechnology that would appeal to free and enterprising people, that would require no coercion, and, most crucially, that would satisfy widespread human desires. Sorting out and dealing with the ethical and social issues of such practices will prove vastly more difficult since they will be intimately connected with goals that go with, rather than against, the human grain. For these reasons, we confine our attention to those well-meaning and strictly voluntary uses of biomedical technology through which the user is seeking some improvement or augmentation of his or her own capacities, or, from similar benevolent motives, of those of his or her children. Such use of biotechnical powers to pursue "improvements" or "perfections," whether of body, mind, performance, or sense of well-being, is at once both the most seductive and the most disquieting temptation. It reflects humankind's deep dissatisfaction with natural limits and its ardent desire to overcome them. It also embodies what is genuinely novel and worrisome in the biotechnical revolution, beyond the so-called "life issues" of abortion and embryo destruction, important though these are. What's at issue is not the crude old power to kill the creature made in God's image but the attractive science-based power to remake ourselves after images of our own devising. As a result, it gives unexpected practical urgency to ancient philosophical questions: What is a good life? What is a good community?

IV. ENDS AND MEANS

Such a dream of human perfectibility by means of science and technology has, in fact, been present from the start of modern science in the seventeenth century. When René Descartes, in his famous *Discourse on Method,* set forth the practical purpose for the new science he was founding, he spoke explicitly of our becoming "like masters and owners of nature" and outlined the specific goals such mastery of nature would serve:

> This is desirable not only for the invention of an infinity of artifices which would enable us to enjoy, without any pain, the fruits of the earth and all the commodities to be found there, but also and principally for the conservation of health, which is without doubt the primary good and the foundation of all other goods in this life.

But, as the sequel makes clear, he has more than health in mind:

> For even the mind is so dependent on the temperament and on the disposition of the organs of the body, that if it is possible to find some means that generally renders men *more wise* and *more capable than they have been up to now,* I believe that we must seek for it in medicine. . . . [W]e could be spared an infinity of diseases, of the body as well as of the mind, and *even also perhaps the enfeeblement of old age,* if we had enough knowledge of their causes and all the remedies which nature has provided us. (Emphasis added.)[4]

Descartes foresaw a new medicine, unlike any the world had known, that would not only be able effectively to conserve health, but might also improve human bodies and minds beyond what nature herself had granted us: to make us wiser, more capable and competent, and perhaps even impervious to aging and decay—in a word, to make us healthy and happy, indefinitely. Owing to the powers now and soon to be available to us, Descartes's dream no longer seems a mere fantasy.

What exactly are the self-augmenting capabilities that we are talking about? What kinds of technology make them possible? What sorts of ends are they likely to serve? How soon will they be available? They are powers that potentially affect the capacities and activities of the human body; the capacities and activities of the mind or soul; and the shape of the human life cycle, at both ends and in between. We already have powers to prevent fertility and to promote it; to initiate life in the laboratory; to screen our genes, both as adults and as embryos, and to select (or reject) nascent life based on genetic criteria; to insert new genes into various parts of the adult body, and perhaps someday also into gametes and embryos; to enhance muscle performance and endurance; to alter memory, mood, appetite, libido, and attention through psychoactive drugs; to replace body parts with natural organs, mechanical organs, or tissues derived from stem cells, perhaps soon to wire ourselves using computer chips implanted into the body and brain; and, in the foreseeable future, to pro-long not just the average but also the maximum human life expectancy. The technologies for altering our native capacities are mainly those of genetic screening and genetic engineering; drugs, especially psychoactive ones; and the ability to replace body parts or to insert novel ones. The availability of some of these capacities, using these techniques, has been demonstrated only with animals; but others are already in use in humans.

It bears emphasis that these powers and technologies have not been and are not being developed for the purpose of producing improved, never mind perfect or post-human, beings. They have been produced largely for the purposes of preventing and curing disease, reversing disabilities, and alleviating suffering. Even the prospect of machine-brain interaction and implanted nanotechnological devices starts with therapeutic efforts to enable the blind to see and the deaf to hear. Yet the "dual use" aspect of most of these powers—encouraged by the ineradicable human urge toward "improvement," exploited by the commercial interests that already see vast market opportunities for nontherapeutic uses, and likely welcomed by many people seeking a competitive edge in their strivings to "get ahead"—means that we must not be lulled to sleep by the fact that the originators of these powers were no friends to Brave New World. Once here, techniques and powers can produce desires where none existed before, and things often go where no one ever intended.

V. THE LIMITATIONS OF THE "THERAPY VS. ENHANCEMENT" DISTINCTION

Although, as we have indicated, the topic of the biotechnological pursuit of human improvement has not yet made it onto the agenda of public bioethics, it has received a certain amount of attention in academic bioethical circles under the rubric of "enhancement," understood in contradistinction to "therapy."⁵ Though we shall ourselves go beyond this distinction, it provides a useful starting place from which to enter the discussion of activities that aim "beyond therapy."* "Therapy," on this view as in common understanding, is the use of biotechnical power to treat individuals with known diseases, disabilities, or impairments, in an attempt to restore them to a normal state of health and fitness. "Enhancement," by contrast, is the directed use of biotechnical power to alter, by direct intervention, not disease processes but the "normal" workings of the human body and psyche, to augment or improve their native capacities and performances. Those who introduced this distinction hoped by this means to distinguish between the acceptable and the dubious or unacceptable uses of biomedical technology: therapy is always ethically fine, enhancement

---

* Our choice of "Beyond Therapy" as the title for this report is meant to acknowledge that this notion offers a good point of entry: it reflects the medical milieu in which the questions arise; it exposes the untraditional goals of the new uses for biotechnical power; it hints at the open-ended character of what lies "beyond" the goal of healing. Yet for reasons that should become clear, the notion of "beyond therapy" does not seem to us to define the royal road to understanding. For this, one must adopt an outlook not only "beyond therapy" but also "beyond the distinction between therapy and enhancement." One needs to see the topic less in relation to medicine and its purposes, and more in relation to human beings and *their* purposes.

is, at least prima facie, ethically suspect. Gene therapy for cystic fibrosis or Prozac for major depression is fine; insertion of genes to enhance intelligence or steroids for Olympic athletes is, to say the least, questionable.

At first glance, the distinction between therapy and enhancement makes good sense. Ordinary experience recognizes the difference between "restoring to normal" and "going beyond the normal." Also, as a practical matter, this distinction seems a useful way to distinguish between the central and obligatory task of medicine (healing the sick) and its marginal and extracurricular practices (for example, Botox injections and other merely cosmetic surgical procedures). Because medicine has, at least traditionally, pursued therapy rather than enhancement, the distinction helps to delimit the proper activities of physicians, understood as healers. And because physicians have been given a more-or-less complete monopoly over the prescription and administration of biotechnology to human beings, the distinction, by seeking to circumscribe the proper goals of medicine, indirectly tries to circumscribe also the legitimate uses of biomedical technology. Accordingly, it also helps us decide about health care costs: health providers and insurance companies have for now bought into the distinction, paying for treatment of disease, but not for enhancements. More fundamentally, the idea of enhancement understood as seeking something "better than well" points to the perfectionist, not to say utopian, aspiration of those who would set out to improve upon human nature in general or their own particular share of it.

But although the distinction between therapy and enhancement is a fitting beginning and useful shorthand for calling attention to the problem (and although we shall from time to time make use of it ourselves), it is finally inadequate to the moral analysis. "Enhancement" is, even as a term, highly problematic. In its most ordinary meaning, it is abstract and imprecise.* Moreover, "therapy" and "enhancement" are overlapping categories: all successful therapies are enhancing, even if not all enhancements

---

* According to the *Oxford English Dictionary*, "to enhance," means "to raise in degree, heighten, intensify"; "to make to appear greater"; "to raise in price, value, importance, attractiveness, etc." An "enhancement" would designate a quantitative change, an increase in magnitude or degree.

enhance by being therapeutic. Even if we take "enhancement" to mean "nontherapeutic enhancement," the term is still ambiguous. When referring to a human function, does enhancing mean making more of it, or making it better? Does it refer to bringing something out more fully, or to altering it qualitatively? In what meaning of the term are both improved memory and selective erasure of memory "enhancements"?

Beyond these largely verbal and conceptual ambiguities, there are difficulties owing to the fact that both "enhancement" and "therapy" are bound up with, and absolutely dependent on, the inherently complicated idea of health and the always-controversial idea of normality. The differences between healthy and sick, fit and unfit, are experientially evident to most people, at least regarding themselves, and so are the differences between sickness and other troubles. When we are bothered by cough and high fever, we suspect that we are sick, and we think of consulting a physician, not a clergyman. By contrast, we think neither of sickness nor of doctors when we are bothered by money problems or worried about the threat of terrorist attacks. But there are notorious difficulties in trying to define "healthy" and "impaired," "normal" and "abnormal" (and hence, "super-normal"), especially in the area of "behavioral" or "psychic" functions and activities. Some psychiatric diagnoses—for example, "dysthymia," "oppositional disorder," or "social anxiety disorder"—are rather vague: what is the difference between extreme shyness and social anxiety? And, on the positive side, mental health shades over into peace of mind, which shades over into contentment, which shades over into happiness. If one follows the famous World Health Organization definition of health as "a state of complete physical, mental and social well-being," almost any intervention aimed at enhancement may be seen as health-promoting, and hence "therapeutic," if it serves to promote the enhanced individual's mental well-being by making him happier.

Yet even for those using a narrower definition of health, the distinction between therapy and enhancement will prove problematic. While in some cases—for instance, a chronic disease or a serious injury—it is fairly easy to point to a departure from the standard of health, other cases defy simple classification. Most human capacities fall along a continuum, or a "normal distribution" curve, and individuals who find themselves near the lower end of the normal distribution may be considered disadvantaged and therefore unhealthy in comparison with others. But the average may equally regard themselves as disadvantaged with regard to the above average. If one is responding in both cases to perceived disadvantage, on what principle can we call helping someone at the lower end "therapy" and helping someone who is merely average "enhancement"? In which cases of traits distributed "normally" (for example, height or IQ or cheerfulness) does the average also function as a norm, or is the norm itself appropriately subject to alteration?

Further complications arise when we consider causes of conditions that clamor for modification. Is it therapy to give growth hormone to a genetic dwarf, but not to a short fellow who is just unhappy to be short? And if the short are brought up to the average, the average, now having become short, will have precedent for a claim to growth hormone injections. Since more and more scientists believe that all traits of personality have at least a partial biological basis, how will we distinguish the biological "defect" that yields "disease" from the biological condition that yields shyness or melancholy or irascibility?

For these reasons, among others, relying on the distinction between therapy and enhancement to do the work of moral judgment will not succeed. In addition, protracted arguments about whether or not something is or is not an "enhancement" can often get in the way of the proper ethical questions: What are the good and bad uses of biotechnical power? What makes a use "good," or even just "acceptable"? It does not follow from the fact that a drug is being taken solely to satisfy one's desires—for example, to increase concentration or sexual performance—that its use is objectionable. Conversely, certain interventions to restore functioning wholeness—for example, to enable postmenopausal women to bear children or sixty-year-old men to keep playing professional ice hockey— might well be dubious uses of biotechnical power. The human meaning and moral assessment must be tackled directly; they are unlikely to be settled by the term "enhancement," any more than they are by the nature of the technological intervention itself.

VI. BEYOND NATURAL LIMITS:
DREAMS OF PERFECTION AND HAPPINESS

Reliance on the therapy-versus-enhancement distinction has one advantage in theory that turns out also to be a further disadvantage in practice. The distinction rests on the assumption that there is a natural human "whole" whose healthy functioning is the goal of therapeutic medicine. It sees medicine, in fact, as thoroughly informed by this idea of health and wholeness, taken as the end of the entire medical art. Medical practice, for the most part and up to the present time, appears to embody this self-understanding of its mission. Yet this observation points to the deepest reason why the distinction between healing and enhancing is, finally, of insufficient ethical, and even less practical, value. For the human being whose wholeness or healing is sought or accomplished by biomedical therapy is finite and frail, medicine or no medicine.

The healthy body declines and its parts wear out. The sound mind slows down and has trouble remembering things. The soul has aspirations beyond what even a healthy body can realize, and it becomes weary from frustration. Even at its fittest, the fatigable and limited human body rarely carries out flawlessly even the ordinary desires of the soul. For this reason (among others), the desires of many human beings—for more, for better, for the unlimited, or even for the merely different—will not be satisfied with the average, nor will they take their bearings from the distinction between normal and abnormal, or even between the healthy and the better-than-healthy.

Joining aspirations to overcome common human limitations are comparable aspirations to overcome individual shortfalls in native endowment. For there is wide variation in the natural gifts with which each of us is endowed: some are born with perfect pitch, others are born tone-deaf; some have flypaper memories, others forget immediately what they have just learned. And as with talents, so too with desires and temperaments: some crave immortal fame, others merely comfortable preservation. Some are sanguine, others phlegmatic, still others bilious or melancholic. When nature dispenses her gifts, some receive only at the end of the line. Yet, one should remember that it is often the most gifted and ambitious who most resent their human limitations: Achilles was willing to destroy every-thing around him, so little could he stomach that he was but a heel short of immortality.

As a result of these infirmities, particular and universal, human beings have long dreamed of overcoming limitations of body and soul, in particular the limitations of bodily decay, psychic distress, and the frustration of human aspiration. Dreams of human perfection—and the terrible consequences of pursuing it at all costs—are the themes of Greek tragedy, as well as of "The Birth-mark," the Hawthorne short story with which the President's Council on Bioethics began its work. Until now these dreams have been pure fantasies, and those who pursued them came crashing down in disaster. But the stupendous successes over the past century in all areas of technology, and especially in medicine, have revived the ancient dreams of human perfection. Like Achilles, many of the major beneficiaries of modern medicine seem, by and large, neither grateful nor satisfied with the bounties we have received from existing biomedical technologies. We seem, in fact, less content than we are "worried well," perhaps more aware of hidden ills we might be heir to, or more worried about losing the health we have than we are pleased to have it. Curiously, we may even be more afraid of death than our forebears, who lived before modern medicine began successfully to do battle with it. Unconsciously, but clearly as a result of what we have been given, our desires grow fat for still further gifts. And we regard our remaining limitations with less equanimity, to the point that dreams of getting rid of them can be turned into moral imperatives.* For these reasons, thanks to biomedical technology, people will be increasingly tempted to try to realize these dreams, at least to some extent: ageless and ever-vigorous bodies, happy (or at least not unhappy)

---

* Consider in this connection our attitudes toward organ transplantation. When first introduced into clinical practice some fifty years ago, receiving a life-saving kidney transplant was regarded as a gift, a blessing, a minor miracle, something beyond anything merited or even expected. Today, though the number of such "miracles" increases annually, supply does not equal demand. Expectations have risen to such an extent that people speak and act as if society's failure to meet the need is in fact the cause of death for those who die before they can be transplanted. Who in 1950 could have thought that he was entitled to have his defective and diseased organs replaced? Will people in 2050 think that they are entitled to have any and all their weakened parts replaced, and not just once?

souls, excellent human achievement (with diminished effort or toil), and better endowed and more accomplished children. These dreams have at bottom nothing to do with medicine, other than the fact that it is doctors who will wield the tools that may get them realized. They are, therefore, only accidentally dreams "beyond therapy." They are dreams, in principle and in the limit, of human perfection.

Not everyone interested in the beyond-therapy uses of biotechnology will dream of human perfection. Many people are more or less satisfied, at least for now, with their native human capacities, though they might willingly accept assistance that would make them prettier, stronger, or smarter. The pursuit of happiness and self-esteem—the satisfaction of one's personal desires and recognition of one's personal worth—are much more common human aspirations than the self-conscious quest for perfection. Indeed, the desire for happiness and the love of excellence are, at first glance, independent aspirations. Although happiness is arguably fuller and deeper when rooted in excellent activity, the pursuit of happiness is often undertaken without any regard for excellence or virtue. Many people crave only some extra boost on the path to success; many people seek only to feel better about themselves. Although less radical than the quest for "perfection," the quests for happiness, success, and self-esteem, especially in our society, may prove to be more powerful motives for an interest in using biotechnical power for purposes that lie "beyond therapy." Thus, though some visionaries—beginning with Descartes—may dream of using biotechnologies to perfect human nature, and though many of us might welcome biotechnical assistance in improving our native powers of mind and body, many more people will probably turn to it in search of advancement, contentment, and self-satisfaction—for themselves and for their children.

Why should anyone be worried about these prospects? What could be wrong with efforts to improve upon or perfect human nature, to try, with the help of biomedical technology, to gain better children, higher achievements, ageless bodies, or happy souls? What are the sources of our disquiet?

The answers to these questions cannot be given in the abstract. They will depend on a case-by-case analysis, with special attention to the ends pursued and the means used to pursue them. In some cases, disquiet attaches not only to the individual pursuit of a particular goal, but also to the social consequences that would follow if many people did likewise (for example, selecting the sex of offspring, if practiced widely, could greatly alter a society's sex ratio). In other cases, disquiet attaches mainly to the individual practice itself (for example, drugs that would erase or transform one's memories). Speaking in the abstract and merely for the sake of illustration, concerns can and have been raised about the safety of the techniques used and about whether access to the benefits will be fairly distributed. Regarding the use of performance-enhancing techniques, especially in competitive activities, concerns can be raised about unfair advantage and inauthentic performance. Questions can be raised about coercion, overt and subtle (through peer pressure), should uses of mind-improving drugs become widespread. Other worries include the misuse of society's precious medical resources, the increasing medicalization of human activities, the manipulation of desires, the possible hubris in trying to improve upon human nature, and the consequences for character of getting results "the easy way" through biotechnology, without proper effort or discipline. There is no point here in detailing these further or in indicating additional possible objections. As concerns arise in their appropriate contexts, we shall discuss them further. At the end of this report, we will offer what generalizations seem appropriate. Between now and then, we shall proceed to examine several instances of activities and uses of biotechnical power that look "beyond therapy."

VII. STRUCTURE OF THE INQUIRY: THE PRIMACY OF HUMAN ASPIRATIONS

We have considered several different ways to organize our inquiry. We could begin from the novel *techniques*: genetic screening, gene insertion, or one or another of the various psychotropic drugs. We could begin with the new *powers* or *capacities* these techniques provide: to select the sex (or other traits) of offspring, to influence mood or memory, or to alter the rate of biological aging. We could begin with the *therapeutic uses* these powers might serve—for example, to treat depression or dwarfism—and look next for the enhancement uses that lie beyond therapy. We could begin with those *aspects of human life* that might be affected: our inborn bodily or psychic capacities, our bodily or psychic activities, or the phases and shape of the life cycle—how we are born, how we die, and how we live in the prime of life. Or we could begin with the *desires and goals* that either drive our pursuit of these techniques or that will enlist the available powers they make possible once they are available: desires for longer life, finer looks, stronger bodies, sharper minds, better performance, and happier souls—in short, with our specific aspirations to improve our lot, our activities, or the hand that nature dealt to us or to our children.

In keeping with our goal of "a richer bioethics"—one that seeks to do justice to the full human meaning of biotechnological advance—we will here proceed in the last of these ways. By structuring the inquiry around the desires and goals of human beings, we adopt the perspective of human experience and human aspiration, rather than the perspective of technique and power. By beginning with long-standing and worthy human desires, we avoid premature adverse judgment on using biotechnologies to help satisfy them. We can also see better how the new technological possibilities for going "beyond therapy" fit with previous and present human pursuits and aspirations, including those well represented in the goals of modern medicine. We will also be able critically to assess the desirability of these goals and the significance of any successes in attaining them. What might the successful pursuit of these goals—longer life, stronger bodies, happier souls, superior performance, better children—using biotechnological means do to both the users and the rest of society? Why might these consequences matter?

In Chapter Two, we consider the pursuit of "better children," using techniques of genetic screening and selection to improve their native endowments or drugs that might make them more accomplished, attentive, or docile. In Chapter Three, we consider the pursuit of "superior performance," using genetic or pharmacologic enhancement, taking the domain of athletics as a specially revealing instance. In Chapter Four, we consider the pursuit of "ageless bodies," both modest and bold, using either soon-to-be-available genetic interventions to increase the strength and vigor of muscles, or various efforts, somewhat more futuristic, to retard the general processes of biological senescence. In Chapter Five, we consider the pursuit of "happy (or satisfied) souls," using pharmacologic agents that dull painful memories or that brighten mood. In a final chapter we briefly try to put together what we have learned from the various "case studies." While each of the separate instances will make our concerns concrete, *the full value of the inquiry requires considering all these instances together and seeing them as part of a larger human project—toward perfection and happiness.*

VIII. METHOD AND SPIRIT

We conclude this introduction with a few words about the method and spirit of our inquiry. In preparing ourselves for the analysis of the various topics comprising the four middle chapters, we commissioned presentations from a wide array of scientists working or writing in the pertinent fields of biology and biotechnology: preimplantation genetic diagnosis and genetic enhancement (Gerald Schatten and Francis Collins); choosing sex of children (Arthur Haney and Nicholas Eberstadt); drugs to modify behavior in children (Lawrence Diller and Steven Hyman); genetic enhancement of muscle strength and vigor (H. Lee Sweeney); genetic enhancement of athletic performance (Theodore Friedmann); aging and longevity research (Steven Austad and S. Jay Olshansky); memory, and drugs that might improve or blunt it (James McGaugh and Daniel Schacter); and mood-brightening drugs (Peter Kramer and Carl Elliott). Drawing on these presentations and on outside reading in the various areas, Council staff prepared working papers on nearly all these topics, and these papers were discussed at some length at eight Council meetings between July 2002 and July 2003. Several Council Members contributed original writings (Michael Sandel on superior performance, Gilbert Meilaender on memory, Paul McHugh on "medicalization," Leon Kass on the pursuit of perfection).[6] The final report is the product of drafting by Council staff, reviewed and critiqued by all Members of the Council, and rewritten many times.

The final document is not a research report, but an ethical inquiry. It makes no pretense of comprehensiveness; it does not report exhaustively on the literature, scientific or ethical. Rather, it aspires to thoughtful reflection and represents mainly a (partial) distillation of the Council's own thinking. Not every Member shares every concern here expressed. Different Members care more about different topics. All of us are aware that there are issues not addressed and viewpoints not reflected. Yet, as a Council, we own the document as a whole, offering it as a guide to further thinking on this potentially very important topic.

Each of the four specialized chapters opens with a brief but critical exploration of the goal under consideration (for example, what are "better children" or "happy souls"). In due course we introduce the relevant biotechnologies and the powers they provide for pursuing these goals. We then proceed with our ethical analysis, trying to assess the meaning and possible consequences of pursuing those goals by these means, and considering the implications both for the individuals involved and for the broader society. Because much of what lies "beyond therapy" lies also in the future, our analysis is necessarily speculative, and by raising possible concerns we do not mean to be setting ourselves up as prophets. As we readily acknowledge, which, if any, of our speculative suggestions regarding possible future consequences turn out to be correct will be a matter, in part, for careful empirical research. At the same time, however, we also insist that figuring out which of them will become a reality is not exactly the main point. Far more important, in our opinion, the human goods and principles discussed here can help shape our thinking across the entire range of technological powers (and the attendant ethical dilemmas) that we are likely to face in the future. By raising the questions we do, and by introducing certain matters of possible concern, we seek to identify exactly the sorts of questions and concerns to which researchers, policy makers, and the public at large should be paying attention.

The spirit of this inquiry is educational. In the first instance, we want to help people sort out fact from fiction, real biotechnological possibilities from merely imaginary ones. We want to clarify the ethical and social issues, both for individuals and the larger society. Precisely because we are taking a long-range view, we are primarily interested in opening up questions, not in issuing moral pronouncements or suggesting legislative or regulatory measures. Our first questions are not "Is this good or bad, right or wrong?" or "Should we allow it?" but rather, "What does and will this mean for us—as individuals, as members of American society, and as human beings eager to live well in an age of biotechnology?" If the questions we raise and the observations we offer strike the reader as conveying a cautionary note, he or she should not mistake this for hostility to biotechnology in general or to its many clearly desirable uses. Neither should anyone be surprised by our concern. The benefits from biomedical progress are clear and powerful. The hazards are less well appreciated, precisely because they are attached to an enterprise we all cherish and support and to goals nearly all of us desire. All the more reason to try to articulate the human goods that we seek to defend and the possible threats they may face.

ENDNOTES

[1] National Science Foundation, *Converging Technologies for Improving Human Performance: Nanotechnology, Biotechnology, Information Technology and Cognitive Science*, Arlington, Virginia: National Science Foundation, 2003, p. 6.

[2] Stock, G., *Redesigning Humans: Our Inevitable Genetic Future*, New York: Houghton Mifflin, 2002, p. 200. A similar opinion has been voiced by Lee Silver: "[W]e're going to be able to manipulate and control the genes that we give to our children. It's just over the horizon. . . . All of these new technologies are going to change humankind as we know it." ("Frontline" interview, www.pbs.org.) See also Silver, L., *Remaking Eden: Cloning and Beyond in a Brave New World*, New York: Avon, 1998. Silver's enthusiasm for the post-human future is diluted only by his fear that not everyone will have equal access to its enhancing benefits. For an examination and critique of these views, see Fukuyama, F., *Our Posthuman Future: Consequences of the Biotechnology Revolution*, New York: Farrar Straus & Giroux, 2002.

[3] James D. Watson, quoted in Wheeler, T., "Miracle Molecule, 50 Years On," *Baltimore Sun*, 4 February 2003, p. 8A. At a symposium in Toronto in October 2002, Watson went further in his support of enhancement: "Going for perfection was something I always thought you should do. You always want the perfect girl." (Abraham, C., "Gene Pioneer Urges Human Perfection," *Toronto Globe and Mail*, 26 October 2002.) The article further quotes Watson's response to the charge that he wants to use genetics "to produce pretty babies or perfect people": "What's wrong with that?" he countered. "It's as if there's something wrong with enhancements."

[4] Descartes, *Discourse on the Method of Conducting One's Reason Well and Seeking Truth in the Sciences*, Part VI, para. 2. Private translation by Richard Kennington.

[5] See, for example, Parens, E., ed., *Enhancing Human Traits*, Washington, D.C.: Georgetown University Press, 1998; and Elliott, C., *Better Than Well: American Medicine Meets the American Dream*, New York: Norton, 2003.

[6] The transcripts of all the presentations and Council discussions, as well as the texts of the staff working papers and the papers written by Members, are available on the Council's website: www.bioethics.gov.

2

Better Children

What father or mother does not dream of a good life for his or her child? What parents would not wish to enhance the life of their children, to make them better people, to help them live better lives? Such wishes and intentions guide much of what all parents do for and to their children. To help our children on their way and to make them strong in body and in mind, we feed and clothe them, see that they get rest, fresh air, and exercise, and take great pains regarding their education. Beyond ordinary schooling, we give them swimming and piano lessons, enroll them in Scouts or Little League, and help them acquire a variety of skills—artistic, intellectual, and social. In addition, we try to develop their character, educate their tastes and sensibilities, and nurture their spiritual growth. In all of these efforts we are guided, whether consciously or not, by some notion or other of what it *means* to improve our children, of what it means to make them *better*.

Needless to say, the thing is easier said than done. Rearing children is work only for the brave. Children can be recalcitrant, outside influences can corrupt, and even the best of efforts may not bear good fruit. But even apart from the practical difficulties, the very aspiration of "producing better children" is hardly trouble-free, even for parents and teachers with the best of intentions. For it is easier to *wish* whole-heartedly that our children be improved than it is to *know* what that would mean. For what, exactly, is a good or a better child?

Is it a child who is more able and talented? If so, able in what and talented how? Is it a child with better character? If so, having which traits or virtues? More obedient or more independent? More sensitive or more enduring? More daring or more measured? Better behaved or more assertive? Is it a child with the right attitude and disposition toward the world? If so, should he or she tend more toward reverence or skepticism, high-mindedness or toleration, the love of justice or the love of mercy? As these questions make clear, human goods and good humans come in many forms, and the various goods and virtues are often in tension with one another. Should we therefore aim at balanced and "well-rounded" children, or should we aim also or instead at genuine excellence in some one or a few dimensions? It is not easy to answer. Yet absent knowledge regarding these matters, acting on the laudable intention of producing better children can be a tricky, not to say dangerous, business.

This is especially true because of a second difficulty, one derived not from the ambiguity of "good" or "better" but from the ambiguity that is at the heart of being a *child*. Children much more than adults are, so to speak, double creatures: they are both who they are here-and-now and, at the same time, they are also creatures on the way to maturity and adulthood. To be a child *means* "to-be-not-yet," means to be "on-the-way-up," growing up, maturing, reaching toward one's prime. Yet to be a child is also to enjoy a special time of our lives, with special gifts, possibilities, and opportunities, and—in comparison with adulthood—with a relatively carefree existence. Childhood is that stage of life justly celebrated as most innocent, open, fresh, playful, wondering, unself-conscious, spontaneous, and honest: "out of the mouths of babes." This "doubleness" of childhood is responsible for the notorious paradox of parenthood: we love our children unconditionally, just as they are, yet we are constantly doing everything in our power to get them to be different, to change for the better. Not content just to appreciate them in their childish glory, we labor to educate them, to lead them out of childhood, and to draw from them those latent but still largely dormant powers and virtues they do not as yet have or have not yet expressed. The task is made still more paradoxical once we remember the most important improvement we seek to promote: their ability to do without our educative meddling, to take the reins of their own chariots, and, in the best case, to repay the debt they owe us by doing the same for the next generation.

This delicate process of rearing the young, supporting and savoring them as they are while coaxing and directing them toward what they might well become, requires special attention to the means of improvement. As hard as it may be to say with confidence what we *mean* by "a *better* child," it is equally difficult to select the proper *means*. Even were we to agree that it were desirable that our children be well-behaved, excellent in their studies, or able to handle disappointment, there are tough questions about which means are best suited to these ends. The use of some means might actually undermine the goal, especially if they achieve their effect without demanding effort or engagement of the child himself; having a child do his arithmetic homework with a calculator will get him the right answers without teaching him long division. Also, the availability of new and attractive means that facilitate one-sided pursuits of a partial goal (for example, superior athletic or academic performance) can threaten the overall goal of rearing: to enable our children to flourish as autonomous adults who can think and act for themselves, learn from adversity, and meet life's vicissitudes with resilience and self-confidence.

These enduring perplexities regarding our aspiration for better children now deserve our thematic and heightened attention. The reason: new biotechnologies, present and projected, are providing new and allegedly powerful means for improving our children. Thinking about these possibilities invites us to examine our existing practices and purposes, even as we try to figure out what is new and how it matters.

In most of our efforts to assist our children's development, we proceed through speech and symbolic deed, using praise and blame, reward and punishment, encouragement and admonition, as well as habituation, training, and ritualized activities. Yet nature sets limits on what can be accomplished by education and training alone. No matter how much we try to help, the tone-deaf will need more training to learn to carry a tune, the short will be less likely to excel at basketball, the irascible will have trouble restraining their tempers, and the insufficiently smart will remain handicapped for competitive college admissions. If the inborn "equipment" is faulty, or even only normally limited and hence inadequate for realizing some human purposes, it is inviting to think about improving the native powers or the efficacy of their expression and use. For whether we like it or not, certain desired improvements in our children will be possible, if at all, only by improving their native equipment.

Even before the coming of the present age of biotechnology, we have used technological adjuncts to improve upon nature's gifts. We give our children supplementary vitamins, fluoridated toothpaste, and, where necessary, corrective lenses or hearing aids. We even use biological means of improving their limited human capacity to resist disease: we immunize our children against polio, diphtheria, and measles, among other infectious diseases, by injecting them with attenuated viruses and bacteria in the form of vaccines. But the scope of these now-routine kinds of biomedical improvement has until now been limited to restoring or protecting our children's health in a quite straightforward sense.

It is here where some truly novel biotechnologies enter the picture. According to some predictions, our ability to improve our children's native endowments may soon take a quantum leap, thanks to prospects for genetically engineered improvements of native human powers and drug-assisted improvements in their use. It is these prospects—for so-called "designer babies" and for drug-enhanced children—that we shall consider in the present chapter. The technologies differ widely, so that they are rarely considered together. Yet once seen in the context of the common goal, "better children," they raise overlapping and similarly profound ethical and social issues—especially about the significance of procreation, the nature of parental responsibility, and the meaning of childhood.

I. IMPROVING NATIVE POWERS: GENETIC KNOWLEDGE AND TECHNOLOGY

A. An Overview

The possibility of using genetic knowledge and genetic engineering to improve the human race and its individual members has been discussed for many years, especially in the heady decades immediately following Watson and Crick's discovery, in 1953, of the structure of DNA. New life was breathed into old eugenic dreams, which had been temporarily discredited by the Nazi pursuits of a "superior race." As late as the early

1970s, serious scientists talked optimistically about humankind's new opportunity to take the reins of its own evolution, thanks to the predicted confluence of genetic engineering and reproductive technologies.[1] But as scientists have learned just how difficult it is to engineer precise genetic change—even to treat individuals with genetic diseases caused by a simple one-gene mutation—explicit talk about improving the species has largely faded. Instead recent years have seen, in its place, much talk about coming prospects for "designer babies," children born with improved genetic endowments, the result either of careful screening and selecting of embryos carrying desirable genes, or of directed genetic change ("genetic engineering") in gametes or embryos.

Interest in such possibilities has been fueled by recent developments in a number of related disciplines, beginning with the completion of the Human Genome Project. Knowledge of the complete chemical sequence of all human genes promises greatly increased powers for genetic screening of individuals and embryos. Numerous studies are already seeking to correlate phenotypic traits (and not only those connected with disease) with the presence or absence of certain genetic markers. Scientists have reported early success with directed genetic change in embryos of non-human animals (including primates[2]), though many more attempts have failed. And we are witnessing large increases in the use of assisted reproductive technologies, including for purposes that go beyond the mere treatment of infertility.[3] Extrapolating from these developments, some scientists have predicted that parents, in the not-too-distant future, will be able to exert precise genetic control over many characteristics of their offspring.[4] These predictions have been greeted both with enthusiasm—"At last, we can escape from the tyranny of fortune and bring our inheritance under rational control!"—and with alarm—"What hubris! Scientists are trying to play God!"

It is difficult to know what to make of these predictions, based as they are largely on speculation. In this enormously fertile and rapidly developing field, the future is unknowable. Thus, anyone can claim to be a prophet, and no one should confidently bet against any form of scientific and technological progress. Yet in our view, for reasons that we shall elaborate below, prophecies and predictions of a "new (positive) eugenics" seem greatly exaggerated. In consequence, much of the public disquiet created by loose talk of genetically engineered "designer babies" seems unwarranted. Nevertheless, the public's misgivings may contain a partial wisdom regarding practices in this area that are not far-fetched, indeed, that are already with us, including prenatal and preimplantation genetic screening. For, as we shall see, there is some reason to be concerned both about negative eugenics and about the practice of genetic *selection* of "better" children. Therefore, even as we try to calm down fears about genetic engineering of children, it behooves us to pay careful attention to the reasons behind them and to the human goods at stake. By this means, we may shed light on the meaning not only of things we might be doing in the future but also of things we are already doing in the present.

B. Technical Possibilities

One can distinguish several ways of trying to produce children with better genetic endowments. First is the use of directed mating, either choosing "superior" mating partners or using donor sperm or donor eggs (or both) obtained from "superior" individuals. Assuming that people with some superior natural ability or accomplishment are genetically better endowed, and, further, that such putative genetic excellence is heritable, directed mating of like with like, so the theory goes, would increase the odds of getting superior children. People seeking to initiate a pregnancy using artificial insemination by donor (AID) or in vitro fertilization (IVF) with donor eggs do check the pedigree (and will soon be able to check the genetic profile) of the prospective donor for general health and fitness, as well as for certain desired traits, from height and hair color to intelligence. In some notorious cases, people planning to undergo IVF have advertised in elite college newspapers, offering up to $100,000 for an egg donor with high SAT scores or "proven college-level athletic ability."[5] Yet these approaches to genetic improvement are relatively crude and probably unreliable, since they all involve the uncertain lottery of chance inherent in all sexual reproduction, and they overestimate the degree to which heredity by itself determines traits such as intelligence or athletic ability. Moreover, most couples would rather have their own children than those they might get by using gametes from a "superior" donor.* We will not be discussing this approach further.

We concentrate instead on various powers that depend upon precise genetic knowledge and technique: (a) the ability to screen and select fetuses, embryos, and gametes (egg and sperm) for the presence or absence of specific genetic markers; and (b) the ability to obtain and introduce such genetic material in order to effect a desired genetic "improvement." The first, by itself, leads to two powers that merely select from among genetic endowments conferred by chance, the difference between them being the stage at which screening is done and whether selection is "negative" or "positive." *Prenatal diagnosis* during an established pregnancy (using amniocentesis or chorionic villus sampling) permits the weeding out, through abortion, of those fetuses carrying *undesired* genetic traits.** *Preimplantation genetic screening and selection* of in vitro embryos, in contrast, permits pregnancy to begin using only those embryos that carry *desired* genetic traits.† In contrast to both of these, a third power, *directed genetic change* (or *genetic engineering*), would attempt to go beyond what chance alone has provided, improving in vitro embryos directly by introducing "better" genes.††

In theory, these three prospects offer scientists and prospective parents a range of increasing genetic control, from (1) eliminating the bad ("screening out"), through (2) selecting the good ("choosing in"), to (3) redesigning for the better ("fixing up"). Each activity raises its own ethical

---

* The Repository for Germinal Choice, a California sperm bank accepting deposits only from Nobel Laureates or other comparably accomplished donors, recently closed its doors, having done only minimal business in the roughly twenty-five years of its existence.

** Although a form of "negative" genetic selection, prenatal diagnosis can give reassurance to prospective parents that such traits are absent.

† Of course, the desired trait for which an embryo is selected may in fact be simply the presence of a normal gene, lacking the feared genetic abnormality.

†† Cloning-to-produce-children (if not all human cloning) could be considered yet another form of genetic control of the next generation. After all, the aim of cloning is to secure a new life with a predetermined and preferred genome. Cloning gives genetic control not only of a single trait but of a whole person; the ethical issues attending other forms of genetic control are, if not identical, similarly troubling. Many of these issues are explored in this Council's report, *Human Cloning and Human Dignity: An Ethical Inquiry*, Washington, D.C.: Government Printing Office, 2002.

questions, some of which we shall consider later. But in practice, they are not equally feasible as means of producing better children, and, for reasons discussed below, we believe that the scale of their use *for this purpose* will probably remain low.

We state the conclusion in advance: The first, prenatal diagnosis and selective abortion, widely practiced since the 1970s in order to prevent the birth of children with genetic or chromosomal abnormalities, is a weeding-out procedure; hence its potential to select "better than normal" babies is negligible, and it is unlikely ever to be effective or widely used for such purposes.* The third and most ambitious, genetic engineering of improved children, is—contrary to much loose prediction—a most unlikely prospect, for reasons of both feasibility and safety. The second, selecting IVF embryos genetically predisposed to certain superior or desirable traits, might soon be possible for some relatively uncomplicated traits (for example, height or leanness). Yet even here, as we shall see, there will likely be large—perhaps insurmountable—logistical problems in obtaining a "genetically superior" embryo for any trait to which many different genes contribute. Moreover, absent certain innovations in technology (and greater insurance coverage for assisted reproduction procedures), this is unlikely to be a widespread practice in the near future, save for those who are willing and able to undergo IVF and to pay extra for the genetic screening. Finally, keeping in mind that most traits of interest to parents seeking better children are heavily influenced by environment, even successful genetic screening and embryo selection might not, in many cases, produce the desired result.

We look briefly at each of the alternatives.

1. Prenatal Diagnosis and Screening Out

Genetic screening by amniocentesis or chorionic villus sampling is an established feature of prenatal care in the United States and other economically advanced countries. It is routinely offered to women of advanced

---

* There is one exception that we will consider later, on its own: the use of prenatal diagnosis and abortion for choosing sex of offspring. Such sex selection is widely practiced in some parts of the world and, on a more modest scale, in the United States. Choosing sex of children need not involve genetic testing: a sonogram can make the diagnosis.

maternal age or to parents known to be carriers of heritable disorders. Some prospective parents prefer not to screen and not to know, in many cases because they have decided that they will not abort, no matter what. But the use of the practice is growing, and it will in all likelihood continue to do so. The capacity for screening both parents-to-be and fetuses is certain to increase, thanks to the completed mapping of the human genome and to greatly improved efficiency of testing. In addition to detecting more genetic diseases, new screening powers may also be able to detect a growing number of genetic markers that correlate statistically with the presence (or absence) of certain heritable—and desirable—traits (for example, tallness, leanness, perfect pitch, longevity, and perhaps even temperament and eventually intelligence). For parents willing to abort and try again repeatedly, prenatal screening could in principle be used to try to land a "better"—and not just a disease-free—baby. But, in practice, such an approach—even leaving ethical issues aside—is unfeasible on scientific grounds. No genetic selection can "optimize" beyond what the parents have contributed to the fetus. Moreover, an enormous number of "trial pregnancies" would be needed to get an "optimum baby" for any polygenic trait. For all these reasons this entire approach strikes us as farfetched, and we shall not consider it further as a realistic possibility.

Yet, before leaving this subject, we think it important to observe that the existence and normalization of prenatal diagnosis and abortion for genetic defect have already had significant effects on our thinking: about our genetic endowments, about reproductive choice and responsible parenthood, and about what constitutes a good or "good enough" child. Attitudes and opinions acquired in connection with this practice will certainly influence how we are likely to think about and deal with the coming new techniques for selecting or altering our prospective children. The ethical issues will be discussed in greater detail later, in the section devoted to them. To prepare that discussion, it is worth noting a few salient facts about the current practice of prenatal diagnosis and some of its social implications—regarding medicine, children, and parental prerogative and responsibility.

First, prenatal diagnosis has enabled many couples to avoid the sorrows and burdens of rearing children with severe genetic and chromosomal disorders. Anyone who has been close to families having children with Tay-Sachs disease or anencephaly knows the anguish and misery that are now preventable by such means. Children born with these and comparable abnormalities endure serious and lifelong physical and mental disabilities. With certain of the conditions, postnatal care can restore some hope of a normal life; with others, such care is moderately palliative at best, and the children afflicted by these diseases are often destined to live relatively short lives marked by persistent physical pain and profound mental retardation. Without the option of prenatal screening, many couples at high risk for such genetic abnormalities would choose not to bear children at all; prenatal screening has also enabled women who have already given birth to an affected child or who are past the age of thirty-five (when the risk of chromosomal abnormalities begins to rise sharply) to become pregnant with some confidence of bearing healthy children.

Yet, second, to achieve these benefits prenatal diagnosis adopts a novel approach to preventive medicine: it works by eliminating the prospective patient before he can be born. This kind of preventive medicine is thus in fact a species of negative eugenics—elimination of the genetically unfit and a reduction in the incidence of their genes—albeit carried out voluntarily and on a case-by-case basis. It is true that the tests themselves are value-neutral and that many genetic counselors are committed to non-directive counseling, leaving prospective parents free to exercise their individual choices based on their own value judgments. Yet the very availability of these tests—accompanied in many cases by subtle pressures, applied by counselors (and others) to prospective parents, to abort any abnormal fetus—strongly implies that certain traits are or should be disqualifying qualities of life that justify prevention of birth.

Third, the practice of prenatal screening has established as a cultural norm (or at least as a culturally acceptable norm) a new notion about children: the notion that admission to life is no longer unconditional, that certain conditions or traits are disqualifying. To be sure, parents confronted with the painful decision whether or not to abort an affected fetus may feel deeply divided and moved by considerations on both sides of the issue, but there appears to be a growing consensus, both in the medical community and in society at large, that a child-to-be should meet a certain (for now, minimal) standard to be entitled to be born. Although, at least in the United States, the practice of screening and elimination is likely to remain voluntary, its growing use could have subtly coercive consequences for prospective parents and could increase discrimination against the "unfit." Children born with defects that could have been diagnosed in utero may no longer be looked upon as "Nature's mistakes" but as parental failings.

Finally, the practice of prenatal screening establishes the principle that parents may choose the qualities of their children, and choose them on the basis of genetic knowledge. This new principle, in conjunction with the cultural norm just mentioned, may already be shifting parental and societal attitudes toward prospective children: from simple acceptance to judgment and control, from seeing a child as an unconditionally welcome gift to seeing him as a conditionally acceptable product. If so, these changes in attitude might well carry over beyond choices confined to the presence or absence of genetic diseases, to the presence or absence of other desired qualities. Far from producing contentment and gratitude in the parents, such changes might feed the desire for better—and *still* better—children.

2. Genetic Engineering of Desired Traits ("Fixing Up")

With directed genetic change aimed at producing certain desired improvements, we enter the futuristic realm of "designer babies." Proponents have made this prospect look straightforward, and, on a theory of strict genetic determinism, it is. One would first need to identify all (or enough) of the specific variants of genes whose presence (or absence) correlates with certain desired traits: higher intelligence, better memory, perfect pitch, calmer temperament, sunnier disposition, greater ambitiousness, etc. Once identified, the requisite genes could be isolated, replicated or synthesized, and then inserted into the early embryo (or perhaps into the egg or sperm) in ways that would eventually contribute to the desired phenotypic traits. In the limit, there is talk of babies "made to order," embodying a slew of desirable qualities acquired with such genetic engineering. But in our considered judgment, these dreams of fully designed babies, based on directed genetic change, are for the foreseeable future pure fantasies. There are huge obstacles, both to accurate knowing and to effective doing. One of these obstacles—the reality that these traits are heavily influenced by environment—will not be overcome by better technology.

Most of the traits for which parents might wish to engineer improvements in their children—appearance, intelligence, memory—are most certainly polygenic, that is, traits (or phenotypes) that depend on specific genes or their variants at several, perhaps many, distinct loci. In such cases the relationships and interactions among these genes (and between one's genes and the environment) are certain to be enormously complex.* Isolating all the relevant genetic variants, and knowing how to work with them to produce the desired result, will therefore prove immensely difficult. To be sure, not every trait for which parents might wish to select need turn out to be highly polygenic: for example, height, skin color, eye color, or even the genetic contributions to sexual orientation or basic temperament might be heavily influenced by a very few genes. As we will see more fully in Chapter Four, one mutation in a single gene has been shown to result in enormous increases in the lifespan of flies, worms, and mice, and the same gene has been identified in humans. Yet even here there would be no guarantee that the predisposing genes, even if correctly and safely introduced into the zygote or early embryo, would necessarily express themselves as desired, to yield the sought-for improvement.

Even more of an obstacle to successful genetic engineering is the practical difficulty of inserting genes into embryos (or gametes) in ways that would produce the desired result and *only* the desired result. Getting the genes into the right place in the cell, able to function yet without disturbing regular cellular functions, is an enormously challenging task. Insertion of genes into the host genome can cause abnormalities, either by activating harmful genes or by inactivating useful ones. Recently, for example, children undergoing experimental gene therapy for immune system deficiencies have developed leukemia after retroviral gene transfer into bone marrow stem cells, very likely the result of activation of a cancer-producing

---

* Growing recognition of the complexity of gene interactions, the importance of epigenetic and other environmental influences on gene expression, and the impact of stochastic events is producing a strong challenge to strict genetic determinism. Straightforward genetic engineering of better children may prove impossible, not only in practice but even in principle.

gene by the virus used to transfer the therapeutic genes into the cell.[6] And should introduced genes become inserted into inappropriate locations, normal host genes could be inactivated. Moreover, because many genes are pleiotropic—that is, they influence many traits, not just one—even a properly inserted gene introduced to enhance a particular trait would often have multiple effects, not all of them for the better.

Running such risks might be justified in *gene therapy* efforts for already existing individuals, where the genes hold out the only hope of cure for an otherwise deadly disease. But these safety risks will pose formidable obstacles to all interventions in gametes or embryos, especially *nontherapeutic* interventions aimed at producing children who would allegedly be, in one respect or another, "better than well." It is difficult to see how such an intervention could ever be considered ethical, especially since the negative effects might extend to future generations.

As a possible way around the hazards of gene insertion, some researchers have proposed the assembly and injection of artificial chromosomes: the new "better" genes could be packaged in small, manufactured chromosomal elements that, on introduction into cells, would not integrate into any of the normal forty-six human chromosomes. Such artificial chromosomes could, in theory, be introduced into ova or zygotes without fear of causing new mutations. But methods would have to be found to guarantee the synchronized replication and normal segregation of such artificial chromosomes. Otherwise, the package of improved genes, once introduced into the embryo, would not be conserved in all cells after normal mitotic division. Even more dauntingly, any gene introduced on such a chromosome would now be present in three copies (one from mother, one from father, and one on the extra chromosome) instead of the usual two, throwing off the normal balance of gene copies among all the genes. The consequences of such "triploidy" can be deleterious (for example, Down syndrome). All in all, safety and efficacy standards would seem to preclude doing such experiments with human subjects, at least in the United States, for the foreseeable future.* It is true that research along

---

* The Recombinant DNA Advisory Committee (RAC) of the National Institutes of Health (NIH), responsible for ethical review of all NIH-funded research proposals that involve putting genes into human beings, is, as a matter of policy, not reviewing any proposals that seek to modify gametes or

these lines might be undertaken in other countries (for example, China), by scientists unconstrained by these considerations, with eventual success in effecting directed genetic change in human embryos. But, at least for the time being, we believe that we may set this prospect safely to the side.

3. Selecting Embryos for Desired Traits ("Choosing In")

Unlike the prospect for precise genetic engineering through directed genetic change, the possibility of genetic enhancement of children through embryo selection cannot be easily dismissed. This approach, less radical or complete in its power to control, would not introduce new genes but would merely select positively among those that occur naturally. It depends absolutely on IVF, as augmented by the screening of the early embryos for the presence (or absence) of the desired genetic markers, followed by the selective transfer of those embryos that pass muster. This would amount to an "improvement-seeking" extension of the recently developed practice of preimplantation genetic diagnosis (PGD), now in growing use as a way to detect the presence or absence of genetic or chromosomal abnormalities *before* the start of a pregnancy.

As currently practiced, PGD works as follows: Couples at risk for having a child with a chromosomal or genetic disease undertake IVF to permit embryo screening before transfer, obviating the need for later prenatal diagnosis and possible abortion. A dozen or more eggs are fertilized and the embryos are grown to the four-cell or the eight-to-ten-cell stage. One or two of the embryonic cells (blastomeres) are removed for chromosomal analysis and genetic testing. Using a technique called polymerase chain reaction to amplify the tiny amount of DNA in the blastomere, researchers are able to detect the presence of genes responsible for one or more genetic disorders.[*] Only the embryos free of the genetic or chromo-

embryos. This decision produces an effective moratorium on all such research (at least that supported by federal funding). The Food and Drug Administration (FDA) has recently shut down the practice of ooplasm transfer into eggs undergoing in vitro fertilization, regarding it as a practice of unapproved germ-line genetic engineering because ooplasm contains mitochondrial DNA.

[*] Although scientists are able to identify thousands of human genes and their variants, the fact that at present blastomere testing is done on the minute quantity of DNA present in one or two cells limits the reach of PGD in any given embryo to a handful of genetic variants. However, ongoing research on techniques for whole genome amplification will likely permit PGD in the

somal determinants for the disorders under scrutiny are made eligible for transfer to the woman to initiate a pregnancy.

The use of IVF and PGD to move from disease avoidance to baby improvement is conceptually simple, at least in terms of the techniques of screening, and would require no change in the procedure. Indeed, PGD has already been used to serve two goals unrelated to the health of the child-to-be: to pre-select the sex of a child, and to produce a child who could serve as a compatible bone-marrow or umbilical-cord-blood donor for a desperately ill sibling. (In the former case, chromosomal analysis of the blastomere identifies the embryo's sex; in the latter case, genetic analysis identifies which embryos are immunocompatible with the needy recipient.) It is certainly likely that blastomere testing can be adapted to look for specific genetic variants at *any* locus of the human genome. And even without knowing the precise function of specific genes, statistical correlation of the presence of certain genetic variants with certain phenotypic traits (say, with an increase in IQ points or with perfect pitch) could lead to testing for these genetic variants, with selection following on this basis. As Dr. Francis Collins, director of the National Human Genome Research Institute, noted in his presentation to the Council, the time may soon arrive in which PGD is practiced for the purpose of selecting embryos with desired genotypes, even in the absence of elevated risk of particular genetic disorders.[7] Dr. Yury Verlinsky, director of the Reproductive Genetics Institute in Chicago, has recently predicted that soon "there will be no IVF without PGD."[8] Over the years, more and more traits will presumably become identifiable with the aid of PGD, including desirable genetic markers for intelligence, musicality, and so on, as well as undesirable markers for obesity, nearsightedness, color-blindness,[*] etc.

Yet, as Dr. Collins also pointed out to the Council, there are numerous practical difficulties with this scenario. For one thing, neither of the

future to test simultaneously for hundreds or even thousands of genetic variants in the same embryo. Of course, because of the complex relationship between genes and traits, the mere ability to screen for multiple genetic variants in no way guarantees that numerous phenotypic traits will soon be detectable.

[*] Color-blindness, a single-gene defect, can already be screened for.

parents may carry the genetic variant they are most interested in selecting for. Also, selecting for highly polygenic traits would require screening a large number of embryos in order to find one that had the desirable complement. With only a dozen or so embryos to choose from, it will not be possible to optimize for the many necessary variants.*

The practice of PGD and selective transfer is still quite new, and fewer than 10,000 children have been born with its aid. How likely or widespread such a practice might become is difficult to predict. As we have already indicated, a number of practical issues would need to be addressed before PGD could be extended to permit selection of desirable traits beyond the absence of genetic disorders. First are questions of possible harm caused by removing blastomeres for testing (up to a sixth or even a quarter of the embryo's cells are taken). Although current evidence (from limited practice) suggests that the procedure inflicts neither any immediately visible harm on the early embryos, nor any obvious harm on the child that results, more attention to long-term risks to the child born following PGD is needed before many people would consider using it for "improvement" purposes only. Because many of the desirable human phenotypic traits are very likely polygenic, the contribution of any single gene identifiable by blastomere testing is likely to be small, and the likelihood of finding all the "desired" genetic variants in a single embryo is exponentially smaller still. Testing for multiple genetic variants using the DNA from a single blastomere is likely to be limited—for a time—by the quantities of DNA available, the sensitivity of the genetic tests, and the ability to perform multiple tests on the same sample. But it seems only a matter of time before techniques are perfected that will permit simultaneous screening of IVF embryos for multiple genetic variants. And should some

---

* If, for example, a desired trait required the concurrence of only seven specific genetic alleles and (to take the simplest case) there were only two alternate variants of each gene, one would need (on the average) 128 embryos (and even more eggs) to get the full complement (2 to the seventh power). (This point is powerfully illustrated in figures VIII.a-c in the recent report of the German National Ethics Council, *Genetic diagnosis before and during pregnancy: opinion*, Berlin: Nationaler Ethikrat, 2003, pp. 158–160.) Today, in the average IVF cycle, twelve to fifteen eggs are obtained by superovulation, and roughly only half make it to the stage where screening could occur. Of course, if the oocyte supply could be increased, say by deriving oocytes from embryonic stem cells, this problem might be soluble.

of the "desirable" genes come grouped in clusters, selection for at least some desired traits might well be possible.

Finally, even if PGD could be used successfully to select an embryo with a number of desirable genetic variants, there is simply no guarantee that the child born after this procedure would grow up with the desired traits. The interplay of nature and nurture (genes and environment) in human development is too complex and too little understood to make such results predictable. Given that IVF combined with PGD is an inconvenient and expensive alternative to normal procreation, and given that success is doubtful at best, the purely elective use of this procedure seems unlikely to become widespread in the foreseeable future. As Professor Steven Pinker put it, in his presentation to the Council:

> The choice that parents would face in a hypothetical future in which even genetic enhancement were possible would not be the one that's popularly portrayed, namely, "Would you opt for a procedure that would give you a happier, more talented child?" When you put it like that, well, who would say no to that question? More realistically, the question that parents would face would be something like this: "Would you opt for a traumatic and expensive procedure that might give you a very slightly happier and more talented child, might give you a less happy, less talented child, might give you a deformed child, and probably would do nothing?" [9]

Nevertheless, we think it would be imprudent to ignore completely this approach to "better children." More and more people are turning to assisted reproduction technologies (ART): in parts of western Europe, roughly five percent of all births involve ART; in the United States, it is roughly one percent and climbing, as the average maternal age of childbirth keeps rising and family size keeps declining. More and more people are using IVF not merely to overcome infertility but to screen and select embryos free of certain genetic defects. Women who plan to delay childbearing are being encouraged to consider early removal and cryopreservation of their own youthful ovarian tissue, to be reintroduced into their bodies at sites easily accessible for egg harvesting when they decide to have children. Other novel methods of obtaining supplies of eggs for IVF—possibly including deriving them in bulk from stem cells[10]—would make the procedure less burdensome, and would, in theory, permit the creation of a large enough population of embryos to make screening for polygenic traits feasible.

The anticipated vast extension of genetic screening will make many more couples aware of the risks they run in natural reproduction, and they may choose to turn to IVF to reduce them—especially if obtaining eggs became easy. Once more and more couples start screening embryos for disease-related concerns, and once scientists have identified those genes that correlate with various admirable traits, the anticipated expansion of improved and more precise screening techniques might enable users of IVF to screen for "desirable genes" as well. People already using PGD to screen for disease markers might seek information also about other traits, as they have with sex or histocompatibility. And if, once screening becomes automated, its cost comes down, or if society decides to reimburse for PGD (regarding it as less expensive than the care of genetically diseased children), the use of this approach toward "better children" might well become the practice of at least a significant minority. Under these circumstances, should genuine and significant improvements be achieved for a few highly desired attributes (say, in maximum lifespan; see Chapter Four), one can easily imagine that there would be an increased demand for the practice, inconvenient or not. In the meantime, we would do well to consider the ethical implications not only of such future prospects but also of our current practices that make use of genetic knowledge.

C. Ethical Analysis

The technologies we have just considered range from the well-established (prenatal "screening out," using amniocentesis and abortion) to the speculative (embryonic "fixing up," using direct genetic modification of embryos or gametes), with special attention to the new and growing ("choosing in," using preimplantation genetic diagnosis followed by selective embryo transfer). It bears emphasis that genetic technologies have been and are being devised mainly with the intention of producing healthier children—not "enhanced children" or "super-babies," but children who are better only in the sense of being free of severe disease and deformity. As we have suggested, we have our doubts whether these powers will soon be widely employed for any other purpose. Yet there are ample reasons why we should not become complacent or take these matters lightly.

Powers to screen and select for one purpose are immediately available to screen and select for another purpose; the same is true for powers of directed genetic change. And, as already noted, it is sometimes hard to distinguish between desirable traits that one would call "healthy" and those that one would call "good in some other way": consider the case of leanness (non-obesity) or perfect pitch (non-tone-deafness) or attentiveness (non-distractibility). Moreover, there is ample reason to take stock of the ethical and social issues related to present and anticipated practices of screening and selection even if, as we have indicated, there is no reason for alarm regarding "designer babies." For the confluence of ever more sophisticated techniques of assisted reproduction with ever greater capacities for genetic screening and manipulation is already increasing the intrusion of science and technology into human procreation, yielding to scientists and parents ever growing powers over the beginnings of human life and the native capacities of the next generation. In addition to welcome consequences for the health of children, such practices may have more ambiguous or worrisome consequences for our ideas about the relation of sex and procreation, parents and children, the requirements of responsible parenthood, and beliefs in the equal worth of all human beings regardless of genetic (or other) disability.

Before one can decide whether these changes should be welcomed enthusiastically, tolerated within limits, or met with disquiet, one must try to think through what they mean—for individuals, for families, and for the larger society. In what follows, we shall examine, first, the reasons why many people welcome these technologies; second, concerns that might be raised about the safety of these procedures and about equality of access to their use; and, finally, more profound ethical questions regarding how these technologies might affect family life and society as a whole.

1. Benefits

There is no question but that assisted reproductive technologies have, over the past few decades, enabled many infertile couples to conceive and bear children, and that the more recent addition of PGD holds the promise of helping couples conceive healthy children when there is a serious risk of heritable disease. The widespread practice of prenatal screening in high-risk pregnancies has enabled numerous couples to terminate pregnancies when severe genetic disorders have been detected. It is the natural aspiration of couples not only to have children, but to have healthy children, and these procedures have in many cases lent crucial assistance to that aspiration. People welcome these technologies for multiple reasons: compassion for the suffering of those afflicted with genetic diseases; the wish to spare families the tragedy and burden of caring for children with deadly and devastating illnesses; sympathy for those couples who might otherwise forego having children, for fear of passing on heritable disorders; an interest in reducing the economic and social costs of caring for the incurable; and hopes for progress in the overall health and fitness of human society.* No one would *wish* to be afflicted, or to have one's child afflicted, by a debilitating genetic disorder, and the new technologies hold out the prospect of eliminating or reducing the prevalence of some of the worst conditions.**

Should it become feasible, many people would have reason to welcome the use of these technologies to select or produce children with improved natural endowments, above and beyond being free of disease. Parents, after all, hope not only for healthy children, but for children best endowed to live fulfilling lives. At some point, if some of the technical challenges are overcome, PGD is likely to present itself as an attractive way to enhance our children's potential in a variety of ways. Assuming that it became possible to select embryos containing genes that conferred

---

* Not all Members of this Council agree that it is obviously and simply good to assist people in avoiding the need to care for children who are not healthy. One Member comments: "It would be good to live in paradise, but, given that we don't, I am not sure that it is necessarily a good not to have to care for children who are not healthy. I would have thought it 'good' to try to produce people who—in a world that is not paradise—are able and willing to shoulder such burdens."

** We know of at least one exception: the case of a deaf couple using genetic screening to produce a deaf child.

certain generic benefits—for example, greater resistance to fatigue, or lowered distractibility, or better memory, or increased longevity—many parents would be eager to secure these advantages for their children. And they would likely regard it as an extension of their reproductive freedom to be able to do so; they might even regard it as their parental obligation. In a word, parents would enjoy enlarged freedom of choice, greater mastery of fortune, and satisfaction of their desires to have "better children." And, if all went well, both parents and children would enjoy the benefits of the enhancements.

2. Questions of Safety

Needless to say, the matter is hardly this simple. As with all biomedical interventions, a primary ethical concern is the matter of safety: the risks of bodily harm incurred by those subject to the procedures involved in genetic screening and manipulation. As with all biomedical interventions in reproductive processes, the safety issue takes on special gravity and difficulty, precisely because some of the hazards will be inflicted on the unconsenting child-to-be, and in the very activities connected with his coming-into-being. The Council has previously dealt at length with this issue in its report on human cloning, *Human Cloning and Human Dignity*, to which the reader is referred.[11]

There are, first of all, hazards connected to the various technological *means* employed in genetic screening and manipulation: risks to the pregnant woman, the egg donor (if different from the mother-to-be), and, most important, to the offspring. In the case of *prenatal screening*, whether by amniocentesis or chorionic villus sampling, there are well known, albeit slight, risks of infection, trauma (to both pregnant woman and fetus), miscarriage, and premature labor. These risks are weighed against the hazards of not screening, when the mother is of advanced reproductive age or when there is other evidence suggesting heightened risk of genetic defects in the fetus. Of course, prenatal screening serves to prevent genetic defects only if it is followed up by abortion, which, besides destroying the fetus, involves some potential health risks to the woman.

Regarding *direct genetic manipulation of the germ line*, we have already examined some of the considerable associated risks and uncertainties in the course of arguing that this technology is unlikely to be applied to humans any time soon.

Regarding the topic of greatest interest here, preimplantation diagnosis and selection, there are questions as to the long-term safety of blastomere biopsy. Although the technique of removing one or two cells from the eight-cell embryo for chromosome or DNA analysis does not appear to harm the embryo (at least in those cases in which it goes on to become a child), there are as yet no studies looking at long-term consequences for children born after blastomere biopsy. Such currently imponderable risks might be thought to recede in importance when severe genetic diseases are in prospect. However, if PGD were to be undertaken, not to screen out genetic defects, but to improve native powers, there should be heightened scrutiny of any possible dangers involved in the procedure.

To date, ethical thinking about the hazards of the techniques of assisted reproduction has often been incomplete, partly as a result of the perceived desirability of the end. IVF and PGD are undertaken with the intention of producing healthy, fit children; put this way, the enterprise would seem to be much like other medical practices and, as such, amenable to the same ethical standards. But a medical procedure designed to *produce* a healthy person has a different character from procedures aimed at safeguarding or healing a patient who is already alive. Yet here our thinking is ill-served owing to a noticeable lacuna in our approach to the ethics of risky therapies and (especially) the ethics of research using human subjects.

Ordinarily, when new technologies are introduced into medical practice or when medical research is undertaken with human subjects, the safety of the patients or subjects is of paramount ethical concern. However, in the case of IVF, with or without PGD, the children who are produced as a result of these procedures are not considered subjects at risk, for the simple reason that the embryos being handled, tested, and manipulated are not regarded as human subjects. Thus, blastomere biopsy performed on a tiny eight-cell embryo is not treated as an experiment on a *human subject* or as diagnosis of a *patient*, even though the future health and well-being of the child are very much at stake. Instead, the ethics of IVF and PGD are generally dealt with as though the only patient involved were the mother.* Whether or not one believes that the embryo here manipulated is a fully human being worthy of moral and legal protection, it is certainly the essential (and fragile) beginnings of the child who will be born and whose health and well-being should therefore be of overriding concern.

A deeper safety question connected with the goal of genetic screening is whether the normal ethical standard—"the best interests of the patient"—can be said to apply if and when PGD is used to select a "better" child. Even when PGD is used only to screen out genetic diseases—and all the more when it is employed to select positive traits—the parents are in effect choosing a particular genotype for their child. The question is, will this unprecedented power in the hands of the parents necessarily be used for the good of the child? Should parents be willing to gamble the safety of their children for the chance to make them "better than well"? What risks to their health and safety are worth taking in pursuit of improvement or perfection?

Ordinarily, in most matters regarding children, our society accepts the principle that each set of parents has authority and responsibility for the well-being of their own children. Yet there are circumstances that lead the state to step in to protect a vulnerable child against abusive or negligent parents. In such cases, the best of parental intentions do not exonerate. How should our society view parental (and biotechnical) discretion to seek to produce "better children" through procedures carrying unknown hazards to those children?

These questions take on greater poignancy once we recognize a novel but morally significant feature of embryo selection using PGD, absent in *prenatal* diagnosis. In intrauterine genetic screening, there is one fetus being tested, and the question at issue is a binary choice of "keep" or "destroy." In contrast, in preimplantation screening a whole array of embryos are scrutinized and tested, and the choice is not the either-or "yes or no" but rather the comparative choice of "best in the class." For if one

---

* In several of its efforts to exercise authority over practices connected with assisted reproduction, such as cloning-to-produce-children or ooplasm transfer, the Food and Drug Administration has had to resort to the fiction that the embryo is a "drug," whose "administration" to the mother is potentially hazardous—to her.

is going to the trouble of doing IVF supplemented by preimplantation diagnosis, why not get "the best"—the healthiest and, perhaps soon, the "better-than-healthiest"? But in order to get the best, or even in order to get a non-diseased child, one must conceptually "bundle" all the separate embryos and regard them as if they were a single precursor. All will be subjected to testing so that the one who is chosen will be disease-free or better. Yet to make sure that the child who is to be born is the fittest, rather than his diseased or inferior brother or sister, the anointed one must bear potential risks (imposed during the testing) *that he would not have borne in the absence of the parental desire for quality control.* For the sake of which benefits *to the child* can we justify imposing on him what kinds and what degrees of risk?

Before leaving the subject of safety and the concern for the health of children, we observe an ironic feature of the search for better babies with the aid of genetic screening. What if, as a result of widespread genetic screening of adults and improvement in diagnostic screening of embryos, the practice of IVF with PGD came to be seen as *superior* to natural procreation in offering a greater probability of obtaining a healthy child? If the procedures became sufficiently routine and inexpensive (to the point, say, where they are covered by ordinary health insurance), prospective parents interested in healthier (or otherwise better) children might increasingly be tempted to consider IVF with PGD. Furthermore, couples who would then elect PGD in order to screen out genetic diseases might well be tempted to engage at the same time in some positive trait selection. In that case, what began modestly as a means to help the infertile bear children and continued as a way to screen out the worst genetic defects might ultimately stand as a competitor to natural reproduction altogether, with significant consequences for the family and for society at large.*

---

* As early as 1971, only two years after the first successful in vitro fertilization of human egg by human sperm (and well before the birth of Louise Brown in 1978), geneticist Bentley Glass, in his presidential address to the American Association for the Advancement of Science, was heralding the eugenic possibilities of IVF. He looked to IVF, coupled with genetic screening of gametes and embryos, not for the relief of infertility but for securing "the right of every child to be born with a sound physical and mental constitution, based on a sound genotype." Glass went on to predict: "No parents will in that future time have a right to burden society with a malformed or a mentally incompetent child." (Glass, B., "Science: Endless Horizons or Golden Age," *Science* 171: 23-29, 1971, p. 28.)

As this discussion indicates, the issue of health and safety proves, on further reflection, to concern more than safety. When biomedical technology permits the substitution, for natural procreation and the rule of chance, of a procedure in which parents begin to control their child's genotype, reproduction becomes to some extent like obtaining or making a product to selected specifications. Even if the parents are guided by their own sense of what would be a good or perfect baby, their selection may serve to satisfy their own interests more than that of the child. The new technologies, even when used only to screen out and get rid of the sick or "imperfect," imply a changed attitude of parents toward their children, a mixture of control and tacit expectations of perfection, an attitude that might grow more pronounced as the relevant techniques grow more sophisticated. Apparently good intentions—to improve the next generation, to enhance the life of our descendants—will not guarantee that genetic screening will be an unqualified blessing for parents and children. (We return to this subject shortly.)

3. Questions of Equality

Many observers have noted with concern that, owing to the sheer expense of IVF and PGD—a successful assisted pregnancy costing, on average, roughly \$20,000–\$30,000[*12]—not all couples who could benefit from these procedures have unfettered access to them. If PGD were to become an established option, but only for the affluent, one envisages the troubling prospect of a society divided between the economically *and* genetically rich, on the one hand, and the economically *and* genetically poor on the other. Severe inherited diseases might disappear except among the poor, while genetic enhancement through screening and selection might be a privilege enjoyed exclusively by the rich. These concerns would, of course, diminish (though they would not disappear) if, as seems likely, the costs of the procedures in question come down and access to these services grows wider.[**]

---

[*] A single reproductive cycle of IVF costs about \$8,000, with roughly a 30 percent chance of producing a baby; PGD adds \$3,000 or more to the cost of an IVF cycle and slightly reduces the chance of producing a baby.

[**] Indeed, one could argue that, under such circumstances, there may be greater relative gains for the poor than for the rich, since the former can, to some degree, "catch up genetically." Even if genetic inequality persisted, the genetically poor might be better off than they are now.

Yet these legitimate concerns about equality of access rest, ironically, on certain *inegalitarian* assumptions that need to be brought to light. First, the goal of eliminating embryos and fetuses with genetic defects carries the unspoken implication that certain "inferior" kinds of human beings—for example, those with Down syndrome—do not deserve to live. The assumption that the genetically unfit ought to be prevented from being born embodies and invites a profoundly denigrating and worrisome attitude toward those who *do* get to be born. How will we come to regard the many people alive today who carry genetic defects that in the future will be screened out, or the many people, even in a future age of more widespread screening, who will still be born with the abhorred disabilities and diseases? The worry over unequal access to PGD is, in effect, a worry about the inability of the *economically* poor to practice the ultimate discrimination against the *genetically* poor.

Second, when new techniques permit parents to be the partial authors of their child's genetic makeup, the inequality between parents and children is substantially increased. Parents thereby acquire the power, not just of giving life to their children, but of shaping (or trying to shape) the character of that life. Of course, through education and upbringing parents have always had an enormous influence on the lives of their children; but inasmuch as the consequences of genetic screening are imposed before birth and are carried as the child's permanent biological destiny, the inegalitarian effect of the new technology is unprecedented and irreversible.

In response to these concerns, it will be pointed out, rightly, that genes are not exactly destiny, and that it will prove very difficult to intervene genetically at the embryonic stage in ways that will guarantee the appearance of the desired "improvements" in one's children. But much mischief can be done to a child simply from the enhanced parental expectations, all the more so if the child fails to attain the superior native gifts for which he was selected. And as we shall soon see, we are already witnessing certain subtle forms of genetic discrimination even though the technology of screening is still very undeveloped.

4. Consequences for Families and Society

Beyond questions of safety and equal access, there is reason to believe that the advent of expanded genetic screening and its uses in reproduction could have a profound impact on human procreation, family life, and society as a whole. At present, fewer than 10,000 children have been born following PGD, and the screening procedure itself is being used to diagnose only a limited number of chromosomal and genetic ailments. For these reasons, it is both difficult to predict and also easy to underestimate the societal import of marrying genomic knowledge with established techniques of assisted reproduction, should the practice become widespread.

To make vivid the possible implications, it may therefore be helpful to imagine a future time at which all external barriers to the use of these procedures have been largely removed.* Suppose that, a decade from now, IVF and PGD have been perfected to the point where preimplantation screening is safe and effective, not prohibitively expensive, and capable of identifying a wide range of markers for heritable disorders. Suppose, in other words, that prospective parents (perfectly fertile) routinely have the option of using these technologies in order to select an essentially disease-free embryo for transfer to the mother's womb.**

Under such circumstances—admittedly quite hypothetical—might not the practice become moderately widespread? Could many people come to regard using IVF plus PGD as safer (for the child) than the randomness of sex, and therefore preferable to natural procreation even when there is no particular history of genetic disease? In societies in which people are limited—or limit themselves—to only one child, might they not increasingly turn to these techniques to ensure that their child might be as "perfect" as possible? And, should this procedure begin to compete

---

* The discussion that follows is frankly speculative, and only time may tell how accurate it is. Yet because the stakes are potentially very high, this thought experiment is useful in clarifying what such innovation could mean for human procreation and our attitudes toward children.

** The desire for a "disease-free" inheritance will be, of course, difficult if not impossible to realize. All of us carry genetic variants that predispose to illness; perhaps a few dozen for each of us. It is highly unlikely that all of these can ever be screened out.

with or even to supplant sex as the more common route to conceiving children, in what ways would the meaning of childbearing be altered?

The hypothetical case just sketched may seem like science fiction, but the important questions it raises are, in fact, implicated in the current practice of genetic screening. Even though the practice of PGD is still in its infancy, its availability has begun to influence our thinking about childbearing. Already the goals of assisted reproductive technologies are changing, from the original modest aim of providing children for the infertile to the novel and more ambitious aim of producing healthy children for whoever needs extra assistance in obtaining them.* Anticipating the coming of augmented powers of genetic screening and selection, people are expanding the idea of "a healthy child" and therewith almost certainly the aspirations of prospective parents. In his presentation to the Council, Dr. Gerald Schatten, a leading researcher in the field of reproductive biology, stated that the overall goal of assisted reproductive technology is "to help prospective parents *realize their own dreams* of having a *disease-free legacy*" (emphasis added).[13] The dream of a disease-free legacy—as stated, a goal that looks beyond merely the next generation—seems rather different from the merely hopeful wish for a healthy child. And even without such a broad ambition, the intervention of rigorous genetic screening into the order of childbearing will likely involve raising the standard for what counts as an acceptable birth. The likely significance of this fact is subtle but profound. The attitude of parents toward their child may be quietly shifted from unconditional acceptance to critical scrutiny: the very first act of parenting now becomes not the unreserved welcoming of an arriving child, but the judging of his or her fitness, while still an embryo, to become their child, all by the standards of

---

* A significant and growing fraction of Americans now using assisted reproductive technologies are not infertile or seeking treatment for infertility. Dr. Gerald Schatten informed the Council that up to a third of couples who undergo IVF with PGD choose to do so without a history of infertility. (See Dr. Schatten's presentation cited in endnote 3.) In Europe, according to a 2001 survey by the European Society of Human Reproduction and Embryology, as many as three-quarters of PGD procedures are performed on couples without a prior history of infertility or subfertility. ("ESHRE PGD Consortium: data collection III [May 2001]," *Human Reproduction*, 17[1]: 233-246, 2002. See especially Table II: Reasons for preimplantation genetic diagnosis.) At present we know nothing about the children born as a result, or how they fare in their families.

contemporary genetic screening. Moreover, as the screening technology itself grows more refined, more able to pick out serious but not life-threatening genetic conditions (from dwarfism and deafness to dyslexia and asthma) and then genetic markers for desirable traits, the standards for what constitutes an acceptable birth may grow more exacting.

With genetic screening, procreation begins to take on certain aspects of the *idea*—if not the practice—of manufacture, the making of a product to a specified standard. The parent—in partnership with the IVF doctor or genetic counselor—becomes in some measure the master of the child's fate, in ways that are without precedent. This leads to the question of what it might mean for a child to live with a chosen genotype: he may feel grateful to his parents for having gone to such trouble to spare him the burden of various genetic defects; but he might also have to deal with the sense that he is not just a gift born of his parents' love but also, in some degree, a product of their will.

These questions of family dynamics could become even more complicated when preimplantation genetic screening is used to select embryos for some desirable traits. While current negative screening is guided by the standard of a healthy or disease-free baby, the goals of prospective positive use are in theory unlimited, governed only by the parents' ideas of what they want in their child. Today, parents using PGD take responsibility for selecting for birth children who will not be chronically sick or severely disabled; in the future, they might also bear responsibility for picking and choosing which "advantages" their children shall enjoy. Such an enlarged degree of parental control over the genetic endowments of their children cannot fail to alter the parent-child relationship. Selecting against disease merely relieves the parents of the fear of specific ailments afflicting their child; selecting for desired traits inevitably plants specific hopes and expectations as to how their child might excel. More than any child does now, the "better" child may bear the burden of living up to the standards he was "designed" to meet. The oppressive weight of his parents' expectations—resting in this case on what they believe to be undeniable biological facts—may impinge upon the child's freedom to make his own way in the world. Here we see one of the ethically paradoxical consequences of the new screening technologies: designed to free us from the tyranny of our genes, they may end up narrowing our freedoms as individuals even further.

In addition to changes in the parent-child relationship, there are reasons to be concerned about the wider social effects of an increased use of genetic screening and selection. There is, first of all, the prospect of diminished tolerance for the "imperfect," especially those born with genetic disorders that could have been screened out. It is offensive to think that children, suffering from "preventable" genetic diseases, should be directly asked, "Why were you born?" (or their parents asked, "Why did you let him live?"). Yet it is almost as troubling to contemplate that "defective" children and their parents may be treated contemptuously and unfairly in light of such prejudices, even if they go unspoken. Already, parents who have a child with Down syndrome are sometimes asked, "Well, didn't you have an amnio? How did this happen?" Many of these parents are people who, for their own ethical reasons, have chosen to proceed with the pregnancy even after learning the results of genetic screening, electing to love and care for the children that it has been given to them to love. Yet as the range of detectable disorders increases, as adult screening becomes ubiquitous and every pregnancy is tested, and as the economic cost of caring for the afflicted remains high, it may become difficult for parents to resist the pressure, both social and economic, of the "consensus" that children with sufficiently severe and detectable disabilities must not be born.

In all likelihood parents will increasingly feel pressure to conform to shifting social standards of what is genetically fit. Along with the freedoms bequeathed by the new technologies comes a certain danger of social coercion and tyranny of public opinion. Furthermore, as our table of detectable genetic markers grows more complete, there is the prospect of using genetic screening to weed out not only the most devastating genetic disorders but also heritable conditions that are bad but manageable, or even merely inconvenient. In practice, it is likely to prove very hard to draw a bright line between identifiable defects that might justify discarding an embryo or preventing a birth and those defects that parents might (or should) be able to find acceptable. It is not clear what resources our society will be able to draw upon to assist parents in making such important decisions.

Should PGD and IVF, contrary to current expectations, ever become widely used for positive screening of desirable traits, the impact on society could be even greater. Our knowledge of the human genome and our powers of genetic selection might grow so great as to unleash competition among parents eager to bear children who are biologically destined to be taller, thinner, brighter, or better-looking than their peers.

It should be noted that the social consequences of the widespread use of genetic screening alone are likely to outstrip the actual biological enhancements: those "unfortunate" enough to be born with genetic "defects" that might have been detected by screening might well be subject to discrimination, even without waiting to see how they turn out. The thoughtful (if not quite scientifically accurate) film *Gattaca* explores some of the chilling social implications of a human future in which genetic screening of children has become the norm. To the careful observer of current practices, the risks of such discriminatory implications are already evident.

II. CHOOSING SEX OF CHILDREN

There is one area in which parents are today already able to choose an important inborn characteristic of their children: sex selection and control. This practice is widespread in many countries around the world, and there is some evidence that it is being used with growing frequency in the United States.[14] Strictly speaking, choosing the sex of children is not exactly a choice for a "better" child, save in those cultures in which one sex (usually male) is held to be superior or privileged (or more rewarding to the family economically). But, if "good" means "that which is desired," it is a choice for a child thought by the parents to be "better" in the limited, but significant, sense of "more wanted." In choosing a child of the preferred sex, the parents are acting to satisfy their own desire for what, to them, is better (at least here and now).

While it is true that *what* is being chosen here is nothing new or different—selection is confined to one or the other of the eternal alternatives, male or female—the choice is not for that reason trivial or free from moral implications. Parents choose a supremely important aspect of their child's lifelong identity, yet in most cases they do so not for the child's sake. They choose not because they think that the child will be better off being male rather than female, or the reverse, but because they now want a boy or a girl, or because they want to balance a family now lacking in one sex or the other.*

The seemingly innocent practice of sex selection in fact raises many of the larger ethical concerns introduced above: about changing the relations between parents and children, moving procreation toward manufacture, and expanding parental choice and mastery over the next generation. Moreover, what happens in the area of sex-selection may have implications for other, more far-reaching efforts to choose or control the genetic makeup of our offspring, if and when that becomes possible. Both for itself and as a precedent, it is worth considering on its own this more modest form of seeking "better children."

In considering the ethical implications of sex selection, we must attend especially to the social consequences not just of the *fact* of choice but of the *choices made.* For the private choices made by individuals, once aggregated, could produce major changes in a society's sex ratio, with profound implications for the entire community—and also its neighbors. Over the past several decades, disturbing evidence has accumulated of the widespread use of various medical technologies to choose the sex of one's child, with a strong preference for the male sex. The natural sex ratio at birth is 105 baby boys born for every 100 baby girls. But in several countries today the ratio approaches or even exceeds 120 baby boys born for every 100 girls. There is also evidence that the ratio at birth of boys to girls is rising among certain ethnic groups in the United States.

---

* Of course, some parents may believe that a balanced family, with both sons and daughters, is better not only for them but for all their children. Alternatively, they might believe that boys need brothers and girls need sisters, or that they (as parents) are better suited to raising a child of one sex rather than the other. And, in societies with a deep cultural belief in the superiority of males, parents might well think they are doing their child a favor by selecting for maleness.

This phenomenon especially calls out for our attention and demands a broad-ranging ethical and social evaluation.*

A. Ends and Means

Sex selection offers a stark example of the marriage that can occur between modern technique, on the one hand, and ancient custom or primordial desire, on the other. For the human desire to choose the sex of one's off-spring—usually to have a son rather than a daughter, but also on occasion a daughter rather than a son—is hardly new. The folk wisdom of times gone by attests to the enduring power of this human want, found in mothers and fathers alike. In ancient Greece, it was believed that if men had sex while on their right side, a boy would result; and in eighteenth-century France, it was recommended to men who wanted sons to tie off their left testicle during intercourse. In our own time, books that claim to reveal the secrets of having a boy or a girl abound, with one bestseller recounting myriad methods but recommending the timing of sexual intercourse as the key. Indeed, the importance to all of us of a baby's sex is revealed in the first question we nearly always ask upon news of a newborn (assuming that we have not already found out by sonogram): "Is it a boy or a girl?"

If the central importance of a baby's sex and our desires to choose it are old, the medical techniques for realizing our desires are new. The principal means for doing so are, first, prenatal diagnosis (either using a

---

* Our focus here is on the *nonmedical* use of sex selection—that is, sex selection for purposes of choosing sex unrelated to the treatment or prevention of disease. Sex selection can also be used to prevent the transmission of sex-linked genetic diseases. For example, in the case of families carrying the gene for hemophilia—an X-linked recessive disease, affecting only males—detection and abortion of all male fetuses will prevent the birth of an afflicted child. In such instances, a clear medical goal is being served. While some Members of Council would question whether sex selection for this purpose is legitimate, or even whether the prevention of disease by selecting for sex is the same as treating a patient for disease, this discussion will not take up these more general issues. Our goal is to examine sex selection for itself and to understand what might be troubling about the practice apart from the issues of elective abortion or the destruction of embryos. It is also worth noting that "sex selection for medical reasons" is a misnomer. It is only incidentally a selection for sex, but uses sex as the criterion for selecting against a sex-based disease. Should genetic tests become available that would distinguish the afflicted male fetus from the non-afflicted one, selection would no longer be based on maleness, but solely on the presence or absence of the mutant gene.

sonogram to disclose the genitalia or using amniocentesis or chorionic villus sampling to disclose whether the karyotype is XX, female, or XY, male), followed by abortion of fetuses having the unwanted sex. Second, preimplantation genetic diagnosis (PGD) followed by selective transfer of embryos having the desired sex. And third, a less certain technique, prefertilization separation of sperm into X- and Y-bearing spermatozoa,* followed by artificial insemination or in vitro fertilization. The first two techniques select post-conception; the last seeks to produce the desired sex at the time of conception.

These methods were developed (or at least the first two were) to prevent disease. However, as with many other medical technologies, nontherapeutic uses were quickly discovered and put into practice. The techniques of amniocentesis and sonograms have been available respectively since the 1970s and 1980s and have become increasingly widespread. Amniocentesis can make a determination of sex at 16 to 18 weeks of gestation; sonograms at 15 to 16 weeks. PGD, the procedure (described earlier) to screen IVF embryos for chromosomal abnormalities and genetic diseases, has been available for about ten years. The newer and less tested sperm-sorting technology was originally a creation of the U.S. government, invented by a Department of Agriculture scientist in the 1980s for the purposes of selecting sex in livestock. The Genetics and IVF Institute in Fairfax, Virginia, developed the technology for humans and currently has an exclusive license on it—the technology is known as "MicroSort." The Institute charges about $2,300 per try, and currently claims a 90 percent success rate for girls and 73 percent success rate for boys. It offers this service only for the purpose of "family balancing"—that is, for achieving a mix of boys and girls in a family.

Even in just the short time that these various methods of sex selection have been available, they have had dramatic effects on sex ratios in many parts of the world. Generally, any variation in the sex ratio exceeding 106 boys born per 100 girls born can be assumed to be evidence of the prac-

---

* For the time being, the separation is physical. But researchers are also interested in finding immunological techniques that might differentially find X- and Y-bearing sperm and destroy or deactivate the undesired ones.

tice of sex selection. Here, from the most recent figures available, are just a few examples of skewed sex ratios around the world today. The sex ratio at birth of boys to 100 girls in Venezuela is 107.5; in Yugoslavia 108.6; in Egypt 108.7; in Hong Kong 109.7; in South Korea 110; in Pakistan 110.9; in Delhi, India, 117; in China 117; in Cuba 118; and in the Caucasus nations of Azerbaijan, Armenia, and Georgia, the sex ratio has reached as high as 120.* While the sex ratio in the United States has remained stable at 104.8, certain American ethnic groups have seen a statistically significant rise in their sex ratios. In 1984 the sex ratio for Chinese-Americans was 104.6 and for Japanese Americans 102.6; in 2000, these ratios had risen respectively to 107.7 and 106.4.[15]

Imbalances in the sex ratio are certainly not evenly spread across every region of the globe. However, one cannot but be impressed by the fact that distortions in the sex ratio afflict developed as well as underdeveloped nations, Hindu and Moslem populations as well as Christian populations, Western as well as non-Western nations, wealthy and educated regions as well as those that are less so. Although the practice is, for now, greater outside than within the United States, the other nations are mainly using technologies that we have developed (albeit for other purposes). One can only expect in the future that technologies of sex selection will be further refined and that new and cheaper technologies will emerge on the market. In the absence of some system of regulation, nothing stands in the way of a continuation and expansion of substantial distortions in the sex ratio, at least in some parts of the world and among some communities in the United States.**

B. Preliminary Ethical Analysis

Previous public discussions of the ethics of sex selection, conducted largely in terms of "sex bias" and "reproductive freedom," have been oddly ambivalent. On the one hand, despite the widespread and growing practice of sex

---

* Although data is lacking regarding the techniques people in these countries use to produce these large shifts in the sex ratio, we suspect that sonography-plus-abortion is by far the most common.

** If sex selection in the United States were practiced largely for family balancing (the use of sex selection to help a couple with at least one child to have another child of the less represented sex in the family), it is unlikely that we would experience major distortions in the sex ratio.

selection, it has attracted few overt defenders or partisans, at least in the United States. Almost no one argues openly in its favor, and those who do rarely offer up the single most important reason for its spread—the desire for sons over daughters (though, as we shall see, this taboo may be changing). To date, several special panels and advisory bodies in the United States have considered the ethics of sex selection.[16] None of these has condoned the practice; all have raised serious ethical concerns. Yet, on the other hand, all have insisted that sex selection should not be made illegal and may at least in some instances be defensible. Even those who condemn the practice urge that there is nothing we can do about it without violating our most cherished principles of reproductive freedom and individual autonomy.

Typifying this approach, the one previous presidential commission to consider the topic gave several reasons to support its judgment that the use of amniocentesis and abortion for sex selection was "morally suspect." First, such a practice was "an expression of sex prejudice." Second, it was incompatible with the findings of developmental psychology that the parent-child relationship depends upon "the attitude of virtually unconditional acceptance." Third, sex selection treated the child "as an artifact and the reproductive process as a chance to design and produce human beings according to parental standards of excellence"—an attitude that the commission condemned.[17] Yet despite these powerful objections, the commission did not see the matter in black-and-white terms either, and its policy recommendations were mild:

> This is not to say that every decision to undergo amniocentesis solely for purposes of sex selection is subject to moral criticism. Nonetheless, widespread use of amniocentesis for sex selection would be a matter of serious moral concern. Therefore, the Commission concludes that although individual physicians are free to follow the dictates of conscience, public policy should discourage the use of amniocentesis for sex selection. The Commission recognizes, however, that a legal prohibition would probably be ineffective and, worse, offensive to important social values (because vigorous enforcement of any such statute might depend on coercive state inquiries into private motivations).[18]

One factor distorting the ethical discussions of sex selection in America is that it has become entangled—as has the debate over stem cells and human cloning—in the controversy over abortion. Certain widely accepted political and ethical principles, such as individual autonomy, equality, the right to choose, and "non-directiveness," are thought to be threatened by any thoroughgoing critique of sex selection. In the early years, when post-conception determination of sex followed by abortion was the only means of sex selection, it was widely argued by many feminist-oriented scholars, as well as other liberal thinkers, that any legal or policy actions taken against abortion for sex selection would put the abortion right itself at risk.

The practice of sex selection also throws other cherished principles into disarray. Since the end of World War II, genetic counselors have adhered to the ethical norm of "nondirectiveness." It was hoped that by this principle they would avoid the coercive eugenic policies of the past, from forced sterilization to genocide. Yet by mandating the moral neutrality of genetic counselors, nondirectiveness in fact makes it easier for individual couples to practice sex selection as a matter of personal choice. And here too the culture wars over abortion play a part. In one study it was found that genetic counselors were reluctant to recommend against sex selection since they considered it a "logical extension of parents' rights to control the number, timing, spacing, and quality of their offspring."[19]

But three new developments conspire to invite a serious reexamination of this matter. First, there is the growing cultural heterogeneity of American society, with a rise in subgroups with distinct preferences for males. Second, there are growing commercial prospects for these services. Although the sex-selection technologies were originally developed within the moral framework of medicine and were directed towards disease prevention, the commercial possibilities of these technologies are becoming increasingly evident. Sex-selection services are openly advertised on the Internet, and sex selection could in the future become a big business.* Third, perhaps related to

---

* Here's how *Fortune* magazine recently summed up the potential market just for MicroSort alone: "Each year, some 3.9 million babies are born in the U.S. In surveys, a consistent 25 percent to 35 percent of parents and prospective parents say they would use sex selection if it were available. If just 2 percent of the 25 percent were to use MicroSort, that's 20,000 customers . . . [and] a $200-

the second, resistance to this practice is weakening, including among those who are keepers and purveyors of the technologies.

In 1999, the American Society for Reproductive Medicine (ASRM) criticized the use of PGD and sperm sorting for sex selection, fearing that such practices might contribute to gender stereotyping and discrimination.[20] In 2001, however, the ASRM relaxed its opposition to sperm sorting if used for the purpose of "family balancing,"[21] and, later that year, the chairman of ASRM's ethics committee appeared to endorse the use of PGD for the same purpose. When this produced considerable public controversy, in part based on concern over the destruction of embryos involved in PGD, the ASRM reaffirmed its position that PGD for sex selection should be discouraged, in deference to concerns about gender bias as well as about the moral status of the embryo. But the Society's recommendations are not enforced, and several of its members are openly offering sex selection to their clients.

In sum, although the practice of sex selection continues to grow, the American public debate over sex selection has never been aired in full. The new impetus to the growth of this practice, from multiculturalism to commercial interests, will make it difficult to slow its future spread. All the more reason to try now to evaluate its significance, beginning with the most common arguments for and against the practice.

There are a number of reasons given to support the practice of sex selection. The most common rationale today for sex selection is that it permits family balancing, enabling a couple to achieve its as-yet-unfulfilled wish to raise both sons and daughters. Many parents have had three or four girls (or boys) in a row, and really want a boy (or girl); effective sex selection would satisfy this wish without any risk of continued "failure." More generally, sex selection is defended on grounds that it could increase the happiness of the parents by enabling them to fulfill their desire for one or more sons or daughters. Sex selection is also supported because it may help to slow population growth (since many families continue to have children only to

---

million-a-year business in the U.S. alone." (Wadman, M., "So You Want a Girl?" *Fortune,* 9 February, 2001.)

achieve a particular balance of boys and girls); because it may enable parents to fulfill religious or cultural expectations (since some cultures attach great importance to or impose special obligations on male heirs); and because it may make children feel more wanted and comfortable with their sex (since they will know that they were in fact chosen to be whichever sex they are).

In certain cultures, the desire of parents for sons is extremely powerful; in traditional Islam, for example, parents are expected to continue bearing children until they have at least one son. A strong preference for sons also appears prevalent in most (though not all) of the countries of Asia. Sex selection can therefore be defended on "multicultural grounds," as helping parents to achieve not merely individual preferences but also traditional and religious aims.

A common objection voiced against sex selection is that, in its most prevalent practice today, it almost always involves the abortion of (otherwise healthy) fetuses of the unwanted sex.* However, sex selection by IVF with PGD involves instead the selective transfer of embryos of the desired sex and the discarding of any embryos of the other sex; some people, for this reason, regard this approach as less morally objectionable than the one that requires abortion, while others see no moral difference. No such stigma attaches to the practice, still nascent, of sex selection by sperm sorting; whether used with artificial insemination or in conjunction with IVF, sperm sorting reduces the need to discard embryos of the unwanted sex. Should ongoing research eventually produce selective spermicides that would permit sex selection via natural intercourse, all such objections to the means would be much diminished or even disappear. We would be left to evaluate only the end itself.

The objection most often raised to sex selection, especially as it is practiced throughout the world today, is that it reflects and contributes to bias or discrimination against women. Sex selection has involved the abortion of female fetuses on a massive scale, or, in a few cases only, the selection of male embryos over female ones for implantation. As we have seen, sex ratios in some communities have been altered sharply in a very

---

* Note that this is not an objection to the activity of sex selection as such, but only to an aspect of the means used. Other objections, considered below, address the thing itself: the *choosing* of sex, the choosing of *sex*, and the *social consequences* of the choices made.

short period of time. Yet, criticism of this phenomenon has tended to be muted because of the connection between sex selection and abortion; those who support the right to an abortion have generally been reluctant to argue that abortion for the sake of sex selection should be restricted. The "pro-choice" idea of "every child a wanted child" establishes the rule in reproductive matters of the supremacy of parental "wants." Ironically, the "right to choose," which was and is defended in the name of equality for women, has in this way made permissible the disproportionate choice of aborting female fetuses. It is open to question whether the cause of equality has been well served by this development.

Paradoxically, the anti-female bias thought by critics to be implicit in sex selection might in fact redound to the advantage of women, at least regarding marriage: their relative scarcity could give them greater selectivity, choice, and control of partners. In certain Asian countries for example, where the ratio of boys to girls at birth has been severely skewed by sex selection, young men of marriageable age are already facing a severe shortage of young women to marry. Thus one might oppose sex selection as much for the actual harm it does to men as for the prejudice it expresses against women.

But sex selection is ethically troubling for reasons that go beyond both its potentially discriminatory use and the necessity, under current procedures, of destroying fetuses or embryos of the unwanted sex. One of the fundamental issues has to do with the limits of liberty.

C. The Limits of Liberty

As we noted earlier, few policy makers or opinion leaders argue openly in favor of sex selection. Rather, the assumption is made that our most cherished ideals of individual autonomy and the right to choose preclude an unambiguous condemnation of sex selection or public polices that might curtail it. Yet this assumption is questionable.

Our society, to be sure, deeply cherishes liberty and rightfully gives a wide berth to its exercise. But liberty is never without its limits. In the case of actions that are purely self-regarding—that is, actions that affect only ourselves—society tends to give the greatest protections to personal freedom. But as we move outward, away from purely self-regarding actions to those actions that affect others, our liberty is necessarily more liable to societal and governmental oversight and restraint. Sex selection clearly does not belong in the category of purely self-regarding action. The parents' actions (their choice of a boy or a girl) are directed not only toward themselves but also toward the child-to-be.

One might argue that, since each child must be either a girl or a boy, the parents' actions in selecting the sex do not constitute much of an intrusion on the prospective child's freedom and well-being. But the binary choice among highly natural and familiar types hardly makes the choice a trivial one. And having one's sex foreordained by another is different from having it determined by the lottery of sexual union. There is thus at least a prima facie case for suggesting that the power to foreordain or control the nature of one's child's sexual identity is not encompassed in the protected sphere of inviolable reproductive liberty. It is far from clear that either the moral or the legal right to procreate includes the right to choose the sex—or other traits—of one's children.

But it is not only that sex selection affects the individual child-to-be that puts it in a class of actions fit for oversight, regulation, and (perhaps) curtailment. Sex selection, if practiced widely, can also have powerful societal effects that reach far beyond individuals and their families to the nation as a whole. The dramatic alteration in sex ratios in such countries as South Korea and Cuba bear this out. Whether or not one views the preference of individuals for sons over daughters as rational, taken together these individual preferences could and do have serious society-wide effects. The males may have diminished chances of finding an acceptable mate, while the broader society may suffer from higher crime, greater social unrest, increased incidence of prostitution, etc.—social troubles closely associated with an abnormally high incidence of men, especially unmarried men.[*]

---

[*] At the same time, the preponderance of males may encourage marriage, discourage cohabitation, and increase the proportion of two-parent families, given that women, being scarce, could exert greater control over the marriage market. See, for example, chapter 3 of the recent book on marriage by Council Member James Q. Wilson (Wilson, J.Q., *The Marriage Problem: How Our Culture Has Weakened Families,* New York: HarperCollins, 2002). But a high incidence of marriage in sex-imbalanced societies does not solve the social problem of the large number of unmarried and unmarriable males.

One could argue that the choice of a male child is individually rational for parents, given the strong preference in certain cultures for males. But such individual choices may be socially costly—a case where individual parental eugenic choices do not yield a social optimum. Indeed, unrestricted sex selection offers a classic example of the Tragedy of the Commons, in which advantages sought by individuals are nullified, or worse, owing to the social costs of allowing them to everyone.[22] In such cases, it is acceptable (and arguably necessary) for a liberal polity to place limits on individual liberty.

D. The Meaning of Sexuality and Procreation

The two aspects of sex control—it is control of *sex*, and it is a form of *control* of offspring—locate the deeper significance of this practice in two important human contexts: the meaning of sexuality, and the nature of procreation and family relations. A discussion of these matters shows why there is more at stake here than personal liberty.

The arguments previously advanced against sex selection, based on concerns regarding sexual bias, have been less than satisfactory. Some have argued, for example, that sex selection would reinforce gender stereotypes and threaten gender equality—presumably because it would manifest preferences for boys. Yet these critics do not specify what they mean by "gender stereotypes" and "gender equality." Sometimes it seems that they are worried that expressed preference for males would lead to a return to the world of 1950s-style stereotypes, with men and women playing distinct social roles. But it sometimes seems that they are also worried that sex selection would threaten a positive goal, a movement toward a more genuinely gender-neutral or socially androgynous society, one in which our socially constructed human identities would triumph over the mere biology of sexual difference. But in such a gender-indifferent society, it would presumably make no difference whether you are a girl or a boy, a woman or a man. And thus the choice of parents of a boy rather than a girl, or vice versa, would have no negative implications of gender stereotyping and would not threaten the equality of the sexes. The choice between a girl and a boy would be purely an aesthetic choice—as between pink and blue. And who could then object to letting parents choose? The very logic and language of gender equality, taken in its androgynous direction, would seem to soften opposition to sex selection. Further, there seems to be a contradiction between arguing that "sex should not count" in opposing the right of parents to choose boys rather than girls, while at the same time implying that "sex counts plenty" in approving sex selection for "family balancing." If, as the critics say, sex does not or should not count, why could they think a sexually balanced family humanly better than an unbalanced one? By selecting sex *for any reason*, does one not in fact acknowledge that it is very important?

As one of its arguments against the use of PGD for sex selection, the ASRM has suggested that it might "trivialize human reproduction by making it depend on the selection of nonessential features of offspring."[23] But if sexual identity is non-essential for many purposes (for example, at least in theory, in employment or other areas where the law forbids discrimination), for other purposes it is central to who and what we are. Humanity exists as a sexually differentiated species; it is *constituted* in part by the sexual difference. The reason is that our bodies are integral to our humanity. There is no generic or androgynous human "self" to which, as a kind of accidental addition, either a male or female body is then appended. Were that the case, sexual identity really would be "nonessential" or "inessential" to our self. It would not in any sense help to *constitute* a person's identity.

If, however, we do not accept that kind of dualism in which the real self simply is attached to and makes use of a (male or female) body, then we will have to take sexual identity seriously as given with our body. Every cell of the body and the entire body plan and form mark us as either male or female, and it is hard to imagine any more fundamental or essential characteristic of a person. It is surely odd, to say the least, to deny the importance of sexual identity in the very activity of initiating a life.

Seeing this, we can understand why it often seems so important to people that they have either a boy or a girl. Indeed, it would be surprising if people did not care about a difference so fundamental. But acknowledging this, we can also understand why we should be reluctant to see ourselves as people who may appropriately dictate such a crucial part of the identity of our child. Many prospective parents will say quite honestly that they don't care whether their baby is a boy or a girl; they'll be happy to have either. That attitude is desirable not because the sex of the child is a matter of indifference but because it counts for so much. Far too much to be seen as their responsibility to determine.

In a previous Council report, on human cloning,[24] we emphasized how cloning-to-produce-children alters the very nature and meaning of human procreation, implicitly turning it (at least in concept) into a form of manufacture and opening the door to a new eugenics. Sex selection raises related concerns.

The salient fact about human procreation in its natural context is that children are not *made* but *begotten*. By this we mean that children are the issue of our love, not the product of our wills. A man and a woman do not produce or choose a *particular* child, as they might buy a particular brand of soap; rather, they stand in relation to their child as recipients of a gift. Gifts and blessings we learn to accept as gratefully as we can; products of our wills we try to shape in accordance with our wants and desires. Procreation as traditionally understood invites acceptance, not reshaping or engineering. It encourages us to see that we do not own our children and that our children exist not simply for our fulfillment. Of course, parents seek to shape and nurture their children in a variety of ways; but being a parent also means being open to the *unbidden* and *unelected* in life.

Sex selection challenges this fundamental understanding of procreation and parenthood. When we select for sex we are, consciously or not, seeking to design our children according to our wants and desires. The choice is never merely innocent or indifferent, since a host of powerful expectations goes into the selection of a boy or a girl. In choosing one sex over the other, we are necessarily making a statement about what we expect of that child—even if it is nothing more than that the child should provide sexual balance in the family. As fathers, we may want a son to go fishing with; or as mothers, we may want a daughter to dress for the prom. The problem goes deeper than sexual stereotyping, however. For it could also be the case that we may want a daughter who will become president to show that women are the equal of men. But in making this kind of selection we have hardly escaped the problem, for the child's sexual identity would be determined by us in order to fulfill some particular desire of our own. If this were not the case then there would be no felt need to choose the sex of our child in the first place. And thus does it happen that in practicing sex selection our acceptance of our children becomes conditional—a stance that is fundamentally incompatible with the deeper meanings of procreation and parenthood.

The truth of this matter is paradoxically displayed by a small fact connected with current American practices of sex-selection. The assisted reproduction clinics that offer elective sex selection (through sperm sorting or PGD) require their clients to agree in advance that they will accept whatever child results, even if the child is not of the sought-for sex. The clinics are no doubt mainly protecting themselves against legal liability for a wrong result. Yet their need to insist on accepting an undesired "product" shows how the practice itself must make into a matter of compulsory agreement what the idea of parenthood should take for granted: that each child is ours to love and care for, from the start, unconditionally, and regardless of any special merit of theirs or special wishes of ours.

III. IMPROVING CHILDREN'S BEHAVIOR: PSYCHOTROPIC DRUGS

In addition to trying to enhance or control the inborn capacities of their children, parents can try to improve what their children do with the capacities they have. They can help them improve specific native gifts (musical, artistic, athletic, etc.) through practice or training. They can stimulate interest, develop tastes, and enlarge horizons through reading, travel, and exposure to culture. They can try to improve their moods, attitudes, and, of course, their behavior: how they act at home and school, how they respond to authority, how they comport themselves with family and friends. They can try to improve their ability and willingness to be considerate, show respect, pay attention, carry out assignments, accept responsibility, deal with stress and disappointment, and practice self-control. In these efforts, parents continue to use, as they always have, our time-honored methods for child rearing and education. But they may be acquiring extra help from biotechnology and the novel approaches to behavior modification that make use of drugs and devices that work directly on the brain.

Opportunities to modify behavior in children using psychotropic drugs are growing rapidly, and the young but expanding field of neuroscience promises vast increases in understanding the genetic and neurochemical contributions to behavior and comparable increases in our ability to alter it, safely and effectively. The variety of available drugs and the range of conditions for which they are now or may soon be used is large and growing. Today, stimulants (Ritalin, amphetamine, and the like) are the class of behavior-modifying drugs most frequently prescribed to children, and they are used almost exclusively for the treatment of attention-deficit/hyperactivity disorder (ADHD). Selective serotonin reuptake inhibitors (SSRIs)—such as Prozac and Zoloft—and other antidepressants, widely prescribed for the treatment of mood and anxiety disorders in adults, are increasingly being prescribed to children and adolescents for treatment of depression, obsessive-compulsive disorder, tic disorders, and anxiety disorders, including separation anxiety and school refusal. Neuroleptics, long used to treat schizophrenia in adults, are now being used to treat children for tics, schizophrenia and other psychoses, behavioral problems in autism, and nonspecific aggression. Research is actively under way exploring the use of mood stabilizers (for example, lithium) to treat children and adolescents for bipolar disorder, oppositional defiant disorder, conduct disorder, episodic explosiveness, and mood lability.[25] A 2003 study found that the overall use of psychotropic drugs by children tripled during the 1990s, in many cases approaching adult rates of utilization.[*26]

The growing availability of a wide range of behavior-modifying drugs offers an ever-expanding armamentarium for parents (and others) interested in trying to improve their children. Indeed, the mere availability of such powerful new agents and knowledge of their effects will invite many parents at least to consider their use, in order to realize

---

[*] This study does not indicate the conditions for which these drugs are being prescribed. The mere increase in utilization rate, though worthy of notice, does not tell us what we most need to know: why this increase, and is all of it reasonable and proper?

more effectively various aspirations they have for their children. And if other people's children are already using them for similar purposes, many parents may feel pressed to give them a try, in order not to deny to their own child an opportunity for greater success. Competitive behavior of many parents seeking advantages for their children is already widespread in schooling and sports programs; there is no reason to believe that it will stop at the border of psychotropic drugs, should they prove effective and safe.

The wish of parents for "better children" most often takes the form of a desire for children who are more well-adjusted, well-behaved, sociable, attentive, high-performing, and academically adept. Parents are moved not only by reasons of parental pride but also by the belief that children who possess these qualities are more likely to succeed and flourish later in life. These are perfectly fitting desires and proper motives, and we might well find fault with parents who did not share them, at least to some considerable degree. But the power to fulfill these aspirations through the dispensing of drugs forces us to wonder both about the propriety of the means and also about the desire for better children itself: how it should best be understood and most responsibly be acted upon. What are the costs, including costs to good conduct itself, of seeking improved conduct by this means? What are the costs, including costs to flourishing childhood itself, of trying to secure our children's future success in life by overzealous efforts to guarantee their achievements or govern their behavior?

Not surprisingly, the pursuit of better-behaved and more competent children through the use of drugs, like the pursuit of better-endowed children through the use of genetic technologies, has raised considerable public disquiet and debate, both about means and about ends. The arguments have been highly emotional, yet beneath the surface lie deep questions about the meaning and responsibilities of parenthood. Because it involves children already here (rather than children on their way to birth), this use of drugs also confronts us with issues of moral education and character development, the uniquely important yet limited freedom afforded to children, and the complex meaning of childhood. It also challenges us to negotiate the often vague boundary between what seems plainly to be therapeutic medicine and what seems plainly to be parental or social control or performance enhancement. As with behavior-modifying drugs used by adults, there is a potential conflict between personal freedom and the need for prudence and restraint. But because the drugs will often be given to young children incapable of making important decisions for themselves, parents must also shoulder a complex and heavy burden of responsibility—whether they choose to have their children medicated, or to forego the advantages such medication might provide.

A. Behavior Modification in Children Using Stimulants

To consider these questions regarding behavior modification in children, we have at our disposal a rich and illuminating case study. For several decades now, stimulant drugs have been routinely used to alter the behavior of children who are inattentive, impulsive, or hyperactive to an abnormal degree. When the behavior in question is sufficiently severe, chronic, and early in its onset, such children are held to suffer from attention-deficit/hyperactivity disorder (ADHD). These children frequently suffer greatly (as do their parents), especially as a result of failures in school, disruptions at home, and the negative responses their behavior generates from teachers, peers, and family members. Caring for them is often an ordeal, affecting everyone in the vicinity. Fortunately, the symptoms comprising ADHD respond well to prescription stimulants such as Ritalin (methylphenidate) or Adderall (amphetamine). For the worst cases, these drugs have proved a godsend, rescuing many a child from failure in school, trouble with authorities, and general shame and opprobrium. In the great majority of children diagnosed with ADHD, stimulant drugs (frequently used in combination with non-medical efforts to alter behavior) have apparently succeeded in enhancing focus and attention, calming disruptive behavior, and improving performance at school. Moreover, their use by children also appears to be safe, non-addictive, and free of major side effects. Thus, when prescribed for children suffering from properly diagnosed and clear-cut cases of ADHD, stimulants are not only an acceptable but a necessary treatment of choice, and, until now, better than all other available alternatives.

Yet this good news comes with nagging concerns. In recent years the rate at which children are diagnosed with ADHD and treated with stimulants has risen dramatically. Although it is difficult to get precise figures, it is estimated that up to four million American children are taking Ritalin or related drugs on a daily basis.[27] The rapid expansion of both ADHD diagnosis and Ritalin prescription has raised troubling questions in some quarters. Because there is at present no definitive biological marker for ADHD, its diagnosis—especially in borderline cases—can be a matter of subjective judgment. This has aroused some concern about misdiagnosis of ADHD and overprescription of Ritalin, especially in children displaying less acute forms of distractibility and restlessness. The wide variation in the incidence of stimulant prescription in different parts of the United States has generated arguments about whether the drugs are underprescribed (and ADHD underdiagnosed) in some communities or overprescribed (and ADHD overdiagnosed) in others—or whether both may be true. Some observers are also apprehensive because the drugs safely used in small doses in children nonetheless belong to a family of powerful stimulants (amphetamines) that are dangerous and addictive when snorted or otherwise abused by teenagers and adults.

Our interest in this case study, however, is not driven by concerns about the possible misdiagnosis of ADHD in children whose symptoms are relatively mild or whose maladaptive behavior might have other sources. Rather, we are interested in the use of psychotropic drugs to correct *this* behavioral disorder because it provides an opportunity to consider what it means *in general* to seek better or better-behaved children by pharmacological means. For this purpose, several aspects of this case study are especially relevant.

First, even when stimulant drugs are properly used to treat a recognizable disorder, they are acting as agents of behavior modification and control, applied by adults to children. It is aberrant behavior that justifies their use; it is the diminution or elimination of said aberrant behavior that is the measure of their success. Second, there are ambiguities in the set of behaviors being treated: the symptoms clustered together under the diagnosis of ADHD—inattentiveness and distractibility, hyperactivity, impulsiveness—can and do exist separately and in varying degrees of severity, and they are always targets of possible corrective intervention, regardless of diagnosis. Third, these symptoms are continuous with unwanted behaviors found in children who do not have the disorder; indeed, these behaviors are found to some extent in most normal children at some time or another. Fourth, the very safety of these drugs in children increases the temptation of parents to seek and physicians to consider prescribing these agents as remedies for the undesirable behaviors. Fifth, growing socio-economic pressures—from schools, clinics, advertising, and health insurance reimbursement arrangements—are encouraging people to consider such pharmacological approaches to controlling the behavior of children. Finally—and perhaps most importantly—the stimulant drugs used to treat ADHD may also be effective in correcting undesirable behavior and improving performance even in the absence of a full-blown picture of ADHD. It is precisely their effectiveness in improving attentiveness, focus, and steady conduct—coupled with the absence of serious side effects when they are properly administered in small doses—that makes these drugs attractive also for the treatment of inattention, distractibility, and impulsivity in children who do not manifest the full disorder. Indeed, these drugs have the capacity to enhance alertness and concentration in children without any symptoms whatsoever.[28]

All these reasons conspire to make the use of stimulants to control behavior a fascinating and important case study for the pursuit of "better children" through psychopharmacology. None of us on the Council questions the reality of attention-deficit/hyperactivity disorder. All of us believe that children suffering its depredations should receive the best treatment available, including prescription stimulants. Though we worry about misuse and abuse, we are not opposed in principle to using behavior-modifying drugs in children, even very young children, if circumstances require it. Though we worry about the consequences of direct marketing of these drugs to parents, we do not even begin with a decided prejudice against the use of drugs in borderline cases, where the benefits to the child may outweigh the potential harms and hazards. And we have no interest in passing judgment on the practice of medicine in relation to ADHD or on the criteria for its diagnosis adopted by the psychiatric profession.

Our purpose here is different. Taking our bearing from the generalized capacities of these behavior-modifying drugs, we are mainly interested in efforts to use them to achieve improvements in behavior and performance that are independent of desires to heal disease. By considering the implications of present and anticipated practices, we hope to shed light on the promise and peril of a whole array of pharmacological avenues toward improving our children. Given that anticipated advances in neuroscience will almost certainly yield many new psychotropic drugs capable of altering various behaviors, it is crucial that we prepare ourselves in advance to identify and cope with the ethical and social implications of using them as agents of control, enhancement, and behavior modification.

The story of stimulant use by children begins to paint a picture of what it means to seek to modify children's behavior through drugs, both within but especially beyond the realm of therapy, and especially in the light of the powerful social and cultural forces that are encouraging this practice. By drawing some lessons from the story of stimulant use in children, we shall try to add some depth and color to that picture and to suggest some potential concerns that should be kept in mind as the technology advances and its use increases. Should we succeed, this picture could function also as a mirror in which we might be able to scrutinize all of our many efforts to produce "better children."

Before considering some ethical and social implications, we pause to review some important aspects of the treatment and the behavior treated.

1. What Are Stimulant Drugs?

The stimulants in question are, for the most part, two related drugs: methylphenidate (sold under the brand name Ritalin, among others) and amphetamine (sold under the brand name Adderall, among others). The two are chemically similar (methylphenidate is in fact a synthetic derivative of amphetamine), and their effects are analogous.* They were not

---

* The public debate over these drugs has tended to use Ritalin as the generic name for the entire class of stimulants, although Adderall has actually been the most widely prescribed and used of these drugs since at least 1999.

originally developed as agents of behavior modification. They were first used in medicine in order to raise and support blood pressure. Yet their stimulant effects on the central nervous system have been known for many years, and these are today almost the exclusive reason for their use. It is believed that they act primarily on the dopaminergic neurotransmitter pathways of the brain, blocking reuptake at dopamine receptor sites and therefore leading to increased dopamine concentrations between nerve cells. Their effects seem especially focused on the pre-frontal cortex and the locus ceruleus region of the brain, centers which are believed to be associated with impulse control, inhibition, and cognitive functions related to choice and action. Among their effects are diminished fatigue, improved concentration, decreased distraction and restlessness, and enhanced effort on demand, as well as increased blood pressure and greater physical strength, speed, and endurance.

Such drugs can therefore have a powerful effect on behavior and performance: concentrating the mind, calming the nerves, enhancing focus and attentiveness. And indeed, behavior modification with the aid of stimulants, including in children, is nothing new. Such drugs have been used by physicians to temper hyperactive children since at least the 1930s,[29] though such uses appear to have been extremely rare until the early 1960s. Over time, the effectiveness of the drugs and the duration of their action have been substantially increased, and their side effects have been decreased. Although this class of stimulants can be prescribed for the treatment of narcolepsy, and as an augmenter for certain antidepressants, they are by far most commonly prescribed for the treatment of hyperactivity and disorders of attention. But they are also used for their stimulant and performance-enhancing effects by high school and college students, pilots and soldiers, and others eager to enhance their alertness and attentiveness, say, for example, during test-taking or combat.

Although they might be successful if tried, such drugs are, of course, not just routinely used today to quiet any restless child. Because of their addictive effects in adults, stimulants like Ritalin and Adderall are not only prescription drugs; since 1971 they have been classified as Schedule II controlled substances. This means their production is strictly monitored and regulated by the federal Drug Enforcement Administration

(DEA). Yet, closer to the ground of action, their prescription and actual use by pediatricians and other physicians are unregulated, and there is no scrutiny of off-label uses. Moreover, because the drugs are so prevalent in most communities, owing to the high incidence of ADHD, they can easily escape from professional control. It is thus extremely difficult to prevent them from being shuttled around from children being treated for ADHD to other users for other purposes.

2. Behaviors Inviting Improvement Through Stimulant Drugs

Compared with adults, many children, at many times, might be described by those around them as restless, jumpy, impulsive, inattentive, distractible, fidgety, overactive, and unruly. When persistent and severe, these characteristics can be distressing to everyone in the vicinity, whether at home, school, church, or playground. People begin to suspect that these aberrant behaviors may be symptoms of some underlying disorder, neurological or psychological. In order to help parents, teachers, and general pediatricians sort out what degree and combinations of aberrant behaviors or symptoms deserve medical or psychiatric intervention, behavioral and pharmacologic, psychiatrists have set down diagnostic criteria for a family of attention deficit and hyperactivity disorders.

The criteria for ADHD are set forth in the *Diagnostic and Statistical Manual of Mental Disorders,* the standard American reference for diagnosis of psychiatric disorders (now in its fourth edition, and often called by a shorthand title, "DSM-IV"). They include serious symptoms of inattention, impulsivity, or hyperactivity that persist for at least six months and that cause significant impairment of function in more than one setting, whether familial, social, academic, or occupational. The criteria further require that at least some of the symptoms must have begun before the age of seven; as defined, ADHD is thus a childhood disorder.* (Readers are encouraged to examine the full text of the DSM-IV criteria, presented in the appendix to this chapter.)

---

* Notwithstanding this conclusion, there has been much recent discussion about "adult ADHD," and pharmaceutical companies are aggressively advertising remedies for this "disorder" on television.

The causes of ADHD are not fully understood, yet the current consensus appears to be that it is brought about by some combination of genetic susceptibility and environmental factors.* Recent studies have shown that genetic factors contribute substantially, "with most estimates of heritability exceeding 0.70,"[30] and one study has located a major susceptibility locus for ADHD on a specific portion of chromosome 16.[31] Environmental risk factors seem to include traumatic brain injury, stroke, severe early emotional deprivation, familial psychosocial adversity, and maternal smoking during pregnancy. Yet despite the generic genetic and environmental correlations, there is at present no clear biological marker or physiological test for ADHD. The disorder is diagnosed solely on the basis of observed and reported symptoms.

In florid cases, a symptom-based diagnosis is easy to make. But the symptoms themselves shade over along a continuum into normal levels of childish distractibility or impulsiveness, and, in all cases, evaluation is unavoidably subjective. Degrees of attentiveness or self-command in children distribute themselves normally, which is to say, around a bell-shaped curve. And there is good reason to believe that the population of children who have ADHD overlaps with children who appear in the low-end tail of the curve. As a result, the purely symptomatic diagnosis of ADHD, even when made by experienced experts after the requisite thoroughgoing examinations in home and school settings, is always at risk of scooping up children who lack the disorder but who are nonetheless comparably handicapped. Where the symptoms are less clear-cut and less severe, diagnosis is fraught with difficulty.** Even the codified

---

* In this respect, too, the behavioral disorders being treated may be seen as paradigmatic. For very few behavioral disorders is there likely to be a purely genetic cause.

** Dr. Lawrence Diller, a pediatrician specializing in behavior problems whose referral practice gets mostly hard-to-diagnose cases, estimates that in his experience less than half of the children for whom he prescribes Ritalin are genuine cases of ADHD. See Diller, L., "Prescription Stimulant Use in Children: Ethical Issues," presentation to the President's Council on Bioethics (www.bioethics.gov), Washington, D.C., 12 December 2002. If diagnostic difficulties obtain even where experienced and careful experts spend several hours, involving separate visits also to school and home, to evaluate the child, one can readily see the risks of misdiagnosis where evaluation is made during a 10-15 minute visit to the family doctor's office.

guidelines of DSM-IV reveal the difficulty: the *Manual*'s classification of the types of ADHD lists, as an additional diagnostic category, "ADHD, not otherwise specified," a type of ADHD defined by "prominent symptoms of inattention or hyperactivity-impulsivity *that do not meet the criteria for ADHD*"[32] (emphasis added).

This unavoidable vagueness in diagnosis tends to create uncertainty with regard to appropriate treatment. In extreme cases, it is easy to conclude that a child desperately needs a trial of treatment with prescription stimulants. But in the cases of children who barely meet the diagnostic criteria, or who barely fail to meet them, the challenge confronting the child's physician and parents is far more complicated, and the question of whether to prescribe stimulants can be quite vexing.

Although estimates of how many children suffer from ADHD vary widely, there seems to be little doubt that the numbers are rising. Conservative estimates range between 3 and 7 percent of school-age children, though only slightly more permissive criteria yield estimates as high as 17 percent.[33] There is also disagreement concerning the cause of the increasing incidence of the diagnosis. Have children always suffered this disorder in comparable numbers, but without being either diagnosed or treated? Or is the increased emergence of symptoms a reaction of today's children to the peculiar stresses of modern life, the changing expectations we have for our children, and the tenuous character of many families and other institutions that should be supporting them? How much of the increase is due to "diagnostic creep," the tendency of diagnoses to expand in accordance with the growing use of effective behavior modification?

Although the DSM criteria are carefully set forth by pediatric psychiatrists, many of the actual diagnoses are made by family physicians lacking specialized training in these disorders, often on the basis of brief visits and incomplete work-ups. Studies reveal widespread regional differences in the frequency of diagnosis, as well as big differences among various ethnic and racial groups. The true incidence of ADHD in children cannot be determined from prescription stimulant use alone, since, for all of the noted reasons, it is highly likely that Ritalin and similar drugs are both over-prescribed and under-prescribed. Some children who receive the drugs likely do not require them, while many children who are in need of treatment are likely not receiving it.*

What is clear, however, is that stimulant prescriptions have skyrocketed in recent years. The DEA attempts to calibrate its production quotas to meet demand, so that production levels roughly correlate with prescription levels. In the decade between 1990 and 2000, annual production of methylphenidate increased by 730 percent, and annual production of amphetamine increased by an even more astounding 2,500 percent.[34] The overwhelming majority of those taking these medications are children, though adult use has been growing rapidly. Estimates of the number of American children taking Ritalin-like stimulants hover around three to four million.** Recent reports also suggest that increasing numbers of very young children—as young as two years old—are receiving prescription stimulants.[35]

These levels of prescription and use have created an entire network of rules, procedures, and institutions within the American educational system charged with identifying and accommodating those children who need or use stimulant medications. In countless schools around the country, distribution of the drugs to those students is a familiar daily routine, and a generation of American students has grown up accustomed to the

---

* A recent study of the use of stimulants to treat children for ADHD in a rural North Carolina community is instructive. The authors found that about a quarter of children with unequivocal symptoms of ADHD were not receiving stimulant medication. Girls and older children with ADHD were less likely to receive such treatment. On the other hand, the authors also found that most of the children receiving stimulants did not actually meet the diagnostic criteria for ADHD and had never been reported by their parents as having impairing ADHD symptoms. The authors concluded that, at least in this community, stimulants were being used in ways "substantially inconsistent with current diagnostic guidelines"—underprescribed in some cases and overprescribed in others. (Angold, A., et al., "Stimulant treatment for children: A community perspective," *Journal of the American Academy of Child and Adolescent Psychiatry* 39: 975-984, 2000.) Commenting on the North Carolina study, Dr. Benedetto Vitiello of the National Institute of Mental Health emphasized that "research is urgently needed to elucidate the most common pathways leading to children's referral, diagnosis and treatment" (*loc. cit.*, pp. 992-994).

** We lack comparable data for other countries. In his presentation to the Council, Dr. Lawrence Diller reported that the United States uses 80 percent of the world's Ritalin. See Diller, L., "Prescription Stimulant Use in Children: Ethical Issues," presentation to the President's Council on Bioethics (www.bioethics.gov), Washington, D.C., 12 December 2002.

presence of Ritalin and similar drugs in their schools and, if not in their own lives, in the lives of their fellow students.

3. The "Universal Enhancer"

The continuity of ADHD symptoms with ordinary behaviors, the range of their severity, and the resultant difficulty of diagnosis is only part of what opens the door to widespread use of stimulant drugs to control behavior. The less-than-precise specificity of the behavioral problems is more than matched by the non-specific enhancing effects of the drugs. As first demonstrated by a groundbreaking NIH study in the 1970s, Ritalin has similar effects on all children, regardless of whether they meet the criteria for ADHD. Researchers found that normal boys (and normal adult men) and boys diagnosed with ADHD had similar rates of improvement in performing certain mental tasks when given Ritalin.[*] The stimulants brought the performance of the ADHD patients up to normal or near-normal levels, and brought those of the normal subjects to above-normal levels.[36]

Stimulants of this sort have therefore been called "universal enhancers," capable of modifying the behavior and improving the performance of anyone who takes them. They will calm an unruly child, whether the child suffers from a recognized psychiatric disorder or not, and they will enhance the concentration and alertness of any user.

Herein lies the rub, and a chief source of our interest in this subject in the present report. The fact that Ritalin and similar stimulants can be, and quite possibly are being, used to mollify or improve children who suffer no disorder except childhood and childishness suggests to us another way in which biotechnology may affect future attitudes toward rearing the young. Leaving aside all questions about the way in which ADHD is understood and approached, we can learn a great deal from the public debates concerning Ritalin use in children about the forces and pressures that accompany the emergence and growth of the power to modify children's behavior. As the ability to modify and pacify behavior has increased,

---

[*] Thus, the effectiveness of Ritalin and similar drugs in calming rowdy children or concentrating unfocused minds does not prove that those being treated have ADHD.

a network of pressures, incentives, and attitudes in medicine, corporate America, the educational system, the political system, and the general culture has formed that tends to push in the direction of greater use of drugs—these and many others. The deep desire for better children has for some found an outlet in prescription stimulant use.

We have no doubt that, in most cases, parents, teachers, and physicians are acting in what they sincerely deem the best interest of the child. But anecdotes abound of schools and teachers pressuring parents to medicate their children, often as a condition of continued enrollment; of doctors, pushed by hectic schedules and distorted insurance rules, prescribing stimulants to children they have not fully examined; and of parents seeking a quick way to calm their unruly child or pressuring their doctors to give their son the same medication that is helping his schoolmates.[37] Powerful social pressures to compete, prominent in schools and felt by parents and students alike, may play a role in encouraging extra stimulant use. The Individuals with Disabilities Education Act, without intending to do so, has created financial incentives for schools—and parallel incentives for parents—to push for an ADHD diagnosis and treatment.[*†] Insurance requirements that tie reimbursement to diagnosis (rather than to need) also conspire to push for more diagnosis and more drug treatment; so do insurance rules that base doctors' fee schedules on the number of visits with patients and provide greater compensation for short visits offering drug treatment than for longer sessions exploring behavior-changing approaches.

---

[*] In 1990, Congress passed the Individuals with Disabilities Education Act (IDEA), which mandates special education and related services for (among others) children diagnosed with ADHD. Compared to other alternatives, according to Dr. Lawrence Diller, "savvy parents prefer to win IDEA eligibility for their child; it offers a wider range of options, access to special-education classrooms and programs that are guaranteed funding, and stricter procedural safeguards." (Diller, L., *Running on Ritalin: A Physician Reflects on Children, Society and Performance on a Pill*, New York: Bantam Books, 1998, p. 149.)

[†] In addition, a doctor's diagnosis of ADHD (or learning disability) will permit college-bound students extra time in taking the all-important SAT exam, and, since 2001, without any notice of this fact reported with the results. It will be interesting to discover whether more students now declare themselves victims of ADHD, eligible not only for extra time on exams but also for stimulant drugs that could improve their attention and performance. Already the annual production quotas for Ritalin almost tripled between 1992 and 1995 (and doubled again between 1995 and 2002). The 2002 quota of 20,967 kg is sufficient to produce a little over one billion Ritalin pills containing 20 mg of methylphenidate.

In a major (and worrisome) change from previous practice, drug companies have taken to marketing drugs directly to parents, with spot ads depicting miraculous transformations of anxious, lonely, or troublesome children into cheerful, confident, honor-roll students. The presence in virtually every community of children known to be gaining advantages from stimulants creates a temptation for other parents to offer similar advantages to their own children. In addition, strong evidence suggests the growing illicit and self-medicating use of Ritalin and similar stimulants by high school and college students, taken (often by snorting and at higher doses) to enhance focus and concentration before important exams or while writing term papers. Anecdotes do not make a trend or a rule, and we do not mean to suggest that this is how Ritalin and similar drugs are usually used. But there is more than ample cause for concern.

For it is clear that the potential for controlling and modifying the behavior of children with such drugs already coincides with the deeply felt desire for better-behaved, well-adjusted, sociable, high-performing, happier children. This desire is felt not only by parents of children who suffer from psychiatric disorders, but by every decent, well-meaning parent of even the healthiest child. It is the desire to do what is best for one's child and to secure his or her present contentment and future success. But when this desire is joined with the power to affect behavior directly through biotechnology, its consequences may not serve the best interests of children and parents. Indeed, the power to mold better children through biotechnical interventions raises serious concerns.

B. Ethical and Social Concerns

Any use of behavior-modifying drugs by children calls for special attention, not only because drugs might do damage to the body or brain of the developing child, but also because the causes of human behavior, perhaps especially in children, are always ambiguous and because a child's behavior is inherently transitory. If the targeted behavior occurred only in cases clearly linked to an underlying medical abnormality, there would be no need for discussion. But human conduct has so many intertwined roots— native biological conditions, environmental factors, specific experiences, habits, beliefs, moods, etc.—that it is rarely possible to pin down the exact source of a particular "maladaptive" behavior. Even when an underlying disorder is unequivocally present, it is hard to say with confidence that its presence alone made someone act the way he did. Then, too, children are constantly changing as they grow, and they complete the journey to adulthood by paths many and varied. In children especially it can be difficult to distinguish between temporary behavior problems that will resolve themselves later in life and long-term or permanent aberrations that will respond only to medical treatment.

The crucial ethical and social issues therefore concern not so much any possible harms to the brain or body produced directly or indirectly by the medications—a problem shared with all drug use. What should concern us most are the implications of inserting the novel and precedent-setting use of drugs into child-rearing and educational practices, and what this means for the character of childhood and the nature of responsible parenting. Yet responsible analysis cannot omit a brief discussion of the safety of the drugs themselves. For these are, as has been noted, dangerous and addicting chemicals.

1. Safety First

No drug is entirely without risk of bodily harm, even when used as directed. And common sense suggests that any drug whose brain effects are powerful enough to alter behavior is powerful enough to do damage, perhaps even as a result of its direct and immediate cerebral effects. Yet the preponderance of the evidence shows a remarkably low incidence of side effects when the stimulants are used, in low doses, in treatment of ADHD and allied conditions. Unlike adolescents and adults who are often attracted by the hepped-up feeling produced by amphetamines (appropriately named "Speed"), small children do not like it. They are thus little tempted to move to the higher, potentially addicting doses. While some have expressed the concern that children who use stimulants when young might be more likely to become drug abusers in their teens and beyond, there is evidence that the opposite is true.[38] By avoiding the dismay and frustration of failure attached to untreated ADHD, effective drug treatment early is thought to reduce the incidence of later drug abuse (and other troubles with the law) in the afflicted population. Yet while the benefits—both direct and indirect—of the treatment are well known, there is not yet sufficient data regarding long-term and late-onset effects of having been on stimulants for several years during childhood. We raise this matter not to cast doubt on the reasonableness of drug treatment in clear-cut cases of need where the benefits are great, but to raise a cautionary flag regarding any behavior-improving uses that are purely "elective" and nontherapeutic.*

2. Rearing Children: The Human Context

Rearing children is a uniquely complicated, difficult, and important task. As we noted at the start of this chapter, parents must guide and instruct their children while at the same time allowing them to develop to their own potential and, to an extent, to follow their own path. The child has his or her own wishes, wants, and inclinations, and a parent must discern which of these are detrimental and should be corrected or countered, and which are expressions of distinctive personality or identity that should be abided, met, or encouraged. Parents know that their children must come to learn certain difficult lessons, and that sometimes the learning is as important as the lesson. But they also want to shield them from this world's difficulties and to make their path in life as free of burdens and dangers as possible. Parents must navigate the narrow way between oppressive control of their children's lives and negligent deference to their children's freedom. They know that sometimes their own desire to do what is best for their child can run to excess, and do harm inadvertently. This difficult balancing act often comes down to allowing one's good intentions to moderate one another.

---

* Special safety concerns have been raised about the growing practice of prescribing stimulants "off label" to toddlers as young as two years old. One concern is that, between the ages of two and four, the brains of children are still undergoing important biological development that might be adversely affected by the use of psychotropic drugs. At present, stimulants are approved by the FDA only for treatment of children age six and above. The National Institute of Mental Health is currently sponsoring a large study of the safety and efficacy of stimulants among preschoolers who exhibit ADHD-like behavior. See Coyle, J., "Psychotropic drug use in very young children," *Journal of the American Medical Association* 283(8): 1059–1060, 2000, and Vitiello, B., "Psychopharmacology for young children: Clinical needs and research opportunities," *Pediatrics* 108(4): 983-989, 2001.

The biotechnical capacity to modify children's behavior threatens to introduce an element into the mix that is so powerful as to be very difficult to moderate. In an effective, safe, and relatively inexpensive way, it would seemingly allow parents to help their otherwise healthy children behave better, learn better, interact better, and perform better.* So why should any parent refrain from making use of behavior-modifying drugs? In light of our above reflections, the following principal reasons or worries present themselves: social control and conformity; moral education and medicalization; and the meaning of performance.

3. Social Control and Conformity **

Behavior-modifying agents would allow parents, teachers, or others to intervene directly in a child's neurochemistry when that child behaves in a way that defies their standards of conduct. In some cases, the children clearly benefit; in other cases, they do not. In all cases, the use of such drugs to shape behavior raises serious questions concerning the liberty of children.

The liberty of children is, of course, a complicated and controversial concept. Children are not sufficiently mature, responsible, or knowledgeable to make for themselves the most important decisions regarding their lives. Choices about their health, their education, their activities, their environment, and their future are made for them by others. And yet, we all recognize certain limits to the degree to which they may be coerced or restricted. If we take the trouble to think about it, we remember that chil-

---

* We say "seemingly," for there may be reasons to question or doubt whether the use of stimulants by normal, healthy, or even above-average children would in fact improve performance in the ways that matter most, or whether the drugs might enhance certain powers and faculties at the expense of other powers and faculties. As far as we know, there have been no major studies on the long-term effect of sustained stimulant use simply as a performance-enhancer or behavior-improver. There is evidence that stimulants do improve performance in immediate and specific tasks such as test-taking. But this is hardly sufficient evidence of long-term educational benefit.

** The phrase "social control" may raise for some readers the specter of Soviet-style oppression masquerading as psychiatry. We imply no such prospect. Yet even without any government policy, people often act to control the social behavior of children. Drugs offer them a new and potentially powerful way to do so. Our discussion in this section considers the whole panoply of behavior-modifying drugs, not just stimulants.

dren are not just little adults and that their native gifts and dispositions come in all shapes and sizes. Some are bold while others are cautious; some are outgoing while others are shy; some are docile while others are seemingly unteachable; some are independent and like their own company, others are dependent and insist on sociability. We recognize that children, even very young ones, display certain traits of personality and forces of will that ought not simply to be repressed by others. Present and emerging psychopharmaceuticals may increasingly enable us to affect and control these traits in our children, and therefore to significantly restrict that liberty that nature and society usually afford them. And whereas the overt behavior of today's overbearing parents may elicit a friendly reminder or a rebuke from grandparents or neighbors—"Take it easy on him; he's just a kid!"—the use of drugs to attain similar goals proceeds out of sight, immune to the correcting eyes of others.

Individual differences notwithstanding, childhood is generally marked by a spirited rambunctiousness that, especially in the case of young boys, often borders on sheer unruliness and hyperactivity. Curbing the latter may too easily stifle the former, and with it an important part of growing up. This would not only restrict the freedom of children, but alter the very character of childhood. Because schooling is crucial (today perhaps more so than before) to later success in a world that demands high cognitive skills, we tend to forget that the temperaments selected over eons of evolution—perhaps especially in males—are not obviously well-suited to sitting quietly in classrooms or to the quiet demeanor that classrooms require. And because our society insists that all children receive more or less the same kind of education ("No child left behind"), we tend to ignore important individual differences and instead tend to treat difficult or non-conforming children as problems. We fail to consider that their spiritedness might be part of a more ambitious nature, their lack of attention part of an artistic temperament, or their restlessness a fitting response of genuinely eager students to uninteresting or poorly taught classes.

A well-meaning teacher, confronted by an oversized class of excitable second graders, might judge the most restless and disruptive among them to be simply uncontrollable and potentially in need of treatment. The busy, tired parents of an especially fidgety and energetic eight-year-old might be tempted to seek pharmacological ways to help their child be more sociable and attentive or do better in class. In some cases such children really will need medical treatment to be able to perform even minimally. But in some cases they won't, and the increasing availability and popularity of the treatment may diminish our ability to tell the two apart; or, more importantly, it may alter our standards of when a child is in need of psychopharmaceutical intervention. Using psychotropic drugs might become, for an increasing number of children, a social necessity or expectation—merely to keep up.

This enhanced ability to make children conform to conventional standards could also diminish our openness to the diversity of human temperaments. As we will find with other biotechnologies with a potential for use beyond therapy, behavior-modifying drugs offer us an unprecedented power to enforce our standards of normality. Human societies have always had such standards, but most societies (and certainly our own) have in practice tolerated fairly significant deviations from them, and have greatly benefited from such tolerance. Some proponents of the new biotechnologies suggest that they will offer us new options and enlarge our capacity to exercise our individual desires. Far from restricting variety, they contend that these new empowerments would serve and increase the diversity of our society. The point is not without merit. Yet diversity is not only a matter of options and choice, but also a matter of innate inclination and temperament, strength of desire and aspiration, and cultivated character. The power to stifle these latter traits in the name of better behavior and elementary education seems likely to diminish both the range of human types in our society and the range of the choices we will finally make. This danger seems especially great with regard to techniques of exercising control over children, since parents are more likely to desire to help their children fit the mold and conform to the conventional pattern than to seek social conformity for themselves. As the physician-bioethicist Carl Elliott put it:

> [T]he very changes that some people may think of as unqualified
> "enhancements" (i.e., becoming more attentive and mindful) are

not quite as unqualified as they may initially think; . . . moreover, these enhancements may well be changes critical to a person's identity, a person's sense of who he or she is.[39]

In an age of routine and widely used agents of behavior modification, the power to control our children would therefore raise significant worries about the prospects for benevolently enforced conformity, restriction of freedom, and perhaps even for the decline of genuine excellence.

4. Moral Education and Medicalization
A further concern has to do with the substitution of the language and methods of medicine for the language and methods of moral education. Children suffering from ADHD and similar disorders genuinely lack some degree of the capacity to impose their will on their behavior. If a child has poor impulse-control equipment in his brain, repeated failure will not produce self-command, but rather a loathing of it. Drugs could help get him to the "level playing field," after which time he might have a fighting chance to enjoy a normal course of learning self-command. Yet most children whose behavior is restless and unruly could (and eventually do) learn to behave better, through instruction and example, and by maturing over time. Praise and blame from parents and teachers, patient instruction and extra attention, as well as the experience of performing poorly or well, can help strengthen the will of the child, which slowly increases the child's ability to control his or her impulses and behavior.

Behavior-modifying agents circumvent that process, and act directly on the brain to affect the child's behavior without the intervening learning process. If what matters is only the child's outward behavior, then this is simply a more effective and efficient means of achieving the desired result. But because moral education is typically more about the shaping of the agent's character than about the outward act, the process of learning to behave appropriately matters most of all. If the development of character depends on effort to choose and act appropriately, often in the face of resisting desires and impulses, then the more direct pharmacological approach bypasses a crucial element. The beneficiaries of drug-induced good conduct may not really be learning self-control; they may be learning to think it is not necessary. As Dr. Steven Hyman put it in his presentation to this Council:

> There are symbolic messages to children about self-efficacy. Behavioral control comes from a bottle. We have the problem of anabolic steroids for the soul.[40]

By slowly learning to master his or her impulses, a child not only comes to behave well, but also learns to exercise genuine self-control and some degree of self-mastery. The child grows more mature. By treating the restlessness of youth as a medical, rather than a moral, challenge, those resorting to behavior-modifying drugs might not only deprive that child of an essential part of this education. They might also encourage him to change his self-understanding, by coming to look upon himself as governed largely by chemical impulses and not by moral decisions grounded in some sense of what is right and appropriate.

This concern arises with a number of the biotechnologies we will consider in this report. By medicalizing key elements of our life through biotechnical interventions, we may weaken our sense of responsibility and agency. And, technologies aside, merely regarding ourselves and our activities in largely genetic or neurochemical terms may diminish our sense of ourselves as moral actors faced with genuine choices and options in life. These concerns are especially serious with regard to children, where those who are treated are not the ones making the choice to seek treatment. Children learn by their elders' example, and in this instance they may learn from those whose opinions matter most to them that behavior is simply a matter of chemistry, and that responsibility for their actions falls not to themselves but to their pills. They may behave better, but they will not have learned why, or even quite how.

5. The Meaning of Performance

A distinct but closely related concern has to do with the lesson taught to children about the significance of their abilities. Agents of behavior modification, like Ritalin, Adderall, and future generations of such drugs, are at the same time also agents of performance enhancement. We will take up performance enhancement in its own terms in the next chapter, but our interest here is in the modification of a child's behavior by drugs given to him by his elders.

Children's behavior, in the limited context in which we have been discussing it, is largely a matter of impulse control and self-restraint. But performance is a matter of ability and skill, and (sometimes) of one's standing in competition with others. One's assessment of one's own achievement and worth often has to do with how one performs in the face of various physical and mental challenges. Building our abilities and self-confidence—through study and practice over time—is an important part of all of our lives, and an especially crucial element of childhood.

Parents understandably want their children to perform at high levels, to stand with or above their peers, and to succeed. They know that such things are crucial for any child's future, and they want their child to do as well as possible. But the introduction of performance-enhancing agents confuses the picture, in this area as in the others. Artificial enhancement can certainly improve a child's abilities and performance (at least of specific tasks, over the short run), *but it does so in a way that separates at least some element of that achievement from the effort of achieving.* It may both rob the child of the edifying features of that effort and teach the child, by parental example, that high performance is to be achieved by artificial, even medical, means. At the very least it sends a confusing message to the child about the meaning of performance: one which at the same time puts too much emphasis on the importance of performance, and too little emphasis on the integrity of genuine ability and unaugmented merit.

The concerns with performance, together with the temptation to seek to improve it through biotechnology, are felt first by parents, and in a sense imposed on children by the parental decision to seek stimulants or similar enhancers. But with time, as a child lives and matures knowing that such agents of behavior modification and performance enhancement have been integral to his life, the child himself may also come to feel the desire to make use of such technologies. Performance enhancement will cease to be imposed, and will come to be a choice, perhaps even more attractive than it is today. In the remaining chapters, we will take up the subject of freely chosen adult use of biotechnologies beyond therapy, and consider the sorts of desires, ends, and means that may shape the human experience in the age of biotechnology.

IV. CONCLUSION: THE MEANING OF CHILDHOOD

To this point we have indicated ways that the use of biotechnical means can actually undermine the end of better children. But there are also serious questions to be put to the goal itself, some about "childhood," some about what is "better." Life is not just behaving, performing, achieving. It is also about being, beholding, savoring. It is not only about preparing for future success. It is also about enjoying present blessings. It is not only about school, work, and networking. It is also about leisure, play, and friendship. At no time of life are these truths more evident—and more realizable—than in childhood. Life soon enough becomes serious, driven, and hard. The sweetness, freshness, and spontaneity of life are available in their purest form only to the as-yet-unburdened young.

Some observers of the present scene have commented ruefully about the way in which much of modern life threatens the innocence and the simple joys of childhood. People note with sadness how both a pragmatic concern for their future successes as adults and a precocious introduction to the troubles of the adult world are obtruding themselves into the lives of younger and younger children. It would be paradoxical, not to say perverse, if the desire to produce "better children," armed with the best that biotechnology has to offer, were to succeed in its goal by pulling down the curtain on the "childishness" of childhood. And it would be paradoxical, not to say perverse, if the desire to improve our children's behavior or performance inculcated short-term and shallow notions of success at the expense of those loftier goals and finer sensibilities that might make their adult lives truly better.

APPENDIX

DIAGNOSTIC CRITERIA FOR
ATTENTION-DEFICIT/HYPERACTIVITY DISORDER

According to the American Psychiatric Association, to be diagnosed with ADHD a patient must meet the following five criteria (A-E) (but also see the category, "*ADHD, not otherwise specified*," below):

A. Either 1 or 2:

1. Six (or more) of the following symptoms of inattention have persisted for at least six months to a degree that is maladaptive and inconsistent with developmental level:

Inattention
a. Often fails to give close attention to details or makes careless mistakes in schoolwork, work, or other activities
b. Often has difficulty sustaining attention in tasks or play activities
c. Often does not seem to listen when spoken to directly
d. Often does not follow through on instructions and fails to finish schoolwork, chores, or duties in the workplace (not due to oppositional behavior or failure to understand instructions)
e. Often has difficulty organizing tasks and activities
f. Often avoids, dislikes, or is reluctant to engage in tasks that require sustained mental effort (such as schoolwork or homework)
g. Often loses things necessary for tasks or activities (e.g., toys, school assignments, pencils, books, or tools)
h. Is often easily distracted by extraneous stimuli
i. Is often forgetful in daily activities

2. Six (or more) of the following symptoms of hyperactivity-impulsivity have persisted for at least six months to a degree that is maladaptive and inconsistent with developmental level:

Hyperactivity
a. Often fidgets with hands or feet or squirms in seat
b. Often leaves seat in classroom or in other situations in which remaining seated is expected
c. Often runs about or climbs excessively in situations in which it is inappropriate (in adolescents or adults, may be limited to subjective feelings of restlessness)
d. Often has difficulty playing or engaging in leisure activities quietly
e. Is often "on the go" or often acts as if "driven by a motor"
f. Often talks excessively

Impulsivity
g. Often blurts out answers before questions have been completed
h. Often has difficulty awaiting turn
i. Often interrupts or intrudes on others (e.g., butts into conversations or games)

B. Some hyperactive-impulsive, or inattentive symptoms that caused impairment were present before age seven years.

C. Some impairment from the symptoms is present in two or more settings (e.g., at school [or work] and at home).

D. There must be clear evidence of clinically significant impairment in social, academic, or occupational functioning.

E. The symptoms do not occur exclusively during the course of a Pervasive Developmental Disorder, Schizophrenia, or other Psychotic Disorder and are not better accounted for by another mental disorder (e.g., Mood Disorder, Anxiety Disorder, Dissociative Disorder, or a Personality Disorder).

TYPES OF ADHD USING DSM-IV CRITERIA

ADHD, predominantly inattentive type
If Criterion A1 is met but Criterion A2 is not met for the past six months.

ADHD, predominantly hyperactive-impulsive type
If Criterion A2 is met but Criterion A1 is not met for the past six months.

ADHD, combined type
If both Criteria A1 and A2 are met for the past six months.

ADHD, not otherwise specified
This category is for disorders with prominent symptoms of inattention or hyperactivity-impulsivity that do not meet the criteria for Attention-Deficit/Hyperactivity Disorder. Examples include:

1. Individuals whose symptoms and impairment meet the criteria for Attention-Deficit/Hyperactivity Disorder but whose age at onset is seven years or after;

2. Individuals with clinically significant impairment who present with inattention and whose symptom pattern does not meet the full criteria for the disorder but have a behavioral pattern marked by sluggishness, daydreaming, and hypoactivity.

Source: American Psychiatric Association, *Diagnostic and Statistical Manual of Mental Disorders, Fourth Edition, Text Revision*, Washington, D.C.: American Psychiatric Association, 2000, pp. 92-93. Reprinted with permission of the American Psychiatric Association, copyright 2000.

ENDNOTES

[1] Glass, B., "Science: Endless Horizons or Golden Age?" *Science* 171: 23-29, 1971, and Sinsheimer, R., "The Prospect of Designed Genetic Change," *Engineering and Science Magazine,* California Institute of Technology, April 1969.

[2] Chan, A., et al., "Foreign DNA transmission by ICSI: injection of spermatozoa bound with exogenous DNA results in embryonic GFP expression and live rhesus monkey births," *Molecular Human Reproduction* 6(1): 26-33, 2000.

[3] Schatten, G., "Assisted Reproductive Technologies in the Genomics Era," Presentation at the December 2002 meeting of the President's Council on Bioethics, Washington, D.C. Transcript available on the Council's website at www.bioethics.gov.

[4] Silver, L., *Remaking Eden,* New York: Avon, 1998, and Stock, G., *Redesigning Humans: Our Inevitable Genetic Future,* New York: Houghton Mifflin, 2002.

[5] Enge, M., "Ad Seeks Donor Eggs for $100,000, Possible New High," *Chicago Tribune,* 10 February 2000.

[6] Marshall, E., "Gene Therapy a Suspect in Leukemia-like Disease," *Science,* 298: 34, 2002, and "Second Child in French Trial is Found to Have Leukemia," *Science,* 299: 320, 2003.

[7] Collins, F., "Genetic Enhancements: Current and Future Prospects," Presentation at the December 2002 meeting of the President's Council on Bioethics, Washington, D.C. Transcript available on the Council's website at www.bioethics.gov.

[8] Mandavilli, A., "Fertility's new frontier takes shape in the test tube," *Nature Medicine* 9(8): 1095, 2003.

[9] Pinker, S., "Human Nature and Its Future," Presentation at the March 2003 meeting of the President's Council on Bioethics, Washington, D.C. Transcript available on the Council's website at www.bioethics.gov.

[10] Hübner, K., et al., "Derivation of oocytes from mouse embryonic stem cells," *Science* 300(5620): 1251-1256, 2003.

[11] The President's Council on Bioethics, *Human Cloning and Human Dignity: An Ethical Inquiry,* Washington, D.C.: Government Printing Office, 2002. The relevant discussion is found in Chapter Five, "The Ethics of Cloning-to-Produce-Children," pp. 87-99.

[12] *Human Reproduction Update,* 8(3): 65-277, 2002.

[13] Schatten, G., 2002, *op. cit.*

[14] Eberstadt, N., "Choosing the Sex of Children: Demographics," Presentation at the October 2002 meeting of the President's Council on Bioethics, Washington, D.C. Transcript available on the Council's website at www.bioethics.gov.

[15] *Ibid.*

[16] The earliest of these are *Assessing Biomedical Technologies: An Inquiry into the Nature of the Process,* Committee on Life Sciences and Social Policy, National Research Council/National Academy of Sciences, Washington, D.C., 1975; and Powledge, T. M. and J. C. Fletcher, "A Report from the Genetics Research Group of the Hastings Center, Institute of Society, Ethics, and Life Sciences," *New England Journal of Medicine* 300(4): 168-172, 1979.

[17] President's Commission for the Study of Ethical Problems in Medicine and Biomedical and Behavioral Research, *Screening and Counseling for Genetic Conditions: A Report on the Ethical, Social, and Legal Implications of Genetic Screening, Counseling, and Education Programs,* Washington, D.C.: Government Printing Office, 1983, pp. 57-58.

[18] *Ibid.,* p. 58.

[19] Davis, D., *Genetic Dilemmas: Reproductive Technology, Parental Choices, and Children's Futures,* New York: Routledge, 2001, p. 98.

[20] The Ethics Committee of the ASRM, "Sex Selection and Preimplantation Genetic Diagnosis," *Fertility and Sterility,* 72: 4, 1999.

[21] The Ethics Committee of the ASRM, "Preconception Gender Selection for Nonmedical Reasons," *Fertility and Sterility,* 75: 5, 2001.

[22] See Hardin, G., "The Tragedy of the Commons," *Science* 162: 1243-1248, 1968.

[23] The Ethics Committee of the ASRM 1999, *op. cit.*

[24] President's Council on Bioethics, *Human Cloning and Human Dignity: An Ethical Inquiry, op. cit.*

[25] Riddle, M., et al., "Pediatric Psychopharmacology," *Journal of Child Psychology and Psychiatry* 42(1): 73-90, 2001.

[26] Zito, J., et al., "Psychotropic Practice Patterns for Youth: A 10-Year Perspective," *Archives of Pediatric and Adolescent Medicine* 157: 17-25, 2003.

[27] Diller, L., "Prescription Stimulant Use in American Children: Ethical Issues," Presentation at the December 2002 meeting of the President's Council on Bioethics, Washington, D.C. Transcript available on the Council's website, www.bioethics.gov.

[28] Rapoport, J., et al., "Dextroamphetamine: its cognitive and behavioral effects in normal and hyperactive boys and normal men," *Archives of General Psychiatry* 37: 933-943, 1980.

[29] Bradley, C., "The Behavior of Children Receiving Benzedrine," *American Journal of Psychiatry* 94: 577-585, 1937.

[30] Castellanos, F., et al., "Neuroscience of Attention Deficit/Hyperactivity Disorder: The Search for Endophenotypes," *Nature Reviews Neuroscience* 3: 617-628, 2002.

[31] Smalley, S., et al., "Genetic linkage of attention-deficit/hyperactivity disorder on chromosome 16p13, in a region implicated in autism," *American Journal of Human Genetics* 71: 959-963, 2002.

[32] *Diagnostic and Statistical Manual of Mental Disorders, Fourth Edition, Text Revision*, Washington, D.C.: American Psychiatric Association, 2000, p. 93; see also the appendix to this chapter.

[33] Barbaresi, W. J., et al., "How common is attention-deficit/hyperactivity disorder? Incidence in a population-based birth cohort in Rochester, Minnesota," *Archives of Pediatric and Adolescent Medicine* 156: 217-224, 2002.

[34] United States Drug Enforcement Administration, *Methylphenidate/amphetamine yearly production quotas*. Washington, D.C.: Department of Justice, 2000.

[35] Zito, J. M., et al., "Trends in the prescribing of psychotropic medications to preschoolers," *Journal of the American Medical Association*, 283: 1025-1030, 2000.

[36] Rapoport, *op. cit.*

[37] See, for example, Eberstadt, M., "Why Ritalin Rules," *Policy Review* 94, April/May 1999; DeGrandpre, R., *Ritalin Nation: Rapid-Fire Culture and the Transformation of Human Consciousness*, New York: Norton, 1999; and Hancock, L., "Mother's Little Helper," *Newsweek*, 18 March 1996.

[38] Biederman, J., et al., "Pharmacotherapy of Attention-Deficit Hyperactivity Disorder Reduces Risk for Substance Use Disorder," *Pediatrics* 104: e20, 1999.

[39] Elliott, C., *Better Than Well*, New York: Norton, 2003, pp. 257-258.

[40] Hyman, S., "Pediatric Psychopharmacology," Presentation at the March 2003 meeting of the President's Council on Bioethics, Washington, D.C. Transcript available on the Council's website at www.bioethics.gov. Dr. Hyman concluded his presentation to the Council with these remarks.

3

Superior Performance

Human beings desire not only "better children," we desire also to be better ourselves. Aspiration, born of the attractiveness of some human good and the energizing awareness that we do not yet possess it, is at the heart of much that we do and much that is admirable about us. We strive to be better human beings and citizens, better friends and lovers, better parents and neighbors, better students and teachers, better followers of our faiths. Many of us aspire also to excel in the specific activities to which we devote ourselves; and nearly all of us admire superior performance whenever we encounter it, even in areas where we ourselves are only mediocre.

Superior performance is pursued in a myriad of human activities. The athlete strives to run faster, the student to know more, the soldier to shoot more accurately, the vocalist to sing more musically, the chess-player to play with greater mastery. Our motives for seeking superior performance are varied and complex, as human desire and human aspiration always are. We seek to win in competition, to advance in rank and status, to increase our earnings, to please others and ourselves, to gain honor and fame, or simply to flourish and fulfill ourselves by being excellent in doing what we love. In pursuing superior performance, human beings have long sought advantages obtainable from better tools and equipment, better training and practice, and better nutrition and exercise. Today, and increasingly tomorrow, we may also find help in new technological capacities for directly improving our bodies and minds—both their native powers and their activities—capacities provided by drugs, genetic modifications, and surgical procedures (including the implantation of mechanical devices).

What should we think about obtaining superior performance through the use of such biotechnologies? That is the theme of this chapter. But before turning to the question raised by the novel means, we must begin with questions about the goal itself: "What is superior performance?"

I. THE MEANING OF "SUPERIOR PERFORMANCE"

The words themselves—"superior performance"—have many meanings, both individually and together, each of them suggestive and important. "Superior" can mean "better than I have done before," or "better than my opponent," or "better than the best." It can describe something that is universally or indisputably outstanding or something that is better only in relation to the alternatives. It can also mean—and this is especially relevant in this context—"better than I would have done without some 'extra edge' or 'performance enhancement.'" Because superiority, on whatever meaning, is time-bound and precarious, we not only seek to do better than we have done before. We also seek to maintain abilities that seem to be slipping away and to regain powers and abilities that we have lost. We want to become superior and stay superior.

Even more central to our analysis is the meaning (or meanings) of "performance." It denotes the *active* doing of *what we do* and the active expression of *what we are: living embodied* beings or agents, individually at-work in the world. To be alive at all means that certain organic systems are *performing* their functions. In the human case, active performance includes not only the autonomic activity of a well-working organism functioning without conscious choice and direction (for example, in heart beating, digesting, and normal breathing). It also includes the self-directed performance of various *chosen* human activities (for example, walking, running, dancing, thinking). To "*per*form" an activity is not just to do it, but to do it thoroughly, "through and through," to do it to completion and fullness. The idea of performance also suggests a relationship with other performers and spectators: performance before others, with others, and against others. Yet it is also possible to perform certain activities *without* others, on one's own and for oneself, manifesting who we are for our own enjoyment alone. Temporally speaking, a performance is both that which is done "in-the-moment" (a great shot to win the game, a great musical performance) and that which is done "over time" (a great career, writing a great symphony). It embraces that which is done effortlessly or seemingly effortlessly (Joe DiMaggio swinging the bat) and that which is done with great and obvious exertion (Pete Rose hustling to turn a single into a double). Finally, and most pertinent to this inquiry, the word "performance" sometimes means a brilliant illusion, a skilled simulation of reality, or the separation of what one does from who one is: performance as the make-believe acting of actors rather than the self-revealing doings of genuine doers. "Performance" suggests both real activity and real agency, but also the possibility of being or seeming to be something other than who and what we are.

At the core of the notion of "superior performance"—understood as an object of noble aspiration—is the idea of *excellent human activity*: excellent, not inferior; human, not inhuman or nonhuman; active and not passive, at-work and not idling. The reason we spend much of our lives trying to "better ourselves"—not just materially, but as athletes, musicians, soldiers, or lovers—is that we know or believe that not all performances are equal: some are higher and some are lower, some are more worthy and some are less worthy, some are excellent and some are average. But we desire to excel *as human* beings; we want to exercise our distinctively human powers both excellently and in our peculiarly human way. We know or believe that some performances will reveal who we are capable of being when we are at our best.*

The striving for superior performance is, as noted, central to our humanity. But it also raises a series of questions and dilemmas, and sometimes unease and concern, not only about the means we employ, but also about the goal itself. We worry that the desire to become better could deform elements of human life that are not properly measured according to the standard of "superiority," or that our improvements will be achieved only at the price of our integrity and dignity. We worry that

---

* This chapter is, accordingly, about both the excellence and the humanity of "superior performance," and about whether improvements in performance do or do not compromise the humanity or individuality of the agent.

pressures to excel will overwhelm us, or that the desire to be the best will tempt us to "cheat" our way to the top. We worry that putting such a high premium on excellence will crowd out the disadvantaged, or lead us to mistreat those who are "failures." In short, we worry about balance, fairness, and charity—but also, and perhaps more profoundly, we worry about pursuing the wrong goals in the wrong way, or posing as something we are not.

These enduring questions about the pursuit of superior performance acquire heightened visibility and greater salience as a result of emerging new biotechnological powers, present and projected, that promise to help us in our efforts. These powers are surgical, genetic, and pharmacological. Some are familiar—like steroids used to enhance athletic performance and amphetamines used to enhance mental performance. Others are novel—such as the genetic modification of human muscles. And still others are imaginary rather than real—such as genetically engineered Michael Jordans or drugs that would give us perfect memory.

Most of the performance-enhancing technologies of the future, like those in use today, will probably be developed less to aid superior performance than to treat disease and relieve suffering. Yet the broad powers of many drugs and devices make them readily adaptable to uses for which they were not originally intended. Our biotechnical armamentarium for aiding superior performance is still extremely limited. Yet we are already witnessing the wide range of activities that might be biologically enhanced. Modafinil, a drug that combats narcolepsy and induces wakefulness more generally, has been shown to enhance the performance of airplane pilots, commercial and military. Ritalin, the amphetamine-like stimulant whose use in children we discussed in the previous chapter, is also widely used by high school and college students to improve their concentration while taking the SATs or writing final exams. Viagra, a remedy devised for male impotence, is increasingly used by the non-impotent to enhance sexual performance. Growth hormone, the body's natural promoter of skeletal growth, is now being used not only to treat dwarfism but also to help the normally short to become taller. Other drugs are used to calm the nerves or to steady and dry the hands of neurosurgeons and concert pianists. These examples constitute but a small preview of coming attractions.

To fully understand the meaning of using these new biotechnical powers, in all their variety of effects and possible uses, we would need to inquire more deeply into the meaning of "superior performance" itself. We would need to explore the reasons we seek to become better, the abilities we seek to enhance, the different means we might use to enhance them, and the true character of the different activities in which we engage. We would need to pay attention both to the ends we seek and the means and manner by which we seek them, as well as the differences between given human activities, their various excellences and what it takes to attain them. And, attending to the special issues raised by the use of *bio-engineered* enhancements, we would need to address these central questions: As we discover new and better ways to "improve" our given bodies, minds, and performance, are we changing or compromising the dignity of human activity? Are we becoming too reliant on "expert chemists" for our achievements? Do such potential enhancements alter the identity of the doer? Whose performance is it, and is it really better? Is the enhanced person still fully *me*, and are my *achievements* still fully mine? Have I been enhanced in ways that are in fact genuinely *better* and *humanly* better? And, beyond these questions regarding individuals, we would need to consider the implications for society should such uses of biotechnology become widespread—in school, at work, or in athletics, warfare, or other competitive activities.

Needless to say, such a comprehensive examination is beyond the possible scope of this discussion. There are too many different kinds of superior performance and too many conceivable biotechnical means of enhancing the performers. To introduce the subject and to illustrate the ethical and social issues involved, we confine ourselves largely to one particular case study in one particular area of human activity: human sport. It is an activity where human excellence is both recognizable and admired, where concerns about wrongfully enhancing performance are familiar, and where disquiet about the use of "performance-enhancing drugs" is widely shared if not always fully understood. As we shall see, many of the larger questions readily emerge from this case study, and the relevance of the present analysis for other human activities should be plain. Where explicit comparisons with other human activities will prove revealing, we shall not hesitate to bring them into the picture.

II. SPORT AND THE SUPERIOR ATHLETE

A. Why Sport?

At first glance, focusing on athletic excellence may seem strange. True, sports are hugely popular and exciting, and the achievements of our greatest athletes are very impressive. But is sport *important?* Why spend time worrying about the dignity of athletics when there are many more serious problems in the world and when many life and death dilemmas in bioethics are so pressing? Such questions raise a powerful point: many aspects of human life are indeed more significant or more worth worrying about than athletics. Nevertheless, if one is interested not only in combating human misery but also in promoting human excellence, the world of sport is an extremely useful case study. Indeed, what we learn of wider application from thinking about athletics may prove far more significant than it first appears.

For one thing, sport is an area of human endeavor where human excellence is widely admired—where we honor the best for their achievements, and where we admire the striving of those who seek to improve, achieve, and excel.* Athletic excellence appeals partly because it is open, genuine, and publicly visible, inviting thousands of otherwise disconnected individuals to unite in shared appreciation. In perhaps no other contemporary activity is there such a manifestly evident and celebrated display of individual (and group) human excellence.

Second, sport is an activity that invites deeper reflection about our bodily nature, and especially our distinctly human bodily nature. After all, animals and machines can do many things much better than we can—artificial pitching machines can "throw" harder, cheetahs can run faster. But it is the human athlete that we admire. Understanding why this is so has implications far beyond athletics.

Third, sport is an area of life where we have made some effort—both cultural and legal—to preserve the "dignity of the game," so to speak, from "cheating," both biological (for example, steroids) and mechanical

---

* Other areas where this is also true include music, dance, theater, and other performing arts.

(for example, corked bats). But we have done so without always examining precisely how the dignity of the game or the excellence of the performance would be compromised were the use of these enhancing agents to become normal.

Thus, while we begin this analysis by acknowledging that "life is not a game," we also suggest that things essential to sport—such as aspiration, effort, activity, achievement, and excellence—are essential also to many aspects of the good human life.* Examining the significance of performance-enhancing biotechnical powers for human sport may help us understand the significance of such powers for excellent human activity more generally.

B. The Superior Athlete

To be a superior athlete depends on numerous things: native gifts, great desire, hard work, fine coaching, worthy competitors, sound equipment, good luck. The types of talents needed will vary with the sport or, in team sports featuring specialization, with one's position or role. But any superior athlete requires strength, drive, endurance, coordination, agility, vision, quickness, cleverness, discipline, and daring, shared virtues of body and soul that manifest themselves in different ways and degrees depending on the activity and the way one performs it. And, in every sport, at every level of competition, superior performance matters.

Some ways of becoming a superior athlete center on the athlete himself: for example, healthy physical growth, better training, more experience. Others involve outside help: better coaches, better teammates, better competitors. Some involve improving one's equipment: fiberglass vaulting poles, graphite tennis rackets, high-tech high-tops. And others involve improving one's own body: high-protein diets, vitamin supplements, anabolic steroids, genetic modifications. These different approaches can be complementary or overlapping: better diet improves one's capacity to train, and better training

---

* Similarly, the things that can corrupt, tarnish, or merely complicate sports—greed, vanity, the desire to injure or crush a rival—can corrupt, tarnish, or merely complicate most other human activities.

improves one's body and its powers. We intuitively sense, however, that there may be a difference between, for example, lifting weights, eating egg whites, and using a graphite tennis racket, just as there appears to us to be a difference between eating egg whites and taking anabolic steroids. But if so, understanding the true nature and significance of these differences is a complex matter, not easily specified. How do the different *means* of becoming superior differ from one another? Is the excellence or superiority of an activity affected by the *way* it is done or pursued? Do some ways of improving performance change the actual character of the activity? If some performance enhancements are considered "cheating," just who or what is being cheated—one's competitors, one's fans, oneself, or the dignity of the activity itself? These are the sorts of questions we shall try to answer.

C. Different Ways of Enhancing Performance

As already indicated, there are multiple ways to improve athletic performance, from the elementary to the sophisticated, from the old to the new. Consider, for example, competitive running. The ancient Greek runners ran barefoot. Then the use of shoes protected against injury. Cleats gave greater traction. Better nutrition augmented general health and energy. Weight training strengthened muscles. Regimens of practicing wind sprints or fixed-distance runs built up endurance. Competition during training provided motivation and experience. Coaching improved mechanics and strategy. High-tech shoes improved efficiency of motion. Erythropoietin injections increased oxygen carrying capacity. Anabolic steroids permitted greater weight training leading to enlarged muscle mass. Stimulant drugs aided alertness and concentration. Someday, insertion of synthetic muscle-enhancing genes may make muscles stronger, quicker, and less prone to damage.* Where in this sequence of devices to improve running do we acquire any disquiet regarding the means used? *Why*, if we are disquieted, are we bothered?

---

* We leave out of the account some further enhancements of "running," such as the use of wheels, or even motors, on the soles of shoes. Such changes, of course, would transform the activity into something other than running.

To prepare for the answers to these questions, let us look more closely at a number of different ways of improving athletic performance—some celebrated and some not, some already here and some on the horizon. They fall generally into three categories: better equipment, better training, and better native powers.

1. Better Equipment

Examples of superior performance through better equipment are ubiquitous. Pole-vaulting used to be done with rigid bamboo poles and vaults of fifteen feet high seemed virtually superhuman; now flexible fiberglass poles are used, and vaults go over nineteen feet. Baseball gloves were once little more than shaped padding for the hand; now, more than twice their original size, they resemble small bushel baskets. Curved hockey sticks, replacing the straight ones, make possible greater puck control and faster shots. Graphite tennis rackets yield greater racket speed and power. With such equipment now an accepted part of the sport, used by virtually everyone in competitive and professional athletics, players who did not use them would be looked upon as foolish, and they would likely never make it to the highest levels of competition.

Yet not all performance-enhancing equipment is welcomed into sport. Corked baseball bats, for example, are believed to permit increased bat speed and thus hitting power. Yet they are considered an unacceptable form of cheating and are illegal in professional baseball. Players who use them are looked down upon by many fans as "cheaters" or seen as fools for believing they could get such an unfair advantage without getting caught. Were someone to propose that the rules be changed, so that everyone could use corked bats, many people would probably still object. Owing to the importance of history and statistics in the glamour of baseball and the desire of fans to be able to make valid comparisons of superior performance across the generations, their wish to see more home runs does not—at least for now—trump their wish to preserve the "integrity of the game." Comparing graphite tennis rackets (which we embrace) and corked baseball bats (which we decry) suggests how our objections to performance-enhancing equipment are often conventional, with differences due to traditions, chance histories, or elective decisions about the rules of the game.

Some of these rules are not matters of principle but of taste, while others involve particular discernments about what is best for individual sports that cannot be universalized.

2. Better Training

Better training can take several forms. It could become more rigorous, the athlete working harder and longer than he did before or harder and longer than his teammates or his rivals. Training could be more effective (*better*, not necessarily harder), the athlete training more intelligently or scientifically. And training could be better coached, the athlete practicing under the guidance of someone with superior wisdom or know-how regarding nutrition, general fitness, or specialized skills such as batting or pitching.

All of these forms of improving performance through training proceed through habituation, practice, and instruction, consciously and conscientiously undertaken. Yet the effects of the training are often written into the bodies of the athletes, in the form of increased strength, longer endurance, greater quickness, improved coordination, and smoother performance. Similar bodily changes might also be produced not through active training or active training alone, but by direct biotechnical intervention into the body of the athlete, seeking to improve his native capacities by altering his underlying genetic or biochemical make-up.

3. Better Native Powers

Direct biological means of improving the powers of our bodies range from the small and familiar to the large and novel. Least dramatic are special diets, for example, diets high in protein, known for decreasing body fat and increasing muscle mass. There is laser eye surgery to correct imperfect or "low-performing" eyesight, capable of producing permanent improvements in the patient's vision with a single treatment. Some prominent athletes (including Tiger Woods) have used this surgery to get "better-than-normal" eyesight, a practice that is fully legal and considered by all professional sports to be an acceptable "enhancement."

More invasive, more controversial, and (for now) illegal in competitive athletics are the uses of various drugs to enhance performance: stimulants like amphetamine to produce heightened attention and quicker reactivity; erythropoietin (EPO) to overproduce red blood cells and, hence, to augment the body's carrying capacity for oxygen (so-called "blood doping"); human growth hormone to increase height or generalized vigor; and anabolic steroids to facilitate training that will increase overall muscle mass. Off in the future, but already visible on the drawing board, are prospects of genetic enhancement of bodily strength and resilience through the insertion into muscles of genes for erythropoietin or more specific muscle growth factors. Because so much of athletic excellence is based on strength and swiftness, the muscle-enhancing technologies are under special scrutiny by the sports authorities. They are also of special interest to us. To illustrate how present and prospective biotechnologies can enhance native bodily powers, we turn next to various technological approaches to direct muscle enhancement, both pharmacologic and genetic.

III. MUSCLE ENHANCEMENT THROUGH BIOTECHNOLOGY

A. Muscles and Their Meanings

Our muscles are essential to human life in many ways. They are central agents of physical strength and speed, attributes admired and celebrated in most human cultures. All of our motions—from walking, swimming, and lifting, to writing, chewing, and shaking hands—depend on them. As basic elements of physical vigor, they also play a role in human attractiveness and in our sense of well-being and even our sense of who we are. Our path through the life cycle is displayed most vividly in the changes of our musculature.

When we are young, the active use of our muscles in play and in sports strengthens and develops them. At puberty, production of estrogen and testosterone enhances these processes, so that the peak of human muscular development usually occurs between ages 20 and 30. Thereafter, the strength and size of human muscles usually declines, falling off by about one-third between the ages of 30 and 80.[1] As we age, we gradually lose the ability to do various physical tasks, sometimes in part, sometimes altogether.*

There are, of course, individual variations from this general pattern. Some people suffer from muscle diseases, often caused by specific genetic mutations (for example, muscular dystrophy), that render them unable to develop their muscles to the same extent as the healthy. Others manage through exercise and fitness training to maintain peak muscular strength and endurance much longer than the average. Still others, sedentary and inactive, neglect those maintenance functions altogether and fall weaker earlier than most.

Muscles do not generate human strength and speed in isolation. They need to be physically integrated with, and function harmoniously through their attachments to, nerves, tendons, ligaments, and bones. While our attention will be on enhancing the activities of muscles and their cells, this fact reminds us that any biotechnological intervention that strengthens only muscles may unbalance the interactions with these other body parts, with serious malfunction as a possible consequence.

Though not exactly a matter of athletic performance, the perfection of our musculature and body build is a matter of great concern to many people intent on improving their body image. Muscles have always played a prominent role in the idealizations of male human form. A classical picture of excellence of the youthful male human form is Michelangelo's sculpture of David, completed around 1504. The musculature is well developed and well proportioned but without much articulation of individual muscles; indeed, the integrated physique points not to itself but to some impending action. Yet David's strength and power shine through the marble, and leave us with a mental picture of the classical ideal of muscular development and proportion, poised for graceful and superior performance.

A more contemporary idealization of the male human form is the modern bodybuilding champion, such as Arnold Schwarzenegger.

---

* The age-related loss of muscle size and strength has been named "sarcopenia." (The term "sarcopenia" was first suggested by I. H. Rosenberg in 1989. It is derived from Greek words meaning "poverty of flesh." See Rosenberg, I., "Summary Comments," *American Journal of Clinical Nutrition* 50: 1231-1233, 1989.) We shall consider sarcopenia further in Chapter Four, "Ageless Bodies."

Through specialized weight training, perhaps with the help of anabolic steroids, all the muscles (especially the biceps and pectoral muscles) become much larger than those in the statue of David, and the different groups of skeletal muscles are individually articulated. The picture is less one of measured and proportionate strength in the service of splendid activity, more one of "muscle-bound" power, to be admired for its own sake.* Yet although they differ in proportion and muscle articulation, both the classical and contemporary ideals testify to the importance of muscles in images of male strength and power.**

The body's appearance reveals more than a superficial image. As embodied agents of our innermost will, muscles not only work our purposes on the world, but make manifest the deep qualities of our character, our dispositions and intentions, our self-discipline, self-development, and self-image. We are highly attentive to posture and motion in others, and muscular actions make possible the communication and cooperative coordination essential for human society. All of these qualities are especially evident—and therefore visible for evaluation—in many forms of athletic performance.

B. Muscle Cell Growth and Development

Scientists have learned a great deal about the cellular structure and development of skeletal muscles, as well as about how genes important to muscle cells function and are regulated. The following brief discussion of muscle cell biology will reveal targets for biotechnical interventions aimed at improving muscle strength and resilience.

The major cell type present in skeletal muscle fibers is the multinucleated myotube, a long clylindrical cell that does the contracting. These

---

* The very idea of "muscle-bound" looks away from activity, and implies *restricted freedom* of motion; the hypertrophied muscles cut down somewhat the range of possible motion around some joints.

** Interestingly, female bodybuilders initially pursued the same path as the males. The result was women bodybuilding champions with smaller but similarly individually developed and articulated skeletal muscles. More recently there has been an aesthetic reaction against the resulting female muscle "overdevelopment" and, commercially at least, the more popular and profitable activity today is women's fitness competition.

myotubes arise from precursor cells, mononucleated myoblasts, by means of their fusion with each other and with pre-existing myotubes. Myoblasts, in turn, are formed by differentiation of a particular stem cell found in muscle tissue, called a satellite cell.[2]

The multiplication and differentiation of satellite cells into myoblasts is regulated by several specific protein growth factors (primarily insulin-like growth factor 1 [IGF-1] and hepatocyte [liver cell] growth factor [HGF]). This process is also influenced by hormones such as growth hormone, testosterone, and estrogen. Growth hormone secreted by the pituitary acts on the liver to stimulate synthesis of IGF-1 and its subsequent release into the circulation. (See Figure 1.)

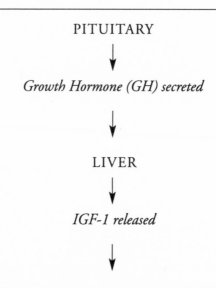

PITUITARY

↓

Growth Hormone (GH) secreted

↓

LIVER

↓

IGF-1 released

↓

SKELETAL MUSCLE GROWTH STIMULATED

Figure 1. Hormone action and muscle growth stimulation.

In muscle tissue, IGF-1 binds to specific receptors on the surface of satellite cells to stimulate their multiplication, producing both differentiation of satellite cells into myoblasts as well as more satellite cells. (See Figure 2.)

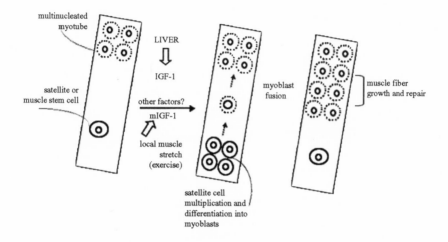

Figure 2. Schematic diagram of some important processes in skeletal muscle fiber growth and repair.

Importantly, a slightly different form of IGF-1 (muscle IGF-1 or mIGF-1) is also produced locally in muscle tissue in response to stretching the muscles during exercise. This form is thought to act the same way as circulating IGF-1 does in stimulating satellite cell multiplication and differentiation. However, because mIGF-1 is slightly different in chemical structure from IGF-1 produced in the liver, mIGF-1 apparently does not enter the circulation, so its effects can be restricted to promoting growth and repair of muscle tissue locally.

C. Opportunities and Techniques for Muscle Enhancement[3]

We can now see how attempts at muscle enhancement might work. As has long been known, exercise increases muscle size and strength. Exercise both transiently damages muscles and, in response, causes them to increase in size and strength. Exercise (muscle stretch) increases the production of a specific locally active form of insulin-like growth factor (mIGF-1), a major mediator of muscle stem cell growth and differentiation. As a consequence of IGF-induced stimulation, muscle stem (satellite) cells multiply, differentiate, and fuse. As a result, the number of muscle fibers increases.

Biotechnological research and development have introduced new possibilities for producing similar muscle proliferation and enhancement, both genetic and pharmacological. The genes for animal and human IGF-1 have been cloned and their DNA sequences determined. Gene expression vectors have been developed that permit the regulated production of IGF-1 proteins (both the liver and muscle forms) for investigation. Thus IGF-1 genes can be introduced into cells and experimental animals—for example, by means of viral vectors—to determine the effect of enhanced IGF-1 (or mIGF-1) production on muscle size and strength. Recent experiments along these lines in animals have yielded very exciting results.

For example, in experiments described by Barton-Davis and coworkers,[4] recombinant viruses[*] containing a rat IGF-1 gene were injected into the anterior compartment of the rear legs of young mice containing the extensor digitorum longus (EDL) muscle. The resulting increased production of IGF-1 promoted an average increase of about 15 percent in EDL muscle mass and strength in young adult mice. Strikingly, such injections led to a 27 percent increase in the strength of the EDL muscles when the mice approached the average lifespan of 27 months. In fact, the continued presence of additional (rat) IGF-1 genes essentially prevented the decline in muscle size and strength observed in untreated old mice.[**†]

---

[*] Recombinant viruses, engineered to express a specific foreign gene, are frequently used to stimulate the production of functionally effective amounts of the foreign protein to treat disease. Recombinant viruses created from genetically engineered human Adenovirus-associated Virus (AAV) have proved to be efficient delivery systems of foreign genes into muscle cells. As AAV is a small virus, only small foreign genes can be used effectively with this virus. Fortunately, the DNA sequence encoding IGF-1 is small enough to function well in AAV-based recombinant viruses.

[**] Professor H. Lee Sweeney, the leader of the team conducting this research, gave a fuller description of his group's recent findings in his presentation to the Council in September 2002. According to Professor Sweeney, the insertion of IGF-1 genes into mouse muscles not only blocked the normal age-related decline of muscle size and strength; in addition, the researchers found, it caused the muscle tissue of older mice to retain the optimal power and speed normally found only in younger mice. It also improved the rate of repair of damaged muscle tissue. Other

An alternate route to genetic enhancement exploits the ability, at embryonic stages of development, to create transgenic animals in which an appropriately regulated foreign gene is expressed throughout embryonic and adult life. Musaro and his colleagues[5] introduced a rat mIGF-1 gene into early-stage mouse embryos, where it became integrated with mouse chromosomal DNA. The resulting transgenic mice produced substantial amounts of rat mIGF-1, in addition to their own mouse IGF-1 and mIGF-1. Embryonic development of these transgenic mice proceeded normally. Yet as early as ten days after birth, the skeletal muscles of the transgenic animals were enlarged, compared to the non-transgenic control mice. Moreover, the skeletal muscle enlargement persisted as the transgenic mice aged. Whereas, in unmodified (wild type) mice, muscle size and strength peaked around six months and decreased considerably by twenty months of age, the size and strength of skeletal muscle in the transgenic mice (containing rat mIGF-1) remained stable at peak levels for up to twenty months.[*]

experiments on rats showed that, when IGF-1 gene injections were accompanied by strenuous exercise, not only did the rats develop bigger and stronger muscles, they also retained those enhanced muscles far longer than they normally would after the exercise had ceased. Should comparable results be attainable with human skeletal muscles, gene insertion would appear to hold great promise, both as therapy for muscular dystrophy and age-related sarcopenia and as a means to enhance athletic performance. See Sweeney, H., "Genetic Enhancement of Muscles," presentation at the September 2002 meeting of the President's Council on Bioethics, Washington, D.C. Transcript available on the Council's website, www.bioethics.gov.

[†] (From previous page.) In this study, approximately 10^{10} recombinant AAV particles in 100 microliters of fluid were injected into a single small muscle compartment of mice. If such treatments were eventually to be applied to humans, large amounts of recombinant AAV containing the human IGF-1 DNA sequence would be required. Assuming such future treatments were shown to be safe and effective, producing sufficient recombinant AAV to treat millions of dystrophic and aging humans would remain a substantial logistical challenge. However, there may be ways around this logistical problem involving the production and transplantation of human muscle stem cells engineered to produce more IGF-1.

[*] The growing understanding of muscle physiology at the molecular level coupled with sophisticated genetic engineering has made it possible to enlarge skeletal muscles selectively, without damaging heart muscles in the process. In previous studies of this type, the IGF-1 transgene was not connected to gene expression regulatory elements that restricted production of mIGF-1 to muscle tissue. This led to overproduction of IGF-1 in the circulation, and eventually to pathological enlargement of the heart muscle. But in the studies with transgenic mice cited here, the rat mIGF-1 transgene was connected to gene expression regulatory elements that restricted production of the rat mIGF-1 protein *only* to muscle tissues containing primarily fast-twitch fibers. Side effects on the heart muscle did not occur.

These and other experimental results stimulate thoughts about possible extensions of these approaches to humans. They hold out the promise of treatments for various diseases of muscle tissue, for sarcopenia and the weaknesses of old age, and for generalized enhancement of muscle strength and fitness in people of all ages, diseased or not. Based on our current understanding, at least three different approaches could be considered. First, one could introduce muscle-enhancing genes directly into the muscles themselves. To do so, one would need to develop recombinant virus vectors containing the human mIGF-1 gene, under the control of appropriate regulatory elements that would limit its expression to muscle cells near the site of injection. Alternatively, one might introduce an appropriately regulated mIGF-1 gene into human embryos, as was done in the experiments with mice. Finally, one might use an approach that combined techniques of stem cell and genetic engineering. After isolating and expanding human muscle stem (satellite) cells in vitro, one could introduce an appropriately regulated human mIGF-1 gene into those cells and then transplant the genetically modified satellite cells back into the muscles of the person being treated.

None of these three approaches has yet been tried in human beings. Each has its advantages and disadvantages.* Developing any

---

* The first approach would be similar to other human gene therapy projects in children and adults. The appropriately regulated human mIGF-1 gene would be combined with a vector capable of efficient delivery to muscle cells, perhaps AAV. This material could be produced in large volumes, carefully characterized by tests in experimental animals, stored frozen and used as needed. While the logistics of producing the large amounts of recombinant AAV that would be required for treatment of thousands or millions of patients are daunting, in principle this would be possible. The advantages of this approach are (1) that it would develop and use a single, well-characterized biological agent; (2) that treatment could be started very slowly by introducing the recombinant mIGF-1 gene-containing AAV into one muscle at a time and evaluating its effects; (3) that treatment could be stopped immediately if untoward side effects developed. Disadvantages include (1) the possibility that a large number of injections would be necessary to treat each of the large number of human skeletal muscles; (2) the possibility that this would not be an effective treatment for humans who had antibodies to AAV as a consequence of a previous infection.

The second approach is a radical proposal, as it envisions treatment of blastocyst-stage human embryos in vitro with a genetic procedure that was intended to change the early development of skeletal muscle size and strength and reduce the rate of loss later in life. This approach shares some advantages with the first approach in that (1) a single biological agent could be prepared and characterized that could treat all embryos; (2) only a single treatment early in embryonic development would be needed, instead of multiple injections into different muscles. The one of them would take a lot of time and money, and many technical and logistical problems would need to be overcome before any treatment could be applied on a large scale. Even before the first genetic treatments to increase muscle size and strength could be tried in humans in the United States, the Food and Drug Administration (FDA) would require demonstrations that the proposed treatment is safe and effective.

Nevertheless, the time may be coming soon for human trials using the first approach, undertaken not to bulk up aspiring athletes but to treat human muscle diseases. Clinical trials of regulated mIGF-1 gene delivery as a treatment for specific forms of muscular dystrophy may begin within the next several years.[6] These clinical trials will likely provide crucial data, en route, on administration, optimal dose, and possible side effects. If efficacy is demonstrated and side effects are small, one can easily imagine the social and economic factors that will favor vast expansions in the use of genetic muscle treatments to enhance muscle size and strength. High school wrestling and football coaches, having learned of the enhancing gene transfer experiments in rats and mice, have already expressed interest in obtaining such treatments for their athletes. Developing a product for which the eventual potential market is up to 100 percent of the human population will be hard to resist.

---

major disadvantages of this approach are the difficult ethical questions it would raise, as well as the difficulty of meeting the safety criteria demanded of any germ-line or embryo genetic engineering (see Chapter Two, "Better Children").

The third approach depends upon the ability to isolate human muscle stem (satellite) cells and expand them in vitro. [This has recently been reported for mice. See Qu-Peterson, Z., et al., "Identification of a novel population of muscle stem cells in mice: potential for muscle regeneration," *Journal of Cell Biology* 157(5): 851-864, 2002.] The isolated human muscle stem cells would then have their mIGF-1 production genetically modified by introducing an appropriately regulated exogenous mIGF-1 gene copy. In theory, this could produce modified muscle stem cells that multiplied continuously in vitro to produce larger numbers of cells, and that differentiated appropriately in vitro. In this case, genetically modified satellite cells would be injected into skeletal muscles. The advantages of this approach include (1) it would develop and use a single, well-characterized biological agent to modify the muscle stem cells in vitro, and (2) the dose of modified stem cells could be varied as necessary to optimize treatment of individual skeletal muscles. The disadvantages include the possibility that a separate preparation of muscle stem cells would have to be made from each patient needing treatment, in order to get around the immune-rejection problem.

Genetic treatments for increasing muscle size and strength are still in the future. But pharmacological means of doing so are already here and in use, and both the desire and the rationale for their use is clear. As noted earlier, various hormones and growth factors play key roles in stimulating muscle stem cells to multiply, differentiate into myoblasts, and then fuse with existing muscle fibers. Growth hormone levels influence the size and strength of muscles, perhaps through the intermediacy of IGF-1. Testosterone levels influence muscle size and strength, helping to explain why men's muscles are generally larger and stronger than women's. Finally, local growth factors like mIGF-1 have important effects as well.

At the present time, three different sorts of drugs are being used to increase (or try to increase) muscle strength. In the newest practice, still on a very small scale, people have begun to use human growth hormone in attempts to enhance muscle size and strength, especially in the elderly. Now that the patent on human growth hormone has expired (2002), the cost of the monthly hormone injections is likely to drop from its steep $1,000. If this occurs, the scale of growth hormone use might very likely increase, as promotion for new uses grows; over the past year, unsolicited e-mail advertisements for human growth hormone have come frequently to the e-mail boxes of Council staff.* Competitive athletes (and others) interested in boosting muscle size and performance have started using growth hormone—though the data suggest that its effectiveness is uncertain.[7]

A second approach to the enhancement of muscle performance works indirectly, not by enlarging muscle size but by increasing muscle endurance.

---

* Earlier this year, the FDA enlarged the domain of approved uses for human growth hormone to include preventive treatment of short stature. To be eligible for approved use, a child's height must be more than 2.25 standard deviations below the mean for age and sex; that is, he or she must be among the shortest 1.2 percent of children. Obviously, successful treatment of this group would automatically create another group of children who were now the shortest 1.2 percent. Even before there was FDA approval, the uses of growth hormone were already expanding, with increasing acceptance of medical intervention for social gains. In an August 1996 article in the *Journal of the American Medical Association,* Leone Cuttler and colleagues report that six out of ten children receiving growth hormone are not actually growth-hormone deficient. Some of these children have other medical problems that stunt growth, but many receive treatment because their parents simply want their children to be taller. (Cuttler, L., et al., "Short stature and growth hormone therapy: a national study of physician recommendation patterns," *Journal of the American Medical Association* 276: 531-537, 1996.)

Known as blood doping, it was originally accomplished by drawing blood from athletes, separating and concentrating the red blood cells, and then re-infusing the red blood cells into the athletes' bloodstream. This raised the amount of hemoglobin (the oxygen-binding protein) in the blood, and thus increased the oxygen-carrying capacity of the blood. Much the same effect can now be obtained by injections of the synthetic protein hormone erythropoietin, which stimulates the body to increase its production of red blood cells. For competitive cyclists, swimmers, and long-distance runners, increased oxygen-carrying capacity in the blood makes possible increased endurance, which in turn improves competitive performance.

The most commonly used chemical means of muscle enhancement are the anabolic steroids, chemical compounds related to hormones like testosterone. Taken orally (for example, "Anadrol" [oxymetholone], "Winstrol" [stanozolol], or "THG" [tetrahydrogestrinone]), or by injection (for example, "Durabolin" [nandrolone] or "Equipoise" [boldenone]), these drugs facilitate bodybuilding. Used in combination with weight training and special diets, they can greatly increase muscle size and strength. It is true that the precise benefits of these drugs for athletic performance are in dispute among scientific researchers, and, for obvious reasons, we have not seen adequate controlled studies to clarify their true effects. Nevertheless, many athletes, trusting their own experience and the testimony of teammates, are not waiting for the scientific evidence. Despite the known health risks and despite official opposition from the professional and college athletic authorities, as information about their effects has diffused throughout American society, more and more professional and amateur athletes are apparently using them. Also believing that they are effective—and that they are dangerous to the athletes—anti-doping sport organizations have banned most of them. At the same time, many (including the ones listed above) are listed as available for sale on the Internet.

Despite the opposition of Olympic and other sports officials to their use, the public attitude toward steroid use by athletes may be changing, at least for sports like baseball, basketball, and football. The recent outcry regarding Sammy Sosa's corked bat seemed to exceed any protests against the multiple revelations of steroid use by professional athletes. Malcolm Gladwell suggests an explanation:

> We have come to prefer a world where the distractible take Ritalin, the depressed take Prozac, and the unattractive get cosmetic surgery to a world ruled, arbitrarily, by those fortunate few who were born focused, happy and beautiful. Cosmetic surgery is not "earned" beauty, but then natural beauty isn't earned, either. One of the principal contributions of the late twentieth century was *the moral deregulation of social competition—the insistence that advantages derived from artificial and extraordinary intervention are no less legitimate than the advantages of nature. All that athletes want, for better or worse, is the chance to play by those same rules.*[8] (Emphasis added.)

It is hard to predict how widely genetic and chemical agents of muscle enhancement would be used, especially should safer versions be developed. Given the popularity of bodybuilding and fitness today, one could imagine that biotechnical agents would be useful for enhancing these activities, both in competitive and non-competitive settings. The commercial and competitive pressures to use genetic muscle treatments to build up, maintain, and repair the muscles of competitive professional athletes in all sports would surely be very strong. And since athletic competition extends down from professional and collegiate ranks to youth soccer and Little League, there would seem to be no place to draw a line against using (safe) genetic or chemical muscle treatments. The incentive to use these treatments during adolescence or young adulthood might increase considerably if it should turn out that treatment during these earlier times of life is also the best means of protecting against the sarcopenia of old age.

Thus, it is not too farfetched to imagine that parents may one day be faced with difficult decisions regarding the development of their children's bodily capacities for athletics. What will and should they do when daughter Jenny's soccer coach tells them she would be a stronger player if they got her genetic muscle treatments, or that she is more likely to make the team if she gets treated? Would untreated children or aspiring athletes become significantly disadvantaged in a society in which many others had genetic or chemical muscle treatments? Conversely, would these new technologies at last provide the remedy for those to whom nature dealt a weaker bodily constitution? Given the difficulty of setting principled limits between the therapeutic uses of these new biotechnical powers and the uses that go "beyond therapy," why might we still seek to set any limits at all?* What is it that such limits would or should seek to defend? It is none too soon to begin to think about these questions, for the future that will make them anything but speculative is now visible on the horizon.

IV. ETHICAL ANALYSIS

To begin the ethical analysis, we must try to distinguish between different ways of achieving superior performance, and how these ways of becoming better might alter, enhance, corrupt, or perfect our different activities. For those performance enhancements that we embrace, are we so sure that they are improvements, if we understand "improvement" to mean enhancing performance in ways that serve, rather than call into question, the dignity or excellence of human activity? And for those performance enhancements that trouble us, what is the nature of our disquiet? Because we want to see the bigger picture, we deliberately take a general approach to these questions, not tying our analysis to any specific means of boosting muscle strength and athletic performance. Rather than spend time on issues peculiar to a particular technique—say, the special safety concerns of genetic transfer, as contrasted with those associated with growth hormone or steroid use—we will concentrate on the larger issues raised by our acquiring and using the new bodily powers that these techniques, each in its own way, supply or promote.

---

* It has been suggested that along with the regular Olympics and the Special Olympics, we have the "Bio-Olympics," where the competition is unconstrained and the athletes are free to use any legal form of pharmaceutical or physiological enhancement.

A. How Is Biotechnical Enhancement Different?

The first task is to try to figure out whether using biotechnological means to gain superior performance is different from using better equipment or engaging in better training. If it is, what might the differences be, and what ethical and social difference do they make? This task is more difficult than it might at first glance seem, for there are similarities as well as differences among these three approaches. Some analysts will try to use such similarities to dismiss expressions of concern regarding drug-mediated improvements: "How are steroids really different from Air Jordan basketball shoes? Special diets and drugs both increase the capacity to train, so why make such a fuss about the drugs?" In response, it is worth emphasizing in advance that *the ethical evaluation of biotechnological enhancements does not finally depend on their being found utterly unique and unprecedented.* The fact that taking anabolic steroids or using genetic muscle enhancers could resemble, in some respects, using special diets or special bodybuilding programs does not by itself dissolve all our moral concerns. On the contrary, it might lead us to think more deeply about the more familiar modes of seeking to promote superior performance. Moreover, as we shall see, a careful examination may reveal that, similarities notwithstanding, the differences are in fact humanly and ethically significant.

In many areas of life, including sports, we take for granted that better equipment makes for better performance. Better gadgets, tools, machines, and devices are both yesterday's news and tomorrow's headlines. We habitually think and act in ways that assume the existence of such equipment, and in many areas of life, we work endlessly and deliberately to make cutting-edge improvements in our "high-performance gear." Unlike training or drugs that change the agent directly, the equipment that boosts our performance does so indirectly, yet it does so quite openly and in plain sight. We can see how the springier running shoes, the lighter tennis racket, and the bigger baseball glove enable their users to go faster, hit harder, and reach the formerly unreachable—yet without apparently changing them in their persons or native powers.

Yet appearances are deceiving. That their effects on our performance are indirect does not mean that they are trivial. And that they remain but visible tools in our hands does not mean that we remain in fact unaltered. Although the alterations, unlike the tools that produce them, are often hard to see, they often go very deep. Not only do we think and act in ways that assume enhanced equipment, we come to take its use for granted. Not only do we come to rely on our better tools; after a while, we have trouble remembering that we could do without them, largely because in truth we *cannot* do without them. This is not to suggest that we *should* do without them or that there is something wrong with accepting the extra edge that they give us in our pursuit of excellence. It is merely to insist that the use of equipment in sports, as in the rest of life, changes and even binds the human users, often without their knowing it.

The point was beautifully made by Rousseau, commenting on how even the earliest human inventors of artful aids to better living "imposed a yoke on themselves without thinking about it":

> For, besides their continuing thus to soften body and mind, as these commodities had lost almost all their pleasantness through habit, and as they had at the same time *degenerated into true needs*, being deprived of them became much more cruel than possessing them was sweet; and people were unhappy to lose them without being happy to possess them.[9] (Emphasis added.)

Our gear (like all our technology) not only improves the way we do things. In the process, it also often changes the very things that we do. It changes the abilities that matter most, and thus the character of our aspirations and the economy of social rewards. Once again, this is not to suggest we should not seek further improvements in our equipment. It is merely to recognize the far-reaching changes, in us and our activities, that the "merely" external equipment can cause—in all that we do, not only in sports. Because of graphite tennis rackets, tennis today is a game of faster serves, stronger strokes, and shorter points, and in consequence requires players of different talents and demeanor than it did only decades ago. Similarly, because of precision-guided weapons and drones, warfare now requires a different and more technical kind of expertise, often less demanding of, and less rewarding to, the physical human powers that served best in hand-to-hand combat. And because of computers, there is a premium on those with habits of mind shaped for programming; indeed, the very way many people think, speak, and write has changed to fit with the possibilities and necessities of the computer age. Adapting Winston Churchill's sage remark about architecture, we might say that we shape our equipment and our equipment shapes us.*

The distinction between better equipment and better training, and even between better equipment and better native powers, is for additional reasons not as sharp as one might wish. For some forms of athletic (and other) equipment are developed not to enhance specific performance as such, but rather to help individuals change or improve themselves precisely through better practice or training. For example, state-of-the-art weight training equipment aims at allowing individuals to make themselves stronger weightlifters and linebackers; state-of-the-art flight simulators allow individuals to make themselves better pilots. Such equipment is a tool that explicitly enables us to change ourselves through our own activity; it is an indirect means to directed and chosen change. Moreover—and more profoundly—the line between person and equipment may be eroding: we already have such therapeutic interventions as artificial limbs and mechanical implants to help blind people to see and deaf people to hear. Mechanical implants of various other kinds are no longer matters merely for science fiction.

Nevertheless, as with night and day in relation to twilight, the blurring of the boundaries between the several approaches does not make the territories themselves indistinct. We can still separate in our mind those means of altering or improving performance that work by giving us tools to perform in new ways, and those interventions that work by changing us directly—whether through self-directed activity and training or through direct biological interventions in the human body and mind. We

---

* Better equipment is thought to be better because it does what old equipment did more effectively. But as it does so, the activities in which the old equipment was used are also altered, and not necessarily improved *as a whole*. We certainly have better tennis rackets—but is the game better now than it was then? We certainly have better weapons—but are the soldiers of today humanly superior to the soldiers of old, and is warfare today "better" than it used to be?

can distinguish using better sneakers from daily running practice for an upcoming race, and both of these from running the race with the benefit of EPO or steroids. In addition, even though our tools change us, they do not necessarily change us irreversibly. We can, if we wish, still try to play baseball with the small, soft gloves of yesteryear, or softball with no gloves at all. Despite the fuzziness at the boundary, it still makes sense to distinguish our tools and equipment from our practice or training, as well as from the more direct biotechnical interventions aimed at improving our native bodily capacities.

In athletics, as in so many other areas of human life, practice and training are the most important means for improving performance, and superior performance is most generally attained through better training: the direct improvement of the specific powers and abilities of the human agent at-work-in-the-world, by means of his self-conscious or self-directed effort, exercise, and activity. To train is to be at work: striving, seeking, pushing, laboring, and developing. It requires self-knowledge or external guidance about the ends worth seeking, and it requires the desire and discipline to pursue those ends through one's own effort. And, most importantly for our purposes, training means acquiring by practice and effort improvements in the very powers and abilities *that training uses*. One gets to run faster by running; one builds up endurance by enduring; one increases one's strength by using it on ever-increasing burdens. *The capacity to be improved is improved by using it; the deed to be perfected is perfected by doing it.*

This insight has some important implications. First, it calls our attention to the very real differences in our natural endowments. If improving through training proceeds as described, certain native abilities are often a prerequisite. In many cases, no amount of training can overcome the unchangeable shortcomings of natural gifts. Second, and more important for present purposes, the source of our different endowments may be mysterious, but our active cultivation of those endowments, whether great or small, is intelligible: we can understand the connection between effort and improvement, between activity and experience, between work and result.

This leads to an important difference between improvements made through training and improvements gained through bioengineering. When and if we use our mastery of biology and biotechnology to alter our native endowments—whether to make the best even better or the below-average more equal—we paradoxically make improvements to our performance less intelligible, in the sense of being less connected to our own self-conscious activity and exertion. The improvements we might once have made through training alone, we now make only with the assistance of artfully inserted IGF-1 genes or anabolic steroids. Though we might be using rational and scientific means to remedy the mysterious inequality or unchosen limits of our native gifts, we would in fact make the individual's agency *less* humanly or experientially intelligible to himself.

The IGF-1-using or steroid-using athlete surely improves: he (or she) develops and becomes superior—and certainly the scientist who produced the biological agents of such improvement can understand in scientific terms the genetic workings or physiochemical processes that make it possible. But from the athlete's perspective, he improves as if by "magic," without the self-conscious or self-directed activity that lies at the heart of better training. True, steroids (or, someday, genetic muscle enhancement) will enable him to perform at a higher level only if he continues to train. True, as he trains, he still tires, perspires, and feels his (altered) body at-work. But as the athlete himself can surely attest, the changes in his body are decisively (albeit not solely) owed to the pills he has popped or the shots he has taken, interventions whose relation to the changes he undergoes are utterly opaque to his direct human experience. He has the advantage of the mastery of modern biology, but he risks a partial alienation from his own doings, as his identity increasingly takes shape at the "molecular" rather than the experiential level. Indeed, the athlete's likely embarrassment proves the point: Even were steroids or stimulants to become legal, one imagines that most athletes would rather not be seen taking their injections right before the race. For there is something shameful about revealing one's own chemical dependence right before demonstrating what is supposed to be one's own personal excellence.

This is not to suggest that changes in the body produced through training and effort are not also molecular, or to ignore the fact that the very purpose of certain biochemical interventions (such as anabolic steroids) is to increase the individual's capacity to train. In expressing this uneasiness about biotechnical enhancement, we are not celebrating some fictitious agency divorced from bodily events and consequences: whenever the body works or is at work, the body's underlying biology changes. Neither are we casting doubts on efforts to improve the body by means that work on it directly; to do so would require us to cast doubts on all of medicine and surgery, not to mention a well-ordered diet. Yet *on the plane of human experience and understanding,* there is a difference between changes in our bodies that proceed through self-direction and those that do not, and between changes that result from our putting our bodies to work and those that result from having our bodies "worked on" by others or altered directly. This is a real difference, one whose importance for the ethical analysis, as we shall see later, may prove decisive.

Yet in trying to preserve the distinction between intelligible agency and unintelligible agency—between getting better because of "what we do" and getting better because of "what is done to us"—we face a dilemma. Many of the basic activities of life—for example, eating, breathing, and sleeping—transform our bodies without our directing the actual work of transformation. Eating the right foods makes our system work better. Science can come to understand why this is so—why protein is "good" and fats are "bad," or how our bodies break them down and to what effect. But these processes of the body, however well understood, can never be made *experientially* intelligible in the same way our self-directed activities are intelligible. We digest and we dance, but digesting and dancing are very differently *our* doings.

We can control the food we eat, but improving our native digestion through practice is beyond our power. We dance by choice, both immediately and self-consciously, with the movements of the body connected to our active desire to dance and our self-awareness of dancing. Over time we can see our dancing improve, at least within the limits of our native capacities, and we can see that it is through our own practice that the superior performance has occurred. Clearly, as with eating, what happens in our bodies as we become better dancers is invisible and mysterious at the organic and molecular levels; it is intelligible, if at all, only in the terms of science, not of human experience. But the lived experience of dancing—of doing the deeds that enable us to do them again and do them better—matters a great deal. When we dance, our improvements are "our own," made possible by and limited by our native biology, but still the result of our own self-directed activity.

And here we begin to understand the complexity: To be a human organism, possessed of a body all of whose activities are mediated by invisible and molecular events, means that our identity is always to some degree independent of all our self-conscious efforts to mold or control it. In important ways, our bodily identity and our bodily capacities are inborn, inherited, and "given," and much of what our bodies do thereafter is shaped by processes and in ways we do not direct or fully grasp at the level of inner human experience. We cannot make our bodies into just anything we like, no matter how hard we try. As human individuals, we are not simply the beings or persons that we *will* ourselves to be, precisely because we are biological beings—with finite capacities and a finite body, which make having an identity possible in the first place. And yet, if there are limits to what we can do, there are also possibilities. We can actively change our bodies and change ourselves in important ways, precisely by trying, doing, working, and performing the very activities we seek to do better.

Even in the most self-directed activities, we remain ignorant, on the level of experience, of what is transpiring chemically in our bodies. This fact has an important implication: The difference between improving the body through training and improving it through diet or drugs is *not absolute but a matter of degree*. Nevertheless, the fact that the difference is one merely of degree does not make it humanly insignificant. Some acts are more, and some acts are less "our own" as human and as individuals. When we seek superior performance through better training, *the way our body works* and our experience and understanding of *our own body at work* are more closely aligned. With interventions that bypass human experience to work their biological "magic" directly—from better nutrition to steroids to genetic muscle enhancements—our silent bodily workings and our conscious agency are more alienated from one another.

The central question becomes: Which biomedical interventions for the sake of superior performance are consistent with (even favorable to) our full flourishing as human beings, including our flourishing as active, self-aware, self-directed agents? And, conversely, when is the alienation of biological process from active experience dehumanizing, compromising the lived humanity of our efforts and thus making our superior performance in some way false—not simply our own, not fully human? Better nutrition seems an obvious good, a way of improving our bodily functioning that serves human flourishing without compromising the "personal" nature or individual agency of what we do with our healthy, well-nourished bodies. But moving outward from there, the puzzle gets more complicated. Where in the progression of possible biological interventions do we lose in our humanity or identity more than we gain in our "performance"? Is there a way to distinguish coffee and caffeine pills to keep us awake from Modafinil to enable us to avoid sleep entirely for several days, from amphetamines to keep us more alert and focused, from human growth hormone, steroids, and EPO to improve strength and endurance, from genetic modifications that make such biological interventions more direct and more lasting? All of them alter our bodily workings; all of them to varying degrees separate self-directed experience from underlying biology.

Does that mean that we are incapable of distinguishing among them, humanly and ethically? Can our disquiet about pharmacological and genetic enhancement withstand rational scrutiny? More deeply, what does the prospect of such interventions tell us about the nature of human activity and the meaning of human identity? These are perhaps the deepest questions for the ethical analysis that follows. But to see why this is so, we must first consider some more familiar sources of ethical disquiet.

B. Fairness and Equality

The most obvious disquiet with performance-enhancing agents in athletics, both equipment like corked bats and biological interventions like steroids, stimulants, or future genetic muscle boosters, concerns fairness: the worry that players using them will have an unfair advantage over other players, the concern that injustice will be perpetrated against one's rivals. Games have rules, and breaking the rules in these ways undermines the fairness of competition and the dignity of the game. This is, of course, a proper concern. But the question of fairness is more complicated than it looks at first.

Athletics, like many other human activities, depend on native gifts that are unequally distributed. Indeed, human sport often highlights and celebrates the very real differences and inequalities in our biological "starting points." In most sports, we do not, in the name of equality, require that our athletes (or others) with special talents assume handicaps so that everyone might compete on an equal footing.* Although we may never settle the ancient and complicated question about how much of our various achievements is due to "nature" and how much to "nurture," there is no question but that gifts of nature have much to do with all sorts of human excellence. Many individuals, lacking certain physical and mental attributes (for example, height, muscle potential, eye-hand coordination), will never achieve the highest levels of human performance in certain activities no matter how hard they strive. At the same time, nature is hardly the whole story. Many individuals, with more limited native powers, will outperform those who are less willing or less able to cultivate their superior gifts.

Some have argued that allowing performance-enhancing drugs would be an acceptable—or even desirable—means of leveling a playing field that is unequal by nature. It could make athletic competition more perfectly fair, allowing winners to become those who *do* the best rather than those who *are* the best. But others argue that such drugs would only exacerbate the naturally unequal endowments rather than correct them. For even were there to be an "enhancement commissar" who calculated what degree of "boost" each person needed in order to get even with the natively gifted, there would be no way to titrate all the relevant gifts.**

---

* This bizarre prospect, the logical extension of a preoccupation with equality, is the ingenious conceit of a short story by Kurt Vonnegut, "Harrison Bergeron," in his collection, *Welcome to the Monkey House.* The goal is accomplished by the work of a "handicapper general" who is charged with weighing down all elevated gifts, physical and mental.

** Even beyond the native gifts, we could never titrate the important advantages of proper nurture, rearing, coaching, encouragement, experience, or faith.

Besides, in a free country there would be no basis for denying the same performance-enhancers also to the more talented. Why, if they wish it, should those destined to be tall or bulky be refused a chance to become taller or bulkier through growth hormone? As a result, those who are "best by nature" would become even better by augmenting nature's gifts with biological enhancements. And whether we allow or disallow such enhancements, we are not likely to alter the inherent biological inequalities that are part of being human, and that are important for human excellence in sports and many other activities. Fairness is always limited, to some degree, by the mysterious gifts of nature, even if such gifts are not solely responsible or even decisive for who will in the end become excellent or who will perform excellently.

The inequality of natural endowments highlights a related dilemma regarding the standards of excellence: to what extent should we judge performances superior for being "the best they can be," rather than simply being the "best"? For example, we celebrate both the real Olympics, which measures the best of the best, and the Special Olympics, which measures the best of those who strive in spite of great natural disadvantages. In the real Olympics, we honor the best human runner, and we appreciate the fact that the excellence of human running is not relative; it can be truthfully and quantitatively measured. At the same time, we judge the Special Olympians according to a different standard. We regard their activity as a kind of excellence—of personal achievement rather than of absolutely superior performance—even as they compete in the same activity with much lower scores. Standards of excellence also change with the times. In some sports, the average professional athlete of today probably has better scores and more physical strength than the greatest champions of yesteryear. But which of these individuals—today's no-name or yesterday's giant—do we judge as "superior" or more excellent?

In sum, there seems to be an "absolute" dimension to human excellence: in certain activities, there is such a thing as the best human performance. And yet, judging human excellence also depends on making sense of nature's unequal allotment of gifts, as well as the way particular human activities, for various reasons, change over time. We need to fit our scales of excellence to the thing being weighed, resisting the twin errors of believing that all excellence is relative or that all excellence can simply be ranked and determined by "score."

Still, there is a danger of sentimentality, as well as of confused thinking, in admiring athletes largely for the excellence of extra effort. The perfectly fitting praise of the resolve, effort, and devotion necessary to perform in the face of serious handicap is praise more for human will and determination, less for superior performance as such. As we shall emphasize below, human performance humanly done does involve human intention, choice, and will; yet it would be strange to celebrate mainly human willfulness in activities such as athletics that display, above all, *bodily grace and beauty*. This observation suggests that, in athletics, it is the harmonious and seemingly seamless fusion of mind and body that is crucial to the athletic ideal of superior performance. Neither the human body regarded as mere animal, nor the human body regarded as recalcitrant slave to be whipped into shape by an unbending will, but the human being displaying in visibly beautiful action the workings of heart, mind, and body united as inseparably as the concave and the convex—that, as we shall argue shortly, is the heart of *humanly* superior performance.

Finally, at least in sports, fairness understood as "playing by the rules" is a matter of convention. When it comes to steroids, EPO, or corked baseball bats, the concern about unfair advantage is to a large degree self-created. It is only because these performance-enhancing agents are disallowed, and because those who use them must do so outside the rules and surreptitiously, that we regard their use as unfair. But if steroids were declared legal in competition, everybody (or nearly everybody) who desired to compete at the highest level in most sports might well use them. The problem of fairness of access and extra advantage would largely disappear—though the problem of natural inequality would remain. It is therefore not enough to defend the rules (no steroids, no corked bats) and decry those who break them. The rules themselves—why they exist and what they are defending—must be understood and supported. This must be done on grounds that go beyond equality and fairness toward others to the nature and meaning of the activity itself.

C. Coercion and Social Pressure

A second source of disquiet centers on issues of freedom and coercion, both overt and subtle. The pride most nations (and schools) take in their athletes is often far from benign, and there are well-known cases in which countries and coaches have forced athletes to use performance-enhancing drugs. In East Germany before the fall of communism, to take just a single example, the young members of the women's Olympic swim team took regular doses of the anabolic steroid known as Oral-Turinabol. This improved their strength and endurance, but it also caused terrible masculinizing side effects (severe acne, uncontrollable libido, gruff voices, abnormal hair growth). Those women who were brave enough to inquire about what they were taking were told that the drugs were simply "vitamin tablets." As one of the swimmers testified years later: "I was fifteen years old when the pills started. . . . The training motto at the pool was, 'You eat the pills, or you die.' It was forbidden to refuse."[10]

But the potential for coercion—or at least intense social pressure—is certainly not limited to tyrannical regimes and despotic coaches. Should the use of an enhancing agent become normal and widespread, anyone who wished to excel in a given activity, from athletics to academics, might "need" to use the same (or better) performance-enhancements in order to "keep up." Anecdotal evidence suggests that this "soft coercion" may already be a problem, given the widespread underground use of illegal substances in many professional sports. True, the individual users, in such circumstances, are still choosing the drugs for themselves. They are free in a way the East German swimmers were not. But their choice is constrained by the fact—or by the belief—that it would be impossible to compete, or compete on an equal playing field, without them. They see the alternative of not using them as a kind of "unilateral disarmament," virtually guaranteeing that only those individuals with every biological advantage would excel or succeed. In professional sports, where not only victory but big money is at stake, the pressures not to disarm oneself pharmacologically will be—are already—enormous.

The point can be generalized beyond athletics, and when this is done, we see additional reasons for concern. In a meritocratic and results-oriented society such as ours, the vast numbers of people caught up in the race "to get ahead" come to feel increasing pressures to enhance their performance. Most are probably moved less by the desire for excellence, more by the love of gain or the wish to beat out the next fellow. As mounting social and economic competition keeps ratcheting up the pressures, people look for any advantage that might win them the more lucrative or higher-status job or that would increase their children's chances of gaining admission to the more prestigious schools. Under these social conditions, with spiraling love of gain conjoined with rising demand for recognition, the temptation in all walks of life to use biotechnologies for some "extra edge" probably rises with the pressure to compete. Today, professional athletes—and those who dream of becoming professional athletes—often succumb to the temptation. Tomorrow, the same might be true in many other areas of human endeavor.

Yet these quite legitimate concerns about pressure and constraint must be examined more closely. For the fact is that athletic (and other) competition is, in important ways, constraining or pressure-filled by nature. By becoming better, our opponents force us to match their improvements or fall behind and fail. By the entirely accepted (and generally laudable) means of training, dieting, or superior coaching, they challenge us to meet or better their improvements. Moreover, the quest for excellence, even in activities (like music or ballet) that are not in essence competitive, typically comes with stiff demands, and anyone who is serious about superior performance has little choice but to yield to or embrace them. The question therefore becomes: Which demands and "necessities" of the pursuit of superior performance are defensible and which are not? Which serve human excellence and which compromise or undermine it?

Seen most clearly, the concern about coercion, as with equality and fairness, turns out to be a pointer to other and deeper concerns, concerns about what gives an individual performer his or her dignity, and what makes an individual performance humanly excellent. If there is a core difficulty here, it is with the biological enhancers themselves, not with the fact that individuals might feel constrained or compelled to use them.

D. Adverse Side Effects: Health, Balance, and the Whole of Life

One of the central concerns about the biotechnical agents themselves is the risk and reality of adverse and undesirable "side effects," in the first instance, on bodily health and safety. The unintended cost of seeking stronger muscles and superior performance through drugs or genetic engineering could well be bodily (or mental) harm. With drugs like steroids, the grave long-term health risks are well known: they include, among others, liver tumors, fluid retention, high blood pressure, infertility, premature cessation of growth in adolescents, and psychological effects from excessive mood swings to drug dependence. With looming biotechnical powers like genetic muscle enhancement, the side effects are for now uncertain. But until proven otherwise, it makes sense to follow this prudent maxim: No biological agent powerful enough to achieve major changes in body or mind is likely to be entirely safe or without side effects. Moreover, targeted interventions aimed at enhancing normally functioning capacities, not repairing broken parts, could produce lopsided "improvements" that throw whole systems out of kilter: monster muscles could threaten unenhanced bones and ligaments.

The concern about safety is a real one: to be an athlete should not mean accepting a sentence of premature death or serious disease or disability, later if not sooner. As admirers of athletes, we should not want to exploit those we most esteem; we should not want to use them up for our own entertainment and satisfaction; and we should not want to treat our fellow human beings as expendable animals. But the concern about safety must also be subjected to scrutiny. Athletic activity is often intrinsically unsafe: Boxing and football, hockey and skiing—such activities require daring, toughness, and sometimes even contempt for "mere safety" as being far less important than victory and achievement. Superior performances in these activities would be less excellent or less genuine if fully stripped of their perils. Inasmuch as risk and sacrifice are part of what it takes to be superior, one might even argue that an athlete's willingness to use such drugs, at so great a personal cost, is not dehumanizing but admirable—a sacrifice of oneself to the game one loves.

Of course, there seems to be a difference between the uncertain dangers of the playing field and the deliberately self-inflicted harm of using performance-enhancing drugs. Playing a game with the risk of great harm seems different from inflicting high-tech, premeditated, long-term damage on oneself to gain a short-term advantage. The hazards intrinsic to the game are generally unavoidable, while those associated with taking the drugs are utterly unnecessary. But again, we must wonder: Why should we value the long-term over the short-term—the long healthy life over the short and glorious one? Isn't part of our admiration for athletics precisely the "gladiator spirit," including the willingness to forego "mere safety" for brief but memorable moments on the field of glory? Absent further analysis, there would seem to be a potential nobility on the part of the athlete who seeks excellence at whatever personal cost. And yet, there also seems to be something perverse, or ignoble, in coming deliberately to abuse one's body for the sake, presumably, of showing off its beautiful and splendid gifts and activities. There seems to be something dehumanizing in coming to rely so heavily on one's chemist to excel, to the point where one might wonder whether such excellence is still "personal" at all.

Some enhancements, both here and coming, may become physically safe, with few side effects that compromise the long-term health of those who use them. Yet there are other consequences "to the side" that deserve our concern, for such enhancements might change the body or mind in ways beyond making them ill. For it stands to reason that drugs sufficiently capable of affecting us in ways we desire are likely to affect us in ways that we do not seek and cannot predict. Perhaps certain hormones that boost training capacity and aggressiveness will make the individual emotionally less "well-balanced" in everyday life. Or perhaps by taking drugs that increase tolerance for physical pain, the individual will decrease his or her experience of other physical pleasures. Part of the problem with certain biological enhancements, in other words, may be that they isolate one set of human powers—the powers that make for a superior runner, linebacker, or weight lifter—at the expense of other areas of life: health, to be sure, but also calmness, balance, equanimity, pleasure, creativity, and so forth. Such enhancements risk creating a distorted form of human excellence—magnifying certain elements of human life while shrinking others.

But the "distortions" of life in pursuit of superior performance cannot be blamed on biotechnical enhancers alone. In any society in which people feel driven by the desire for success, whether measured in terms of wealth, power, or status, many human activities (including athletics) are easily bent out of their natural shape in order to serve these external goals. Yet the difficulty exists even when superior performance is pursued not for outside ends but for its own sake. All human excellence, to some degree, requires at least some distortion: putting aside many activities or aspirations to excel in one; leaving several powers undeveloped to develop a few; sacrificing most human goods to pursue a single one at the highest level; and perhaps becoming so excellent in one particular area of human endeavor that most other human beings only encounter such superior performance at a distance. All excellence, in other words, requires at least some separation from the majority: the separation required by long hours of practice and the separation inherent in performing in the arena or on the stage. We need think only of the strange life lived by Olympic gymnasts, often whisked away from normal childhood at a very early age to enter the all-consuming world of the training camp. Or the women's Olympic volleyball teams that not only practice but live in camp together 365 days a year for nearly the entire four years between the quadrennial events. Sometimes this separation from others and from ordinary life enables individuals to embody the best that human beings are capable of, at least in a particular area of activity. At other times, the separation might be so severe, and the way we pursue our chosen activity so distorting of the human whole, that the dignity of the performer is called into question. He or she might be a great athlete, but only by becoming inhuman in other ways. Viewed more fully, the concern about side effects, beginning with health, gets us to the deepest matters and the greatest "side effect" of all: that we improve performance at the cost of our full humanity; that we become "better" by no longer fully being ourselves.

E. The Dignity of Human Activity

The preceding analysis has considered several sources of our disquiet about different technical and biotechnological agents that might enhance or alter athletic performance: unfairness and inequality, coercion and constraint, and adverse effects on the health and balance of human life. Each has indicated something important; but none gets us to the core issue. The problem is not simply inequality and unfairness, since our natural endowments are unequal to begin with, and the conventions outlawing certain enhancements could be changed to allow everyone equal access to the same technical and biotechnological advantages. The problem is not simply coercive pressure, since only if there is something intrinsically troubling about bioengineered enhancements should we be really troubled by the pressures to use them, especially given that "pressures" are inherent in the pursuit of athletic or any other kind of excellence. And the problem is not simply health hazards and adverse side effects, or the ways that enhancing certain human capacities might limit or endanger other elements of human life. For the pursuit of athletic (and other) excellences necessarily seeks something higher than mere safety, and excellence nearly always requires putting aside some aspirations to pursue others; the individual accepts less excellence in many aspects of life in order to be excellent in this one. Yet the concern about compromising the whole of life for the sake of one isolated part points us closer to the heart of the matter: understanding the true dignity of excellent human activity, and how some new ways of improving performance may distort or undermine it.

Our deepest concerns are tied to the large questions we raised at the start of this chapter: What is a human *performance*, and what is an *excellent* one? And what makes it *excellent as a human* performance? For it seems that some performance-enhancing agents, from stimulants to blood doping to genetic engineering of muscles, call into question the *dignity* of the performance of those who use them. The performance seems less real, less one's own, less worthy of our admiration. Not only do such enhancing agents distort or damage other dimensions of human life—for example, by causing early death or sexual impotence—they also seem to distort the athletic activity itself. It is not simply that our greatest sportsmen could become bad fathers if their enhancements made them uncontrollably aggressive or left them prematurely dead. It is that they are, despite their higher scores and faster times, bad or diminished *as sportsmen*—not simply because they cheated their opponents, but because they also cheated, undermined, or corrupted themselves and the very athletic activity in which they seem to excel.

What is at stake here is the very meaning of human agency, the meaning of being *at-work* in the world, being at-work as *myself,* and being at-work in a *humanly excellent* way. To clarify this claim, we must consider several aspects of human activity and human agency. Before doing so, we must first address the matter of competition and its significance for the things we do.

1. The Meaning of Competition

We have already noted, in the discussion of coercion and constraint, the distortions that social pressures to get ahead introduce into athletics and other human activities. Yet unlike many of our activities—such as learning, doctoring, or even governing—athletics are intrinsically competitive. They involve a contest of single opponents or opposing teams, matching their talents against one another and seeking on that day or in this event to be better than the rest (or better than the best). Sometimes competition is friendly, a playful meeting of fellows who take pleasure in each other's achievements. Sometimes competition is fierce, mixed with a desire not only to see oneself victorious but to see one's opponent roundly defeated. Most often, competition mixes the friendly and the fierce: good friends are often rivals on the playing field, and bitter opponents often have a deep respect for one another as being worthy foes, demanding and evincing one's own best efforts.

But not all human activity, as we have noted, is intrinsically competitive and rivalrous. Consider, as a comparison to human sport, the activity of making music. It is certainly the case that musicians sometimes compete with one another: for first chair in the orchestra, for record contracts, for prizes and public esteem. But strictly speaking, when engaged in these rivalries they are not at work making music. Indeed, it seems misguided to say that music is *in its essence* a competitive activity—in the way Olympic running and professional chess are intrinsically competitive activities. When the string quartet or the symphony orchestra makes music, it has no opponent against whom it is competing. Moreover, no musician's performance or excellence can be "measured" in the same way as the shot-putter's or the runner's when he or she breaks a world record. To be sure, we can judge some musical performances as clearly better than others, and individuals strive to become better musicians than they were before. But the many forms of musical excellence seem to belie final comparative judgments about better and worse: two individuals can play the same sonata or sing the same song very differently but both excellently, each capturing something essential but something different in the music. Runners in the same race may run differently— with different styles, each embodying a different form of excellent running—but in the end we can say, at least in a given race, who is the "best."

And yet, even those activities that are intrinsically competitive, such as sports, are not *simply* competitive in their essence. The dignity of athletic activity is not defined only by winners and losers, faster and slower times, old records and new. Competition can sometimes blind us to the fact that it is not simply the separable, measurable, and comparative *result* that makes a performance excellent—but *who* is performing and *how*. The word "superior" itself captures this dichotomy, meaning both "better than one's competitor" but also denoting a performance or activity that is simply outstanding in itself. Excellent running seems to have a meaning—the human body in action, the grace and rhythm of the moving human form, the striving and exertion of the aspiring human runner—that is separable from competition, even when the runner is running competitively. Even in the most competitive activities, the deepest meaning may not be honorable victory, or beating one's best human opponents in a worthy way, but rather the human agent at-work in the world—especially the lived experience, for both the spectator and doer, of a *humanly cultivated gift, excellently-at-work*.

2. The Relationship Between Doer and Deed

This leads us to the second consideration: the relationship between the doer and the deed, or between the human agent and the human activities he or she engages in. As said above, the dignity of human sport (or any other human activity) is determined not simply or predominantly by the measured and separate *result*, but also by *who* achieves it and *how*. Seen not as a detachable deed but as an activity of an agent, athletic performance depends on both the *doing* of a deed and the *identity* of the *doer*. The purpose of competitive running, for example, is to cover the set distance as quickly as possible. But this is only part of the story. The man on roller skates moves more quickly than the runner. But he obviously engages in a different activity—moving quickly, but not running—and thus should be judged according to a different standard. (Just because we have invented roller skates, cars, and airplanes—all faster ways of moving—does not mean we have stopped competing in running.)

Animals run, often quickly. In contrast with mechanized movement, in animal running doer and deed are seamlessly united. And as already noted, the average cheetah runs much faster than the fastest human being and is beautiful to behold. But we do not honor the cheetah in the same way we honor the Olympic runner, because the Olympian runs in a *human way* as a *human being*. (Of this, more soon.) In a word, in athletic performance seen as a performance of a performer, we cannot separate the "result" (the fastest time) from the "activity" (human running). In assessing athletic performance, we do not in fact separate *what* is done from *how* it is done and *who* is doing it, from the fact that it is *being done by a doer*. And we should not separate the score from the purpose of keeping score in the first place: to honor and promote a given type of human excellence, whose meaning is in the *doing*, not simply in the scored result. Tomorrow's box score is at most a ghostly shadow of today's ballgame.

Consider another example: the best human chess player playing against a chess-playing computer. It is worth asking how or whether man and machine are really "competing" at all, and to what extent we can really compare the superior capacity of a computer to "play" chess with the distinctive excellence of a human chess player. On one level, of course, they are indeed competing: playing the same game according to the same rules. And yet, the computer "plays" the game rather differently—with no uncertainty, no nervousness, no sweaty palms, no active mind, and, most importantly, with no desire or aspiration and no hopes or expectations regarding possible future success. In this new type of competition, our best human being faces off against our best human artifact. But the computer's way of "playing" is really a kind of simulation—the product of genuine human achievement, to be sure, since building such a computer is its own manifestation of human excellence. But is this simulation the real thing—*playing* chess?* And by building computers that "play" perfect chess, do we change the meaning of the activity itself? Do we reorient the very character of our aspiration—from becoming great *human* chess players to becoming better chess-playing *machines*, or, if you prefer, from *becoming* great chess *players* to *producing* the *best-executed game* of chess? Why, if chess is no more than the sum of opposing moves that are in principle calculable by a machine, would human beings wish to play chess at all, especially if the machines can do it better?

The answer is at once simple and complex: We still play chess because only *we* can play chess as *human beings*, as genuine chess *players*. We still run because running, while not as fast as moving on wheels, retains a dignity unique to itself and unique to those who engage in this activity. The runner on steroids or with genetically enhanced muscles is still, of course, a human being who runs. But the doer of the deed is, arguably, less obviously *himself* and less obviously *human* than his unaltered counterpart. He may be faster, but he may also be on the way to becoming "more cheetah" than man, or more like the horses we breed for the racetrack than a self-willing, self-directing, human agent. He does the deed (running), and his resulting time may be measurably superior. But he is also (or increasingly) the passive recipient of outside agents that are at least partly responsible for his achievements.

---

* Would anyone be interested in watching a chess match "played" by two computers? If so, why? Would that be a "chess match" in any ordinary sense?

3. Acts of Humans, Human Acts: Harmony of Mind and Body

This brings us to a third and closely related consideration, the specific difference of a *human* act or performance. For in judging a performance to be genuinely and humanly superior, we care not only that there be an integral connection between doer and excellent deed. We care also that the doer-at-work display those qualities that make us admire the performance as a *human* activity and as *his own* activity. Borrowing a useful distinction from moral philosophy, not all acts done *by* humans are *human* acts, acts that spring from the roots of our humanity. Not all acts done *by* persons are *personal* acts.

One common way of getting at the crucial difference is to talk about "true" and "false" acts, acts that do and acts that do not spring truly from who or what we are. This is what people have in mind when they say that athletes who use steroids or a corked bat to hit the ball farther than they could before are not only breaking the rules, but getting their achievements "on the cheap," performing deeds that *appear* to be, but that are not *in truth*, wholly their own. This makes sense as far as it goes, but it gives rise to the question, "What would make an act of humans genuinely a human act?" "What would make the deed truly one's own?"

Comparison with the doings of animals other than man proves helpful. In the activity of other animals, there is necessarily a unity between doer and deed; acting impulsively and without reflection, an animal—unlike a human being—cannot deliberately feign activity or separate its acts from itself as their immediate source. Yet though a cheetah runs, it does not truly run a race. Though it senses and pursues its prey, it does not seek a goal with full consciousness or with ambitions to surpass previous performances. Though its motion is voluntary (not externally compelled), it does not run by choice. Though it moves in ordered sequence, it has not planned the course. Its beauty and its excellence—and these are not to be disparaged—it owes largely to nature and instinct.

In contrast, the human runner chooses to run a race and sets before himself (herself) his (her) goal. He measures the course and prepares himself precisely for it. He surveys his rivals and plots his strategy. Though constrained by the limits of his flesh, he cultivates and disciplines his body and its natural gifts in pursuit of his goal. The end, the means, and the manner are all matters of conscious awareness and deliberate choice, from start to finish. In a word, what makes the racer's running a human act humanly done is that it is done freely, knowingly, and by conscious choice.

So far so good. But if the humanity of our actions rests solely on their being rooted in knowledge and conscious choice, we face this difficulty: Is not a decision to enhance our bodies through drugs or genetic intervention also a matter of human choice? Why would this not be *precisely* the expression of our rational will, a manifestation of its peculiarly human ability not to be enslaved by the limitations of our animal bodies? If it is the presence of free, knowing, and conscious choice that makes for a human act, then the bulking up of the genetically or drug-enhanced athlete—and derivatively, his drug-assisted superior performance—would seem to be *preeminently* human or even superhuman, a manifestation of our ability to transcend nature's and our personal limitations in a way no animal can.

This welcome objection invites a fuller account, with a three-part response—one regarding the mind (and will), another regarding the body, the third regarding their peculiar interrelations as expressed in athletics and human activity more generally, as well as in human desire and aspiration.* The point about the mind has already been prepared by our earlier discussion of the difference between gaining superior performance through training and practice and gaining superior performance through biotechnological intervention and engineering. We called attention to the difference between perfecting a capacity by using it knowingly and repetitively and perfecting a capacity by means that bear no relation to its use. And we stressed the difference, *on the plane of human experience and understanding*, between changes to our bodies that do and those that do not proceed through intelligible and self-directed action, capable of being informed by the knowledge of human experience. Thus, though the decision to take anabolic steroids to enhance athletic performance can be said

---

*These questions about mind, body, and their interrelation, we are well aware, are deep and difficult philosophical matters. We have no illusion that we have done more here than signal their crucial importance to the ethical analysis at hand.

to be, in one sense of the term, a rational choice, it is a choice to alter oneself by submitting oneself to means that are unintelligible to one's own self-understanding and entirely beyond one's control. In contrast with the choice to adopt a better training regimen, it is a calculating act of will to bypass one's own will and intelligibility altogether.

Yet the problem with biotechnical enhancement lies not merely on the side of exaggerated and self-contradictory willfulness. It lies also with its mistaken identification of the human with the merely rational and its neglect of our embodiment. For the humanity of athletic performance resides not only in the chosenness and intelligibility of the deed. It depends decisively on the performance of a well-tuned and well-working body. The body in question is a living body, not a mere machine; not just any animal body but a human one; not someone else's body but one's own. Each of us is personally embodied. Each of us lives with and because of certain bodily gifts that owe nothing to our rational will. Each of us not only has a body; each of us also *is* a body.

In few activities is this truth more manifest than in sports. When we see the outstanding athlete in action, we do not see—as we do in horse racing—a rational agent riding or whipping a separate animal body. What we mainly see is a body gracefully and harmoniously at work, but at work with discipline and focus, and tacitly obeying the rules and requirements of the game. We can tell immediately that the human runner is engaged in deliberate and goal-directed activity, that he is not running in flight moved by fear or in pursuit moved by hunger. Yet while the peculiarly human character of the running is at once obvious, the "mindedness" of the bodily activity is tacit and unobtrusive. So attuned is the body, and so harmonious is it with heart and mind, that—in the best instance—the whole activity of the athlete appears effortlessly to flow from a unified and undivided being.[*]

---

[*] The perceived "at-one-ness" of the runner can produce a parallel sense of at-one-ness in the spectators, also manifesting mind, body, and heart. Unselfconsciously we spectators are stunned by the manifestation of genuine human excellence: it holds our attention, it takes away our breath; it wins our heart. In appreciating seamless excellence, we have moments of seamless excellence ourselves, sharing reflectively in the glory of the superior human performance we are witnessing. This "superior performance" of the spectators has important implications for the character of the whole society, a matter to which we return in the final section of this chapter.

At such moments the athlete experiences and displays something like the unity of doer and deed one observes in other animals, but for humans that unity is a notable *achievement* which far transcends what mere animals are capable of. A great sprinter may run like a gazelle, a great boxer may fight like a tiger, but one would never mistake their harmony of body and soul for the brute instinct that spurs an animal toward flight or fight.

Athletic activity is not only generically human and manifestly a bodily matter; it is also emphatically the work of particular individuals. This is hardly accidental. Although we are all equally embodied, we are not bodily identical. On the contrary, our differing identities are advertised and displayed in our unique bodily appearance. True, in many gifts of body and mind we are indistinguishable from our fellow human beings; but in some gifts many of us are specially favored. It is the special distribution and assortment of common and particular gifts, allotted to each of us, that constitute the biological beginnings of our individual identity. In pursuing superior athletic (or other) performance, we are cultivating and exercising both our common and our particular gifts, seeking our own individual flourishing. We discipline our gifts through choice and effort in the service of enabling them to shine forth in our own beautiful and splendid activity. We take pleasure in our own performance and achievement. The added bonus of victory and the recognition that follows from it we esteem largely because they confirm that our own embodied excellence has been attained and that our desire for superior performance has been satisfied.

In trying to achieve better bodies through muscle-enhancing agents, pharmacological or genetic, we are not in fact honoring our bodies or cultivating our individual gifts. We are instead, whether we realize it or not, voting with our syringes to have a *different* body, with different native capacities and powers.* We are giving ourselves new and foreign gifts, not

---

* To be sure, these transforming agents do not in fact produce a completely different body. And a steroid-enhanced athlete probably still feels that he is the same person he was before the treatment. But the fans, seeing him for the first time in his new physique, so suddenly acquired, often wonder if the newly minted slugger really has the same body, really is the "same" person. More important, the implicit aspiration, even in these modest transformations, is indeed to have a body more perfect than one could ever acquire simply by cultivating one's own natural gifts. In this sense, using these agents on one's muscles expresses the same desire as having major cosmetic sur-

nature's and not our own, and—exaggerating, but in the direction of the truth—treating ourselves rather as if we were batting machines to be perfected or as superior horses bred for the race and bound to do our bidding. These acts of will do not respect either our own individuality or the dignity of our own embodiment—on which, by the way, our will absolutely depends for its very existence.

At the root of all human activity is desire or aspiration, especially when it aims at excellence. Human aspiration for superior performance, for excellent activity, for something memorable and great, is not, finally, the product of pure reason or pure will. Neither is it merely the product of our animality. It stems rather from that peculiar blending of mind and desire, perhaps peculiar to human beings, called by the Greeks *eros*, the longing for wholeness, perfection, and something transcendent. In one formulation, it is the desire: (1) for the good, (2) to be one's own, (3) always.[11] The root of this longing lies in the awareness that, alas, we are not entirely unified and undivided beings. We are rather frail and finite in body and conflicted in soul. Being conscious of our finitude and self-division, we strive to make of ourselves something less imperfect, something more noble, something fine—something that would be fulfilling as much as is humanly possible. Further, we pursue this aspiration as ourselves and—at least to begin with—for ourselves. We would not seek excellence on condition that, in order to attain it, we would gladly have to become someone or something else.* Not the excellence of god or beast, not even the excellence of some generic human person or disembodied human will, but the excellence of our own embodied allotment of human possibility is our goal. It is doubtful, to say the least, that biotechnical transformations of our bodies—or minds—will contribute to our realizing this goal *for ourselves*.

gery on one's face: to become, to some extent, someone else, someone with a more perfect body. The use of analogous agents on one's psyche—say, to acquire a superior temperament or a different set of memories—is likewise a (tacit) aspiration to become someone else. We shall explore this subject in Chapter Five, "Happy Souls."

* For example: No sane person, we suggest, would choose to be the fastest runner on two legs if it required becoming an ostrich. And few people would choose to acquire someone else's perfections of body or mind on condition of becoming that other person. Who, in the event of such self-transformative improvements, would we say now enjoyed them?

The ironies of biotechnological enhancement of athletic performance should now be painfully clear. First, by turning to biological agents to transform ourselves in the image we choose and will, we in fact compromise our choosing and willing identity itself, since we are choosing to become less than normally the source or the shapers of our own identity. We take a pill or insert a gene that makes us into something we desire, yet only by seeming to compromise the self-directed path toward its attainment. Second, by using these agents to transform our bodies for the sake of better bodily performance, we mock the very excellence of our own individual embodiment that superior performance is meant to display. Finally, by using these technological means to transcend the limits of our natures, we are deforming also the character of human desire and aspiration, settling for externally gauged achievements that are less and less the fruits of our own individual striving and cultivated finite gifts.

There is, we might add, no limit in principle to the desire to transcend the limits of our own nature. The desire to have a perfect body, one that perfectly executes the dictates of the will, is tantamount to a desire to transcend our embodiment altogether, to become as gods, to become something more-than-human. No doubt the longing for perfection has inspired many of the greatest human achievements. But unless guided by some idea of the character of *human* perfection, such longings risk becoming a full-scale revolt against our humanity altogether. Fueled in addition by a thirst not merely to excel but to defeat and surpass our rivals, the desire for superhuman powers easily becomes boundless.

The argument we have offered seems to have landed us in this strange position: We seek to defend human willing or agency, in the sense of defending our being what we really do. But we also seek to recognize the biological limits of the will, in the sense that much that is central about us is not truly our doing. Biotechnology seems to promise the triumph of the will with less willing effort and bodily excellence in bodies not quite ours: we can become what we desire without being the responsible and embodied agents of our own becoming. A more human course, however, might be accepting that we cannot will ourselves into anything we like, but we can still live with the dignity of being willing, self-directed, embodied, and aspiring persons, not biological artifacts, not thoroughbreds or pitching machines. Better, in other words, to be great human runners with permanent limitations than (non)human artifacts bred to break records.

Though our subject has not been athletics as such, but the uses of biotechnical means to enhance athletic performance, our analysis casts light on the ways in which the currently popular view of sports may already be corrupting genuine human excellence and may lead, unless we change our tastes, to enormous pressure to pursue any and all biological performance-enhancers, should they be safe and effective. For we have long since blurred the line between athletics and entertainment. If the baseball-loving public cares mainly about how many homers are hit or how far they go, then it will matter less how much the deeds flow from the unadulterated yet cultivated gifts of the hitter. Only if superiority of performance continues to mean not just the excellence of a detached act, but of the act as displaying the excellence of a superior human being, excellently at-work—in our own mindful and aspiring embodiments— can we preserve the full sense of humanly superior performance.

F. Superior Performance and the Good Society

Much of the above analysis focuses on the excellence of the individual person at-work in the world. But any analysis of superior performance must also take into account the performer's relationship with others: teammates and competitors, teachers and admirers, co-workers and friends, as well as the larger community. It is true that the individual, even when working in tandem with his fellows, is excellent as himself. But excellent human activity is by nature situated within a community, a society, and a culture. The human individual flourishes as himself, but he does not flourish alone. And he rarely flourishes without enormous contributions from others, people near and even far to whom he is indebted for nurture, rearing, coaching, encouragement, employment, and the appreciation and support of the activity in which he gets the opportunity to excel. Likewise, all excellence is particular to time and place, even if particular examples of human excellence are "for all time," and even if we can admire those who perform in activities that we no longer engage in ourselves.

In myriad ways, society has a stake in excellent human activity. It rewards, honors, and nourishes the superior performances of its members. But it also expects, demands, and depends upon them. In many everyday functions—flying airplanes, fixing computers, educating children—we rely on others to "get the job done" or "rise to the occasion" when needed. We need them to perform and perform well, not just occasionally or sporadically, but steadily and reliably. Allowing some leeway to beginners, we expect practice will make perfect, we expect people to improve on the job and through the experience of repeated performance.

Beyond its everyday utility, superior performance also *ennobles* society: it makes everyone better; it raises the spirits of a community; it nourishes the desire to be better and to do better, as individuals and as a people. The example of superior performers gives those who are still developing an image of who or what they might aspire to become themselves. And everyone may be elevated by discovering that human beings—like them in being human, unlike them in the superior ways they perform—can do the beautiful and marvelous things they themselves cannot do, but in which they can surely, if only partially, participate as appreciators and admirers.

Our analysis of human sport sheds light also on the entire range of such socially valuable and excellent performances, both those that adorn our community and those that make it possible. Each of these human activities has its own character and meaning, and hence also its own dignity. In music, as in sport, the body is gracefully at work, but at work in a different way: the fingers striking the keys, the hand and arm moving the bow, the voice singing at perfect pitch. The musician takes inspiration from others—perhaps including rivals—but he does not compete. He *makes* music—arranging notes and melodies as a composer and playing them as a performer. But he also *captures* what is musical—hitting notes and singing harmonies as they were meant to be hit and be sung. He knows the notes and his body knows the movements. And guiding it all is his musical understanding of the musical whole, grasped in both heart and mind, that both inspires the performance and that is, when given life in the playing, its completion.

In a similar way, one might describe a range of other human activities—painting, dancing, building, designing, writing. Each of these activities has a distinct character and excellence, and each retains a dignity unique to itself, demanding and rewarding different human powers and capacities. But each of them, like sport, involves a humanly cultivated gift, a human doer and human deed, a deed performed, at its best, in a humanly excellent way. It is the *human* musician, not the synthesizing machine, whom we admire and defend: the musician with desire and fallibility, who creates what did not exist before and rises to the occasion when the moment most demands it. Most important, while such superior performances are the work of individuals, all of society shares in their excellence, as it always does when taste is receptive to genius. Properly appreciative witnessing *is* participating, and it enables everyone present to experience the surpassing human possibility in a passing human moment.

In addition, even those activities necessary for life in society and devoted to some external result or purpose—for example, human work to produce some useful object or to perform some needed service—can be done in a way that is dignified or undignified, human or dehumanizing. The difference is not simply how many objects are produced, with what efficiency and what effectiveness. What matters is that we produce the given result—the objects that we make—in a human way as human beings, not simply as inputs who produce outputs. Indeed, it is here that the temptation to improve performance—to make workers more focused by giving them Ritalin, less sleepy by giving them Modafinil, more muscular by genetically enhancing their muscles, and so on—is most tempting. If all that matters is getting more out of them—or more out of ourselves, by any means possible—then improving performance by every biotechnical intervention available makes perfect sense. But as we have seen with human sport, more is at stake than simply improving output. What matters is that we do our work and treat our fellow workers in ways that honor all of us as agents and makers, demanding our own best possible performance, to be sure, but our best performance as human beings, not animals or machines.

But there is one further complication. Defending what is humanly good or excellent must not only guard against the possibility of dehumanization; it must defend first against the many threats to personal or communal survival itself. When the very existence of the human agent or human society is at stake, certain special superior performances are not only edifying but urgent: for example, the superior performance of soldiers or doctors. What guidance, if any, does our analysis provide for such moments of extreme peril and consequence, in war or in medicine, when superior performance is a matter of life or death? Are some biotechnical interventions to enhance performance justified in these activities (surgery, war) while not justified in the other activities of human life (sports, music, test-taking)? In these circumstances, might we treat men as alterable artifacts—or willingly become artifacts ourselves—in order to "get the job done"?*

There may indeed be times when we must override certain limits or prohibitions that make sense in other contexts—offering steroids to improve the strength of soldiers while rejecting them for athletes, offering amphetamines to improve the alertness of fighter-pilots while rejecting them for students, offering anti-anxiety agents to steady the hands of surgeons while rejecting them for musicians. When we override our own boundaries, we do so or should do so for the sake of the whole, and only when the whole itself is at stake, when everything human and humanly dignified might be lost. And we should do so only uneasily, *overriding* boundaries rather than abandoning them, and respecting certain ultimate limits to ensure that men remain human even in moments of great crisis. For example: Even if they existed, and even in times of great peril, we might resist drugs that eliminate completely the fear or inhibition of our soldiers, turning them into "killing machines" (or "dying machines"),

---

* Though both are concerned with matters of life and death, soldiering and doctoring are different. The two "wholes" that they serve are different, the community being both more comprehensive and much less intrinsically perishable. The existence of all individual life within a community depends on the survival of that community. An argument could be made to cut soldiers a bit more slack than physicians in doing whatever it takes to "get the job done," precisely because the whole itself is at stake in time of war. A counter-argument could also be made, not on the basis of the superiority of the good being served, but rather the means used (cutting the body to heal it versus cutting the body to kill it), which might justify cutting more slack to surgeons than to soldiers.

without trembling or remorse. Such biotechnical interventions might improve performance in a just cause, but only at the cost of making men no different from the weapons they employ.

This particular case, in short, is the exception that proves the rule: even in moments of great crisis, when superior performance is most necessary, we must never lose sight of the human agency that gives superior performance its dignity. We must live, or try to live, as true men and women, accepting our finite limits, cultivating our given gifts, and performing in ways that are humanly excellent. To do otherwise is to achieve our most desired results at the ultimate cost: getting what we seek or think we seek by no longer being ourselves.

We are well aware that this assessment of human activity and human dignity, highly philosophical, may not be persuasive to some people. And even those who might share the foregoing views of the possible corruptions of using direct biotechnical intervention to gain superior performance might be reluctant to argue against it for others. In a free country, so they might say, people should be allowed to take their muscle enhancers or alertness pills, even if we would not use them ourselves. Where's the harm if some football players here and there take steroids or a few ambitious college-bound students take stimulants before their SATs?

Perhaps none. Human life is complicated, innovations abound, and human activities often change their character without necessarily losing their integrity. But we must at least try to imagine what kind of society we might become if such biotechnical interventions were to become more significant in their effects and more widespread in their use. We might come to see human running and dog races, singers and synthesizers, craftsmen and robots, as little different from one another. Human beings, here mostly for our entertainment or our use, might become little more than props or prop-makers. We might lose sight of the difference between real and false excellence, and eventually not care. And in the process, the very ends we desire might become divorced from any idea of what is humanly superior, and therefore humanly worth seeking or admiring. We would become a society of spectators, and our activities a mere spectacle. Or a society of parasites, needing and taking, but never doing or acting. Worst of all, we would be in danger of turning our would-be heroes into slaves, persons who exist only to entertain us and meet our standards and whose freedom to pursue human excellence has been shackled by the need to perform—and conform—for our amusement and applause.

For a while—perhaps indefinitely—we might relish the superior results that only our biotechnical ingenuity made possible: broken records on the playing fields, more efficient workplaces, improved national SAT scores. But we would have gone very far, potentially, in losing sight of why excellence is worth seeking at all, and hence what excellence really is, and how we pursue it as human beings, not as artifacts.

ENDNOTES

[1] Tzankoff, S., "Effect of Muscle Mass on Age-Related BMR Changes," *Journal of Applied Physiology* 43: 1001-1006, 1977.

[2] Asakura, A., et al., "Muscle satellite cells are multipotential stem cells that exhibit myogenic, osteogenic, and adipogenic differentiation," *Differentiation* 68(4-5): 245-253, 2001; Zammit, P., et al., "The skeletal muscle satellite cell: stem cell or son of stem cell?" *Differentiation* 68(4-5): 193-204, 2001.

[3] This discussion owes much to the work of Professor H. Lee Sweeney and his colleagues at the University of Pennsylvania and elsewhere (see Bibliography), and to his description and discussion of that work at the September 2002 meeting of the President's Council on Bioethics. Transcript available at the Council's website, www.bioethics.gov.

[4] Barton-Davis, E., et al., "Viral mediated expression of insulin-like growth factor I blocks the aging-related loss of skeletal muscle function," *Proceedings of the National Academy of Sciences* 95: 15603-15607, 1998.

[5] Musaro, A., et al., "Localized Igf-1 transgene expression sustains enlargement and regeneration in senescent skeletal muscle," *Nature Genetics* 27: 195-200, 2001.

[6] H. Lee Sweeney, personal communication with Council staff, 2002.

[7] Weber, M., "Effects of growth hormone on skeletal muscle," *Hormone Research* 58(3):43-48, 2002.

[8] Gladwell, M., "The Sporting Scene: Drugstore Athlete," *The New Yorker*, September 10, 2001.

[9] Rousseau, "Discourse on the Origin and Foundations of Inequality (Second Discourse)," transl. Roger D. and Judith R. Masters, in *The First and Second Discourses*, ed. Roger D. Masters, New York: St. Martin's Press, 1964, p. 147.

[10] Gladwell, *op. cit.*

[11] Plato, *Symposium*, 206A.

4

Ageless Bodies

Try as we might to improve or enhance our performance, we all know that it is bound to degrade over time. As the body ages, its abilities decline: we lose strength and speed, flexibility and reaction time, mental and physical agility, memory and recall, immune response, and overall functioning. We know that in the end, and generally as a result of this accumulation of debilities, our bodies will give out, and our lives will end.

The inevitability of aging, and with it the specter of dying, has always haunted human life; and the desire to overcome age, and even to defy death, has long been a human dream. The oldest stories of many civilizations include myths of long lives: of ancients who lived for hundreds of years, of faraway places where even now the barriers of age are broken, or of magical formulas, concoctions, or fountains of youth. And for several centuries now the goal of conquering aging has not been confined to magic and myth; it was central to the aspirations of the founders of modern science, who sought through their project the possibility of mastering nature for the relief of the human condition—decay and death emphatically included. But it is only recently that biotechnology has begun to show real progress toward meeting these goals, and bringing us face to face with the possibility of extended youth and substantially prolonged lives. Using rapidly growing new knowledge about how and why we age, scientists have achieved some success in prolonging lifespans in several animal species. To be sure, there is at present no medical intervention that slows, stops, or reverses human aging, and for *none* of the currently marketed agents said to increase human longevity is there any hard scientific evidence to support the hyped-up claims.[1] Yet the prospect of possible future success along these lines raises high hopes, as well as profound and complicated questions.

To elucidate these hopes, and to introduce these questions, we will examine some of the potential techniques for the extension of longevity and youthfulness, and some of their imaginable consequences. Our aim here, as throughout this report, is not primarily to analyze the details of the scientific prospects, or to predict which techniques might prove most effective in retarding aging. Rather we consider a range of reasonably plausible possibilities in order to discern their potential human and ethical implications.* But before we can begin to examine such possibilities, we must inquire about the underlying desire. What do we wish for when we yearn for "ageless bodies"?

I. THE MEANING OF "AGELESS BODIES"

It may at first seem strange to suggest that we yearn for an "ageless body," not a term commonly heard and certainly not the conscious and explicit longing of very many people. Still, when properly examined, something like a desire for an "ageless body" seems in fact to be commonplace and deeply held; and should our capacities to retard the senescence of our bodies increase, that desire may well become more explicit and strong.

We all know at least something of what it is to age, but perhaps we have not often enough given thought to the full place of aging in human experience, and to the significance of the nearly universal desire to defy or to stop it. We measure our age in terms of years we have lived, and in that sense there is no stopping aging. Time marches on incessantly, and we are ever dragged along right with it. But we experience aging not just as the passage of time, but rather also as the effect of that passage on us: on our bodies, our minds, our souls, and our lives. In this respect, aging has two contradictory faces. Generally speaking, our physical and mental faculties degrade as we age, but often our understanding and judgment can improve.

---

* In doing so, we shall exploit the heuristic value of specific prospects and approaches (that may or may not pan out) because we believe they can most clearly teach us about the significance of any successful program for retarding human aging.

Our bodies grow frail under the weight of the years, but our wisdom—we hope—may grow greater as our store of experience swells.

It is only the former of these facets of aging that we rebel against and seek to push away. We want still to grow wiser or at least less foolish with age, but we wish we could do it without growing weaker. We mean not so much to slow the passing of the years as merely to shield our bodies from brutal bombardment by the silent artillery of time (in Abraham Lincoln's memorable phrase). That way, we might be in a position to make more practical use of our hard-earned wisdom, and youth would not be so carelessly wasted on the young. As C. S. Lewis put it: "I envy youth its stomach, not its heart."

In this sense, it is fundamentally the aging of the *body* we wish to stop. Indeed, we experience bodily decline as in many respects a kind of betrayal, as our body, once youthful and vibrant, seems somehow less responsive to our will, and less capable of executing some once routine demands of daily life. We wonder, together with Shakespeare, "is it not strange that desire should so many years outlive performance?"[2] And this betrayal grows worse with time, and step by step we find ourselves less able and competent in many of life's activities. We feel keenly what we have irreversibly lost, and worse yet, we know that much of the strength that remains will also be lost over time.

But it is more than the dread of decline that motivates us to seek ageless bodies. The corruption of the body brought on by aging points necessarily in the direction of eventual death, and unexpected encounters with new and unfamiliar weaknesses give us glimpses of mortality we would rather avoid. The fear of death, that ultimate and universal fear, surely has a hand (even if only implicitly) in motivating the search for ways to slow the clock. Death is nature's deepest and greatest barrier to total human self-mastery. However much power and control we may come to exercise over our lives and our environments, the time in which we may exercise that power and control is finite, and awareness of that finitude must always make the power feel somehow lacking. Different human societies have had very different conceptions of the divine, but one attribute has almost universally been attached to the gods: immortality. Our subjection to death—and our awareness of this fact—is central to what makes us human ("mortals") rather than divine, and it makes us fearful and weak and constrained.

The scientific quest to slow the aging process is not explicitly aimed at conquering death. But in taking the aging of the body as itself a kind of disorder to be corrected, it treats man's mortal condition as a target for medicine, as if death were indeed rather like one of the specific (fatal) diseases. There is no obvious end-point to the quest for ageless bodies: after all, why should any lifespan, however long, be long enough? In principle, the quest for any age-retardation suggests no inherent stopping point, and therefore, in the extreme case, it is difficult to distinguish it from a quest for endless life. It seeks to overcome the ephemeral nature of the human body, and to replace it with permanent facility and endless youth.*

The finitude of our power, and of our time, is part and parcel of our being embodied living creatures. An ageless body is almost a contradiction in terms, since all physical things necessarily decay over time, and so experience the passing of time in a most immediate way. To escape from time and age would be to escape from our bodily self—and the wish for this escape, too, inheres deeply in at least some forms of the desire for agelessness.

In these fundamental terms, the wish for ageless bodies and its potential fulfillment by biotechnology may be the most radical of the subjects we address in this report. It is not only an aspiration that can carry us past its

---

* Some commentators, including a few members of this Council, raise the legitimate question of whether an interest in retarding aging is, as implied here, an (at least tacit) interest in immortality. One could, after all, hope for a longer and hence more satisfying life or a less burdensome and decrepit old age without ever consciously formulating a wish to live forever. While the point is well taken, it does not refute the connection we have drawn between the open pursuit of ageless bodies and the secret longing to overcome death. Fear of death (however veiled and inchoate) and awareness of mortality (however dim and confused) have long wielded a pervasive influence on much if not all of human experience. And the founders of the modern scientific project brought that fear and that awareness very much into the foreground when they put forward the conquest of nature as mankind's utmost aim. Moreover, some contemporary scientists (though of course by no means all or most aging researchers) do express their aspirations in these terms. For instance, in marking the creation of the Society of Regenerative Medicine, William Hazeltine, head of Human Genome Sciences, declared that "the real goal is to keep people alive forever" (*Science* 290: 2249, 22 December 2000). We shall carry this suggestion—as well as the serious doubts raised—with us as we go forward.

usual and reasonable bounds by means of new technical powers; and it is more than a desire to be always what we are only sometimes. It is, at its core, a desire to overcome the most fundamental bounds of our humanity, and to redefine our bodily relationship with time and with the physical world.

And yet, although supremely radical, it is at the same time a perfectly routine desire, one which absolutely every one of us has often felt: watching helplessly as a loved one weakens and declines; contemplating the limits of our time here on earth; or just hearing an unfamiliar "snap" in our back as we reach up for a rebound on the basketball court or bend over to lift up a grandchild. The possibility that biotechnology might be able to significantly slow the process of aging invites us to consider carefully the meaning of this routine but radical desire.

The retardation of aging is among the most complex—both scientifically and ethically—of the potential "nontherapeutic" or "extra-therapeutic" uses of biotechnology, involving several different scientific avenues and raising deeply complicated questions for individuals and society. The moral case for living longer is very strong, and the desire to live longer speaks powerfully to each and every one of us. But the full consequences of doing so may not be quite so obvious.

II. BASIC TERMS AND CONCEPTS

Though everybody more or less knows what aging means, offering a concrete definition is no simple task. In one sense, aging just refers to the passage of time in relation to us or, put another way, it describes our passage through time. The more years we have lived, the greater our age (and with it our cumulative experience of life). In this sense, of course, it is absurd to speak of age-retardation, for by definition, only death could put a stop to our increasing years. But we mean more than this by "aging." It encompasses not only the passage of time but also (and more so) the biological processes of senescence that accompany that passage, and especially the progressive degeneration that affects the body and mind, beginning in adulthood. To clarify the discussion that follows, we offer some basic definitions for aging and related terms:

Aging. In this chapter we shall use "aging" synonymously with "senescence," rather than merely to describe the increase in the number of years a person has been alive. Aging therefore denotes the gradual and progressive loss of various functions over time, beginning in early adulthood, leading to decreasing health, vigor, and well-being, increasing vulnerability to disease, and increased likelihood of death.*

Life-Extension: An increase in the number of years that a person remains alive. It may be accomplished by a variety of means, including reducing causes of death among the young, combating the diseases of the aged, or the slowing down of aging. It may involve pushing back senescence or merely allowing an individual to survive into longer and deeper senescence.

Age-Retardation: The slowing down of the biological processes involved in aging, resulting in delayed decline and degeneration and perhaps also a longer life. It is one possible route to life-extension.

Lifespan: The verified age at death of an individual, and therefore the strictly chronological duration of life.

Maximum Lifespan: The longest lifespan ever recorded for a species—in humans today it is 122.5 years.

Life Expectancy: The average number of years of life remaining for individuals at a given age, assuming that age-specific mortality risks remain unchanged.

Life Cycle: The series of "stages" through which one passes in the course of life—including, among others, infancy, childhood, adolescence, adult-

---

* There is no clear consensus among scientists on a definition or even a particular physical description of aging. In offering the above "definition" we do not mean to imply a unitary phenomenon of aging, much less a unitary cause. This description is compatible both with the notion that senescence is due to some underlying process called "aging" and with the notion that "aging" is a descriptive term for observable senescence, from whatever cause.

hood, and old age; and the overall form given to the experience of life by the relations of these "stages" and the transitions between them.*

The desire for ageless bodies involves the pursuit not only of longer lives, but also of lives that remain vigorous longer. It seeks not only to add years to life, but also to add life to years. This double purpose is therefore likely to be better served by certain approaches to life-extension than by others. Life-extension may take three broad approaches: (1) efforts to allow more individuals to live to old age by combating the causes of death among the young and middle-aged; (2) efforts to further extend the lives of those who already live to advanced ages by reducing the incidence and severity of diseases and impairments of the elderly (including muscle and memory loss) or by replacing cells, tissues, and organs damaged over time; and (3) efforts to mitigate or retard the effects of senescence more generally by affecting the general process (or processes) of aging, potentially increasing not only the average but also the maximum human lifespan.

The first, particularly in the form of combating infant mortality (mostly through improvements in basic public health, sanitation, and immunization), is largely responsible for the great increase in lifespans in the twentieth century, from an average life expectancy at birth of about 48 years in 1900 to an average of about 78 years in 1999 in the United States (and even higher in some other developed nations—for instance, over 80 years in Japan). But this approach has been so successful that almost no further gains in average lifespan can be expected from efforts to improve the health of the young in the developed world.** In fact, even if, starting today, no one in the United States died before the age of 50, average life expectancy at birth would increase by only about 3.5 years (from just over 78 to 82 years). The increasing lifespans of the twentieth century were an extraordinary achievement, but further significant gains in life expectancy

---

* These "stages" of course come with indistinct boundaries and (with the exception of puberty) without clear biological or experiential markers. In referring to them, we do not mean to suggest that the life trajectory is anything but a continuum.

** Of course, this is very far from true in many less developed nations, where mortality among the young is still very high, and where the methods that served to improve health and increase lifespans in the United States in the twentieth century still stand to do a great deal of good.

would require a much greater feat: extending the lives of people who already make it to old age, and eventually extending the maximum lifespan.

The second approach, extending the life of the elderly by combating particular causes of death or reversing damage done by senescence, has been most actively pursued over the past several decades. In some forms, it has already contributed to the improved health of the elderly and to moderate extensions of life. Extreme old age already is, in many respects, a gift or product of human artifice, and modern medicine seems likely to make it more so and to bring further modest increases in average lifespan. But in most of its forms this approach, too, promises relatively moderate (though surely meaningful and much-desired) life-extension, even if it succeeds far beyond the most optimistic of present expectations.

For instance, if diabetes, all cardiovascular diseases, and all forms of cancer were eliminated today, life expectancy at birth in the United States would rise to about 90 years, from the present 78. This would certainly be a significant increase, but not one so great as to bring about many of the social and moral consequences that might be anticipated with significant age-retardation. It would be a much smaller increase than that achieved in the last century. Also, it would likely not have a serious impact on the maximum lifespan, with few if any people living longer than the current human maximum of 122 years.

The piecemeal character of this disease-by-disease approach contributes to what might be its most important limitation. If (on hypothesis) it would not get at the more general physical and mental deterioration that often comes with old age,* and which we more generally think of as

---

* Until one knows the cause or causes of aging, one cannot be sure that piecemeal improvements would not significantly retard general deterioration and thereby extend lifespan. Consider just one possible explanation of aging that would suggest possible piecemeal interventions at numerous sites. If alpha motor neuron input into muscles declines (for whatever reason), this would lead to muscle weakness, which could lead to a more sedentary lifestyle, which would decrease aerobic exercise, which may cause generalized circulatory decline with a small but significant effect on tissue perfusion (perhaps only during stress or cold), which could result in periodic ischemia (inadequate oxygenation of tissues), which might result in cell damage that causes slight but progressive degeneration to specific organs (for example, kidneys, which influence blood pressure), which would add their own imbalance and deficiencies to overall body coordination of function and

"aging," it would allow individuals to live longer, but often thereby expose them further and for a longer time to the other ravages of the general process of progressive degeneration, including loss of strength, hampered mobility, memory problems, impairments of the senses, and declining mental functions and any other particular age-related declines not specifically addressed by the methods employed. Extensions of life that do not address this general degeneration consign their beneficiaries to the fate of the mythical Tithonus or the Struldbruggs in Swift's *Gulliver's Travels*: degeneration without end. A number of the most promising avenues of cutting-edge aging research—including those involving stem-cell research, tissue and organ replacement, and, potentially some day, nanotechnology—would likely fall into this category, as do current efforts to find treatments for cancers, heart disease, Alzheimer disease, and other ailments. Promising though these may be, their currently foreseeable applications do not seem likely to significantly extend the maximum human lifespan or to fundamentally alter the shape of the human life cycle.

Since aging is itself a major risk-factor for many of these human diseases, if aging could be slowed, the onset of these diseases might be greatly delayed or mitigated. For this reason, among others, it is the third approach—direct and general age-retardation, now being actively pursued on several paths—that, if successful, would have the most significant physical, social, and moral consequences. If successful, age-retardation could not only extend the average lifespan or slow down generalized senescence; it could extend the maximum lifespan, perhaps quite significantly. Should it succeed in doing so, it may involve heretofore-unknown changes throughout the human life cycle. Our discussion will briefly touch on two sorts of piecemeal approaches to combating senescence (muscle enhancement and memory improvement), but will then focus largely on the more generalized approach to the retardation of aging as a whole.

response with other "aging" effects (including maybe further decline in alpha motor neurons). Because the organism is a single interrelated unit, anything that adversely influences cell function can appear to be a "cause" of aging.

III. SCIENTIFIC BACKGROUND

A. Targeting Specific Deficiencies of Old Age

Two piecemeal approaches to opposing or slowing two specific debilities of old age illustrate the potential of targeted techniques of combating the aging of the body, and display their differences from the more holistic efforts to retard bodily aging altogether.

1. Muscle Enhancement

A loss of strength and muscle mass is one of the most noticeable and significant signs of bodily senescence. With aging, we become more sedentary and use our muscles less, and the production of growth hormone and circulating insulin-like growth factor (IGF-1, discussed in the previous chapter) also decreases. There is thus less IGF-1 available to keep the muscles large, and they become smaller, weaker, and less easily repaired when injured. In addition, aged muscle cells are apparently less responsive to the action of IGF-1 and mIGF-1 (muscle IGF-1) so that the impact of even vigorous exercise on muscle size and strength diminishes with age.[3] This age-related muscle diminution has been given a medical-sounding name: sarcopenia.

As we age, several things change that predispose us to the development of sarcopenia. We either reduce the output of, and/or become more resistant to, anabolic stimuli to muscle, such as central nervous system input, growth hormone, estrogen, testosterone, dietary protein, physical activity, and insulin action. The loss of alpha-motor neuron input to muscle that occurs with age[4] is believed to be a critical factor[5] since nerve-cell-to-muscle-cell connections are critical to maintaining muscle mass and strength.

A loss of muscle size and strength is a significant problem for older persons. In addition to slowing movement and hampering some activities, sarcopenia is associated with an increased tendency to fall and break bones, and such falls are major causes of morbidity among the elderly. The techniques of muscle enhancement described in the previous chapter (including the introduction of IGF-1 genes, the use of human growth hormone, and other approaches) seem likely (and in a number of cases have been shown in animals) to significantly reduce age-related loss of strength and of muscle mass.

2. Memory Enhancement

Memory loss is another particularly agonizing consequence of senescence, disjointing the individual from his or her past, and bringing about not only a loss of function but a loss of faith in one's own senses of self and the world. Researchers have been making meaningful strides toward an understanding of memory loss—as a discrete and specific consequence of aging. Much of this work has been a by-product of the effort to understand and to treat Alzheimer disease, which first expresses itself in memory loss.

For example, researchers have discovered that cholinergic cells are "among the first to die in Alzheimer patients and that cholinergic mechanisms may be involved in memory formation."[6] This has led to therapeutic interventions with a class of drugs called acetylcholinesterase inhibitors. These agents block the enzyme that destroys acetylcholine (a neurotransmitter that scientists believe is crucial to forming memories), with the result that acetylcholine, once released, remains in the synapse for a longer period of time. These drugs have had a real but limited effect on improving memory in some Alzheimer patients; they can slow down or moderate the effects of the disease, but they do not reverse the progressive destruction of the brain.

Memory loss is not confined to patients with Alzheimer disease, or even to the elderly. And we should not simply assume that biotechnical interventions that address or counteract the biological causes of specific memory diseases like Alzheimer would have a similar effect on other elderly individuals, or would improve memory in general. As Stephen Rose explains: "The deficits in Alzheimer Disease and other conditions relate to specific biochemical or physiological lesions, and there is no a priori reason, irrespective of any ethical or other arguments, to suppose that, in the absence of pathology, pharmacological enhancement of such processes will necessarily enhance memory or cognition, which may already be 'set' at psychologically optimal levels."[7]

Nonetheless, some evidence suggests that at least some portion of the discoveries made in research on Alzheimer disease could well prove to enhance memory in general. For instance, a recent study tested the effect of donepezil, one of the major acetylcholinesterase inhibitors, on the performance of middle-aged pilots. Pilots conducted seven practice flights on a flight simulator to train them to perform a complex series of instructions. Then half of them took the drug donepezil for thirty days, while the other half took a placebo. When the simulator test was then repeated, the pilots who had taken the drug retained the training better than those who had taken the placebo.[8] There is also a large body of research, mostly in animals, demonstrating that "opiate receptor antagonists" may improve memory formation by stimulating the hormones that are typically released in response to emotionally arousing experiences.[9]

The remarkable complexity of the human body as a whole and the brain in particular makes it very difficult to isolate the functions of memory from other neuro-physiological processes (perception, attention, arousal, etc.) with which it is interconnected. Many "non-memory drugs" or stimulants therefore have a significant effect on memory; and many "memory drugs" have a significant effect on other bodily functions. So, for example, amphetamines, Ritalin, and dunking one's hand in freezing water have a "positive effect" on the capacity to remember new information, at least over the short term. But these drugs or experiences work on memory only indirectly, affecting not the specific memory systems but the other systems of the body that influence how the different memory systems function.[*]

---

[*] The above description draws heavily on Steven Rose (Rose, S., "'Smart drugs': do they work, are they ethical, will they be legal?," *Nature Reviews Neuroscience* 3: 975-979, 2002). As Rose has said: "[M]emory formation requires, amongst other cerebral processes: perception, attention, arousal. All engage both peripheral (hormonal) and central mechanisms. Although the processes involved in recall are less well studied it may be assumed that it makes similar demands. Thus agents that affect any of these concomitant processes may also function to enhance (or inhibit) cognitive performance. Memory formation in simple learning tasks is affected by plasma steroid levels, by adrenaline and even by glucose. At least one agent claimed to function as a nootropic and once widely touted as a smart drug, piracetam, seems to act at least in part via modulation of peripheral steroid levels. Central processes too can affect performance by reducing anxiety, enhancing attention or increasing the salience of the experience to be learned and remembered. Amphetamines, methylphenidate (Ritalin), antidepressants, and anxiolytics probably act in this way. Other agents

Recent research in animals has also improved our understanding of certain molecular and genetic "switches" that control memory. For example, in 1990, Eric Kandel discovered that blocking the molecule CREB (c-AMP [cyclic adenosine monophosphate] Response Element Binding protein) in sea slug nerve cells blocked new long-term memory without affecting short-term memory.[10] A few years later, Tim Tully and Jerry Yin genetically engineered fruit flies with the CREB molecule turned "on"; the resulting flies learned basic tasks in one try, where for normal flies it often took ten tries or more. The hypothesis is that "CREB helps turn on the genes needed to produce new proteins that etch permanent connections between nerve cells," and that it is "in these links that long-term memories are stored."[11] These exciting discoveries have already launched several new pharmaceutical companies formed specifically to develop potential drugs based on this research. In 1999, another group of researchers succeeded in genetically engineering mice that learn tasks much more readily. They inserted into a mouse embryo a gene that caused over-expression of a specific receptor in the outer surface of certain brain cells, "long suspected to be one of the basic mechanisms of memory formation" because it allows the "brain to make an association between two events."[*][12]

Though exciting, all of this work is very preliminary; and its significance for producing biotechnologies that might preserve or enhance human memory remains to be determined. So far, there seems to be no efficacious "silver pill" or "golden gene" for producing better memories, never mind one without any countervailing biological costs. But the work continues, and its potential ought not be dismissed.

regularly cited as potential smart drugs, such as ACTH and vasopressin, may function similarly. Finally, there is evidence from animal studies that endogenous cerebral neuromodulators such as the neurosteroids (e.g., DHEA) and growth factors like BDNF will enhance long-term memory for weakly acquired stimuli." See original for complete list of citations.

[*] The difficulty of simple and direct improvement in complex neurological processes is underscored by the results of this experiment. Together with some improvements in memory the mice experienced other neurological changes, including hypersensitivity to inflammatory pain. See Pinker, S., "Human Nature and Its Future," presentation at the March 2003 meeting of the President's Council on Bioethics, Washington, D.C. Transcript available on the Council's website, www.bioethics.gov.

Piecemeal interventions to combat sarcopenia, memory loss, or any other specific aspect or consequence of aging and senescence may of course have profound implications for the way human beings age. But inasmuch as they mitigate one element of aging while further exposing the individual to others, their overall result may not be simply attractive: Longer life with improved muscles but with unimproved or ever-weaker memories might well be undesirable. In any case, the contribution of these piecemeal interventions to longer, more vigorous life is unlikely to be as profound as that of some potential approaches to the systematic (body-wide) retardation of aging.

B. General (Body-Wide) Age-Retardation

An even more significant potential route to nearly ageless bodies involves the body-wide retardation of the aging process, now being pursued by some researchers. The concept of general age-retardation presumes the existence of a general organism-wide process of aging, as opposed to a series of unconnected processes of degeneration that would have to be treated separately. For aging as a whole to be slowed, there must be such a thing as "aging as a whole." Its existence has been debated by biologists for many years, but over the last two decades experimental evidence has increasingly suggested that a unified process of senescence does indeed exist. There is still no clear empirically supported theoretical concept of just how aging works, but evidence has shown that a number of techniques appear to affect the aging of a wide variety, if not indeed all, of the body's organs and systems. Sharp decreases in caloric intake and a number of genetic interventions in animals (both of which will be discussed in greater detail below) have been shown to have dramatic effects not only on longevity, but on practically every measurable expression of the rate of aging, including the rates of memory loss, muscle loss, declining activity, immune-system response, and a broad range of bodily processes that might not otherwise be conceived of as synchronized.

Even if the way in which these techniques of age-retardation work is not fully understood, it seems increasingly plausible that there just might be a single process (or a small number of processes) of aging on which they do their work. The multiple effects suggest that most, if not all, of the various phenomena of aging are deeply connected and, in principle, could be jointly influenced by the right sorts of interventions. It seems increasingly likely, therefore, that something like age-retardation is in fact possible.

The most prominent techniques of age-retardation currently under investigation fall into the following four general categories: caloric restriction, genetic manipulations, prevention of oxidative damage, and methods of treating the ailments of the aged that might affect age-retardation.

1. Caloric Restriction

It has been known since the mid-1930s that substantial reductions in the food intake of many animals (combined with nutritional supplements to avoid malnutrition) can have a dramatic effect on lifespan. With nearly seven decades of laboratory research, this is by far the most studied and best-described avenue of age-retardation, though scientists still lack a clear understanding of how it works. What is clear, however, from numerous studies in both invertebrates and vertebrates (including mammals), is that a reduction of food intake to about 60 percent of normal has a significant impact not only on lifespan but also on the rate of decline of the animal's neurological activity, muscle functions, immune response, and nearly every other measurable marker of aging. Moreover, it is now clear that the effect is not a product of a diminished metabolism, as was long believed. Calorically restricted animals do become physically smaller, but they process energy at the same levels as members of their species on a normal diet. In fact, studies in mice and rats suggest that caloric restriction appears to result in significantly increased rates of spontaneous activity, including the ability to run greater distances and to maintain a "youthful" level of activity at an age well beyond that of non-restricted animals of the same species. (Importantly, however, caloric restriction in animals also often results in sterility, or reduced fertility.)

The degree of life-extension (and likely age-retardation) achieved through caloric restriction is quite remarkable. In mice and rats, researchers have regularly found lifespan extended by more than 30 percent, and in some studies by more than 50 percent.[13] Studies have also found significant extensions of life and signs of retarded aging in a number of other mammalian species, including, recently, a 16-percent increase in the lifespan of dogs.[14]

Studies of caloric restriction in monkeys, conducted since the late 1980s at the National Institute on Aging, the University of Maryland, and the University of Wisconsin, have shown comparable effects even on some of our nearest evolutionary cousins.[15] Calorically restricted monkeys retain youthful levels of several vital hormones well into late adulthood, have lower blood pressure, and, over a fifteen-year period, suffer substantially less chronic illness than members of their species on normal diets. The effect on lifespan is as yet not known. Monkeys generally live several decades, so it will be years before it is apparent whether calorically restricted monkeys live significantly longer than others.

The biological basis for the dramatic anti-aging effects of caloric restriction is not now well understood, in large part because of the sheer number of changes wrought by a simple reduction in food intake. Hundreds of discretely measurable physiological changes occur in mice and rats on reduced diets, making cause and effect difficult to disentangle and the processes from which age-retardation results difficult to identify. However, researchers in the field believe that a number of new tools and techniques available only in the last decade or so (including DNA microarrays, new types of genetically engineered mice, and others) promise to facilitate a greater understanding of this process, and they believe that, in the foreseeable future, the mechanisms by which it operates might be understood, and techniques for achieving the same ends without a diet of near-starvation may be developed.*

2. Genetic Manipulations

Some of the most startling and extraordinary discoveries in age-retardation research have involved genetic mutations that have significant impact

---

* To reduce food consumption to 60 percent of normal, the average active adult human being would have to lower his daily caloric intake from 2,500 calories a day to 1,500. By any standard, that is a severely restricted diet that few people would want to sustain for long periods. Accordingly, much research is being devoted to the search for pharmaceuticals (known as "caloric restriction mimetics") that might mimic the benefits of caloric restriction without actually forcing people to go hungry. See Lane, M., et al., "The Serious Search for an Anti-Aging Pill," *Scientific American* 287(2): 36-41, 2002.

on lifespan and on the rate of senescence. Over the past few decades, researchers have identified *single* gene alterations that, in a number of species, dramatically extend life. For example, in nematode worms, it appears that changes in any one of at least 50 and potentially as many as 200 genes can significantly extend life.[*] Study of these mutations is enabling scientists to trace with some precision the biochemical pathways responsible for changes in the aging rate; knowledge of these pathways will then provide specific targets for possible age-retarding interventions. In recent years, a few such pathways have been identified in worms, fruit flies, and yeast, with the numerous mutant genes having their effect on one or another of these pathways.[**] More remarkably, a number of life-extending genetic mutations have been identified in mice, whose genetics and physiology are far more complex than those of worms.

As long as life-extending single-gene mutations were known only in worms and fruit flies, there was little reason to expect that they might also occur in humans. But findings that similar biochemical pathways are responsible for this phenomenon in both worms and mice suggest the potential for a similar possibility in humans. For instance, in worms, flies, and mice, an alteration in a receptor for an insulin-like growth factor (present also in humans) has resulted in substantial increases in lifespan. It now seems possible that the rate of aging may be governed by highly conserved general mechanisms across many species, and that single-gene alterations that extend life may ultimately be discovered in humans.

Most remarkable is the magnitude of life-extension that these mutations confer. In worms, where the effect has been most dramatic, a single-gene alteration has been shown to double lifespan, and an alteration in

---

[*] See Austad, S., "Adding Years to Life: Current Knowledge and Future Prospects," presentation at the December 2002 meeting of the President's Council on Bioethics. Transcript available on the Council's website, www.bioethics.gov.

[**] A number of recent studies suggest that there may be three separate pathways affecting normal longevity: an insulin/IGF-1 pathway; a pathway that, during early development, sets the rate of mitochondrial respiration in ways that affect the rate of aging and behavior of the adult; and a poorly defined pathway affected by caloric restriction. Of course, all these pathways may converge at some "downstream" positions. See, for instance, Dillin, A., et al., "Rates of behavior and aging specified by mitochondrial function during development," *Science* 298 (5602): 2398-2401, 2002; and Murphy, C., et al., "Genes that act downstream of DAF-16 to influence the lifespan of Caenorhabditis elegans," *Nature* 424: 277-283, 2003.

two genes has nearly tripled it. In the most extreme cases, involving particular single-gene mutations in male worms, researchers have observed a six-fold increase in lifespan. There are, of course, enormous physiological differences between humans and worms. Most notably, the cells of nematode worms stop dividing in adulthood, a fact that of course has great significance for aging. In mammals, most notably mice, the effects have been less pronounced, but still quite significant. Increases in the normal two-year lifespan of laboratory mice by 25 percent to even 50 percent have been reported, and single-gene mutations combined with caloric restriction have been shown to result in a nearly 75-percent increase in lifespan (or up to nearly three-and-a-half years). That 75-percent extension is, to date, the greatest increased lifespan achieved in mammals.[16]

Some single-gene mutations do, however, have serious side effects, including, most commonly, sterility or reduced fertility—problems also observed with other techniques of age-retardation—though, on the other hand, some recent research suggests that, at least in some organisms, it may be possible to decouple the age-retarding effects of certain mutations from the observed diminution of fertility and reproductive fitness.[17] Some single-gene differences have also been shown to decrease longevity in one sex of a species (most notably in fruit flies) while increasing it in the other. In addition, some of these mutations result in reduced body size and increased susceptibility to cold.

The effects of induced age retardation on fertility and reproductive fitness invite interesting speculation on the possible connection between longevity and reproduction: prolongation of life for the individual may be in tension with renewal of life through generation; conversely, fitness for reproduction is correlated with the process of decline leading to death. The possibility that hormonal events triggering puberty might also be involved in accelerating senescence has also been discussed by researchers on aging.

A different approach to the genetics of age-retardation, this one in humans, begins with knowledge gained from the study of progeria, a very rare genetic condition that leads not to delayed but to precocious senescence. One form of this progressive, fatal disorder, which afflicts approximately one in eight million newborns, is now believed to result from a single DNA base substitution in a gene on chromosome 1. This mutation leads to abnormal formation of the protein lamin A (LMNA), a key component of the membrane surrounding the nucleus of cells. Many victims of progeria carry the defective LMNA gene; others carry a mutation in a gene encoding a protein that repairs DNA damage. These findings will likely lead not only to genetic tests and therapeutic approaches to the treatment of progeria but also, perhaps, to new insights into the normal aging process itself. According to Dr. Francis Collins, director of the National Human Genome Research Institute (NHGRI) and the leader of the research team that found the LMNA gene defect, "Our hypothesis is that LMNA may help us solve some of the great mysteries of aging." Conceivably, future therapies developed to alleviate symptoms of premature aging in progeria patients may prove effective in delaying the aging process in unafflicted human beings as well.[18]

Single-gene differences that affect lifespan have not been studied for as long as caloric restriction. It is not yet clear, in this case, whether what is involved is true age-retardation or a form of more general extension of life. The evidence that does exist, however, suggests a retardation of aging, and a slowing of the loss of function and of the deterioration of tissues and cells.

3. Prevention of Oxidative Damage

For many years, there has been ample (if indirect) evidence that oxygen free radicals—oxygen molecules that have one unpaired electron, and that are therefore chemically very active—produced as inevitable by-products of the body's various functions, cause gradual deterioration of many of the body's cells and tissues. These oxygen free radicals perform some important metabolic functions, but they can also disrupt protein synthesis and repair (especially in mitochondria) and can cause minor errors in DNA replication that accumulate over time. Our body produces, or obtains through our diet, a number of antioxidants (such as superoxide dismutase [SOD], catalase [CAT], vitamin E, vitamin C, coenzyme Q10, and alpha-lipoic acid) that destroy many, but not all, of these oxygen free radicals. The balance of oxygen free radicals and antioxidants seems to be connected to the rate of degeneration of cells and tissues in the body. In fact, antioxidants may be deeply involved in the operation of the other success-ful age-retardation techniques in animals. For instance, the balance between free-radical production and antioxidant activity may modulate the impact of caloric restriction; and one specific antioxidant seems to play a critical role in the operation of nearly all the single-gene life-extending mutations in nematode worms. In addition, a recent study has shown that a synthetic antioxidant can significantly extend the lifespan of mice, and the life-extending effect of antioxidant activity in fruit flies has also been well documented. Researchers are exploring the potential for employing both naturally occurring and synthetic antioxidants in humans, to retard the degeneration of cells, reduce and slow the accumulation of errors in DNA replication, and thereby extend the human lifespan, perhaps significantly. The study of free-radical activity will also likely inform our understanding of the operation of other age-retardation techniques.

4. Methods of Treating the Ailments of the Aged That Might Affect Age-Retardation

A number of techniques that do not themselves fall squarely under the heading of age-retardation may nonetheless offer vital clues to the nature of the aging process, and may have a significant role to play in the opera-tion of age-retardation techniques. These include:

a. Hormone treatments: It has long been known that endocrine fac-tors are closely tied to a number of the most prominent elements of aging. The rates of production of certain hormones (particularly testosterone and estrogen) decline sharply in one's later years, and these declines are closely related to the loss of muscle mass that accompanies aging and to a series of other age-related declines. In the past fifteen years, researchers have been investigating the possi-bility of slowing or, in certain instances, reversing these effects of aging by the replenishment of certain hormones to more youthful levels, with particular focus on human growth hormone, dehy-droepiandrosterone (DHEA), testosterone, estrogen, pregnenolone, progesterone, and melatonin. One prominent study, conducted in 1990 and repeated several times since, showed that men between the ages of 60 and 80 who were injected with human growth hormone over a six-month period developed increased muscle mass, a loss of fat, improved skin elasticity, and decreased cholesterol levels.[19] To this point, however, there has been no verifiable claim of changes in human lifespan as a result of hormone replacement, and some researchers have expressed doubts about the possibility of such changes.[20] This approach in a certain sense falls between what we have called age-retardation and what might be better understood as a treatment of the symptoms of aging. The human growth hormone studies cited above, and most similar efforts, do not appear to slow the general rate of degeneration and loss of function, but they reverse some of their particular effects, on both body and mind. Although the impact of such treatments does not appear to be generalized throughout the body, hormone treatments may play an important role in unlocking the secrets of the aging process, and in future age-retardation techniques. (The same may be said of stem-cell treatments and other forms of regenerative medicine.)

b. Telomere research: Since the mid-1980s, researchers have known that telomeres—which form the tips of chromosomes—can shorten over time as cells divide, and that eventually this shortening causes cells to stop dividing and to die. Certain cells—germ cells, cancer cells, some stem cells, hair follicles, and others—are able to escape this process of degeneration with the help of an enzyme called telomerase, which slows the erosion and shortening of telomeres. Several studies in the 1990s suggested that telomere length correlates with cell aging, so that preventing the shortening of telomeres can slow the aging of cells, and, under certain conditions, might do so without increasing the risk of uncontrolled cell-growth and cancers.[21] The links between cell aging and the general aging of organisms are, however, still quite unclear. A number of particular conditions of the aged—including wrinkling of the skin, age-related muscular degeneration, and atherosclerosis—have been linked, in various degrees, to cellular aging and degeneration. These studies suggest a use for the manipulation of telomeres in counteracting and even preventing certain "symptoms" of aging, but at this point no mechanistic link has been demonstrated between telomere length and the general process of organismal senescence. One recent study, however, has found a statistically significant link between shorter average telomere length and increased rates of mortality (from a number of causes) in the elderly.[22] The appearance of changes in telomere length in experiments with other age-retardation techniques, including caloric restriction and single-gene mutation, also suggests a potential connection, but for the moment the nature of that connection remains unclear. The promise of telomere manipulation appears greatest as a means of combating some afflictions of the aged, rather than retarding aging as such.

These different avenues of age-retardation research are not as clearly distinguished from one another as this classification suggests. In almost all cases, the employment of one technique offers results that are relevant for the understanding of the others. Caloric restriction seems to affect antioxidant production; genetic alterations can affect telomere length. Several of these methods have also been shown to work in tandem. Also, recent developments and advances in the tools of cellular and molecular biology have begun to fuse together these disparate fields. The techniques used for one are often also used in the others.

None of these techniques has been demonstrated to increase human lifespans or to slow the process of aging in humans. Such a demonstration would be quite difficult to undertake, since the human lifespan is on average between seven and eight decades. Experiments seeking to alter it would require a great deal of time and more than one generation of researchers (as the subjects outlived the researchers). Moreover, there are reasons to be cautious about extrapolating from animal models to human beings, for we are not simply more complicated versions of worms, flies, or mice.* Nevertheless, there is much to be learned from animal experi-

* Fruit flies, roundworms, and mice are short-lived species subject to hazardous environments and seasonal exigencies. It may simply make sense biologically that their lifespan would be both constrained and flexibly regulated to coordinate survival and reproduction within favorable circum-

ments, and from planned observational studies of human populations, and the results of such work, combined with the existence of analogous systems and processes in humans, suggest that scientists may indeed in the future be able to retard the human aging process and extend both the maximum and average human lifespan. Even if the prospect is not imminent, it may not be too early to begin considering its potential implications.

IV. ETHICAL ISSUES

That this prospect will be welcomed seems almost self-evident. Who among us would not want more healthy years added to his or her life? No one truly relishes the thought of bodily degeneration or decline, and of one's final years marked, as Shakespeare put it, by "a moist eye, a dry hand, a yellow cheek, a white beard, a decreasing leg, an increasing belly . . . your voice broken, your wind short, your chin double, your wit single, and every part about you blasted with antiquity."[23] We would probably all want to save ourselves, and even more so our loved ones, from the fate we have seen some of our elders endure.

The desire to live longer is also clearly echoed in some ethical ideals. It is surely one form of the true love of life and is driven by a deep commitment to the activities and engagements to which our lives are dedicated. Life's end nearly always finds human beings in the midst of projects still uncompleted, painfully aware that the world is full of wisdom they have yet to gain and experiences they have yet to enjoy. Much that is good about life is the result not of our finitude but of our longevity. Although some of us may live best when we live each day as if it were our last, many of us thrive because we live looking ahead to many days to come—making plans, laying foundations, building our lives with the future in mind. More time to plan, more healthy years in which to build and to enjoy

stances in a way quite different from the human lifespan. Also, they are less complex and more genetically determined than human beings; indeed, they are studied in part because their genetics are so predictable. Human beings have evolved to be much longer-lived and more versatile, and have a different overall biological strategy, one of open indeterminacy and consciously mediated flexibility and freedom, complemented by creativity, communication, and cultural continuity.

what we have built, and in which to contribute to the lives of others, would surely be a great blessing. Not only individuals but society too might benefit, gaining much from the added experience and wisdom of its older members. The case for living longer is, in part, a moral case, and a strong one. Indeed, it may well be strong enough to overwhelm any possible objections or worries.

But to know if it would overwhelm such worries, we must identify those worries and examine them with care. Because the case for longer—even greatly longer—life seems so strong, the worries may at first escape our notice. Finding and pondering them leads us to suggest that any major alteration of the human life cycle is likely to have serious consequences beyond the mere extension of life, and to raise difficult ethical and practical questions, both for individuals and especially for society.

In suggesting some of these questions (and for the sake of discussion), we make several assumptions, both about the availability of age-retarding technology and its likely effects. We assume, first, that technology will be available to significantly retard the process of aging, of both body and mind, and second, that this technology will be widely available and widely used. If the first is correct, the second almost certainly will be. Which consequences of age-retardation are most likely will depend upon the particular techniques that become available and the effect they have on the shape of a life. Different techniques might alter the aging process differently and have different effects on the life cycle. Three general possibilities might be considered: (1) the life cycle would be stretched out like a rubber band, so that aging is slowed more or less equally at all stages of life, and maturation, middle age, and decline extend over a greater period; (2) a holding back of bodily decline, so that both the process of maturation and the process of decline occur roughly in the way they do now, but the period between them—that is, the healthy years of the prime of life—are greatly extended; and (3) a change in the form of decline, so that, for instance, rather than a slow and gradual loss of faculties, bodily degradation comes very quickly, and death comes suddenly following long years of health and vigor. We shall seek to take account of all of these possibilities, pointing to their potentially different ethical implications where they arise.

In listing the three alternatives, we have taken the optimist's view, confining our attention to life-extending outcomes that many people might find attractive. We have done this deliberately, for two reasons. First, only such attractive outcomes are likely to be widely embraced. Second, we wish to stipulate that people will get what they wish for, so that we may then examine whether what they get is likely to turn out in fact to be what they wanted (the Midas problem). Yet before proceeding to the ethical discussion, we should insert some notes of caution. It is possible that age-retarding techniques, like many medical interventions, will have uneven effects: they might work well for some, not well for others, and cause serious side effects in yet others. For example, for some recipients of greater longevity, the result might include a much longer period of decline and debility. Indeed, the period of debility could be lengthened not only absolutely (as it would be on the model of a rubber band being stretched) but also relative to the whole lifespan, and, in either case, virtually everyone who survives past eighty or ninety might come to expect ten to fifteen years of severely diminished capacity. All the scenarios for *happy* life-extension depend on technologies that will keep *all* the body's systems going for roughly the same duration, after which time they will shut down more or less simultaneously. But what if it should turn out that many people experience instead partial or uncoordinated increases in vigor (stronger joints but weaker memory, more ardent desire but diminished potency)? Given that age-retardation sets out to alter not just this organ or that tissue but the entire (putative) coordinated biological clock of a most complex organism, caution and modest expectations are proper leavens for zeal, especially as the love of longer life needs little encouragement to embrace false hopes of greater time on earth.

We divide our discussion of the ethical questions into two sections, dealing with the effects on individuals and the effects on society and its institutions. As will become evident, however, the distinction between them is not always sharp.

A. Effects on the Individual

The question of the effect of age-retardation on our individual lives must begin with a sense of what aging means in those lives.

First we must remember that aging is not just about old age. It is a crucial part of the (nearly) lifelong process by which we reach old age and the end of our lives. Accordingly, its product is not so much old age and death as the life cycle itself: the form and contour of our life experienced in time. Strange as it may seem, from the perspective of personal experience aging defines youth almost as much as it does old age, because each stage of our life is defined relative to the others and to the whole of life. Age-retardation would therefore affect not only our later years, but all of our years, in both immediate and mediated ways. For one thing, if administered early in life, it might quite directly prolong our youthful years by slowing down the processes of maturation. Some of the evidence from animal studies, cited above, suggests that some of the methods that rely upon an alteration at the outset—including genetic alteration or the mimetics of lifelong caloric restriction—might retard aging in the young just as in the old. This might imply an overall "stretching out" of the entire life cycle, as one stretches a rubber band, extending the period we spend in infancy, childhood, adolescence, in our prime and in decline, and profoundly altering our sense of the relation between years lived and stages of life. Slower biological aging (particularly in a culture of faster "social aging" like ours, in which children are increasingly exposed to things that might not so long ago have been deemed exclusively appropriate for adult life) may cause an increasing disjunction between the maturity of the body and mind and the expectations and requirements of life.

Even if the age-retarding technology produces no *direct* bodily effects during youth, an increased maximum lifespan or even only greatly diminished senescence in the old could very likely affect the attitudes of the young along with those of the old. Indeed, age-retardation could affect the young even more than the old, insofar as the attitudes of the young are shaped by a sense of what is to come and what is to be expected of life. The great changes in average life expectancy over the twentieth century may have already influenced ways in which people perceive their own future, though it is a difficult matter after the fact to determine exactly how and why. Yet the changes resulting from those recent increases in *average* life expectancy may not provide precedent for human expectations in an unprecedented world, in which the *maximum* lifespan has increased significantly and many people are living longer than anyone has ever lived before.*

How might such expectations be different? It is not easy to say, and different people will no doubt react differently. But some general observations are in order. The first concerns the "shape" of the life cycle as a whole. Some proponents of age-retardation research use language that suggests an image of life as a "time line," uniform and homogeneous, rather than as a forward-moving drama, composing different acts or stages—infancy, childhood, adolescence, coming-of-age, adulthood, parenthood, ripeness, decline. This would imply an understanding of life as composed of interchangeable and essentially identical units of time, rather than composing a whole with a meaningful form of its own, its meaning derived in part from the stages of the life cycle and the fact that we live as links in the chain of generations. Viewed through the prism of this chronological atomism, the prospect of adding more years to our lives means simply having more time, more of the same. And since life is good, more life is better. But life as lived and experienced does not present itself homogeneously and in discrete uniform bits, and the "time of our lives," informed by experience past and bent toward the future, is not the homogeneous and featureless "dimension" that is the time of physicists. Life as lived in time may be more akin to a symphony, in which a certain temporal order—pacing and procession, meter and momentum—governs the relationship between the parts and the whole and, more important, gives a dynamic process its directed

---

* In this sense, life expectancy turns out to be a uniquely useful measure. Life expectancy is a measurement, based on statistical tables of mortality, of the number of additional years that people of some particular age may expect to live at a given time. This seems better suited for insurance purposes than for capturing a snapshot of longevity. And yet, life expectancy may be distinctly useful to moral reflection and analysis, because it is a measure of the number of years a person may expect to have yet ahead of him or her at any moment. It is therefore a measure of the view ahead, of the expected and anticipated years to come, which has much to do with our attitudes about aging and death and about how to regard and what to do with the time we have available. Many of the most significant consequences of age-retardation could result from an increase in the number of years that people can expect to live, and from the resulting changes in attitudes.

character. Lived time is also shaped by memories of those who came before, and of who we ourselves have been; it is informed by imagined future possibilities, created by our hopes and plans for what we might yet become. The animated shape of a whole life affects how we live every portion, and altering the shape of that whole might therefore have far greater consequences than merely giving us more time.

A second observation concerns the relation between aging and death, and between age-retardation and our attitudes about mortality. Moving the midnight hour of a human lifespan could alter human attitudes and dispositions toward mortality and toward the whole of life. Life-extension does not mean immortality, to be sure—if for no other reason than that the attainment of immortality is scientifically implausible. But the impulse to extend our lives in general, rather than to combat particular diseases or ailments that shorten our lives, is a declaration of opposition to death as such. In addressing aging as a disease to be cured, we are, in principle, and at least tacitly, expressing a desire never to grow old and die, or, in a word, a desire to live forever. There is no reason to suspect that life-extension research would stop were we to achieve some mildly extended human lifespan, say, to 140, or 160, or 180 years. Why would it? Having declared that our present term of life is inadequate, why should we settle for another? A life lived from the start under the influence of age-retarding techniques is a life lived in express opposition to the constraints of mortality. Taken to its extreme, the underlying impulse driving age-retardation research is, at least implicitly, limitless, the equivalent of a desire for immortality.

These two observations are, of course, closely tied, since the boundaries and shape of the life cycle give form and possible meaning to a mortal life. Its virtue consists not so much in that it leads us to death, but in that it reminds us, by its very nature, that we will someday die, and that we must live in a way that takes heed of that reality. If we remained at our prime, in full swing, for decade after decade, and perhaps even for a couple of centuries, the character of our attitudes and our activities might well change significantly. These changes could take at least six principal forms:

1. Greater Freedom from Constraints of Time

First is a potentially positive consequence. A significantly greater lifespan would open up new possibilities and freedoms. Quite simply, longer-lived individuals would have more time in the course of their lives to explore new things and enjoy familiar ones, to gain more and deeper experiences, to complete more projects, to engage in more activities, to start a new course or a new career having gained much valuable experience in earlier ones, to have a second or third or fourth chance at something they deem important. If life is good, more life is in many ways better. Moreover, if the prospect of dying is well out of sight, the fear of death might diminish as well, alleviating many of the distortions this fear can produce in our lives.

2. Commitment and Engagement

On the other hand, the remoteness of the midnight hour might influence negatively how we spend our days. For although the gift of extra time is a boon, the perception of time ahead as less limited or as indefinite may not be. All our activities are, in one way or another, informed by the knowledge that our time is limited, and ultimately that we have only a certain portion of years to use up. The more keenly we are aware of that fact, the more likely we are to aspire to *spend* our lives in the ways we deem most important and vital. The notion of spending a life suggests a finite quantity of available devotion, and as economists are fond of telling us, the scarcity of a commodity contributes to its value. The very experience of spending a life, and of becoming *spent* in doing so—that is, the very experience of *aging*—contributes to our sense of accomplishment and commitment, and to our sense of the meaningfulness of time's passage, and of our passage through it. Being "used up" by our activities reinforces our sense of fully living in the world. Our dedication to our activities, our engagement with life's callings, and our continuing interest in our projects all rely to some degree upon a sense that we are *giving* of ourselves, in a process destined to result in our complete expenditure. A life lived devoid of that sense, or so thoroughly removed from it as to be in practice devoid of it, might well be a life of lesser engagements and weakened commitments—a life other than the one that we have come to understand as fully human. This is not to say it will be worse—but it will very likely be quite different.

3. Aspiration and Urgency

Very much related to our sense of being used up in the course of our lives is the sense of urgency given to life by the prospect of foreseeable death. This may be what the Psalmist means in asking God to "teach us to number our days, that we may get a heart of wisdom." Many of our greatest accomplishments are pushed along, if only subtly and implicitly, by the spur of our finitude and the sense of having only a limited time. A far more distant horizon, a sense of essentially limitless time, might leave us less inclined to act with urgency. Why not leave for tomorrow what you might do today, if there are endless tomorrows before you? Our sense of the size and shape of our future—our "life expectancy"—is a major factor affecting how we act and think in the present.

4. Renewal and Children

Perhaps most significant, and most intriguing, is the deep connection between death and new birth. The link between longevity and fertility is a nexus of profound and mysterious human significance. The link appears again and again, in different forms and different arenas, both in empirical scientific investigation and in any effort at moral analysis. Most of the age-retardation techniques tested in animals to this point appear to result in very significant decreases in fertility (though, as noted earlier, in some cases the effects can be uncoupled). Various theories have been proffered to explain this link, mostly having to do with a relationship between the mechanisms that enable fertility and those that result in degeneration and death. Some have even suggested that the changes connected to puberty may well be linked to those that trigger decline. Fertility and aging may be biologically linked. Moreover, they seem to be linked in terms of human behavior and experience.

Throughout the twentieth century, increases in life expectancy have been accompanied by decreases in the birth rate.* Of course, increased longevity alone does not explain declining birth rates. Increased income and economic opportunity as well as improved methods of contraception surely play a role. But increased longevity and improved health are surely elements of the broader cultural transformation that does explain declining birth rates. Perhaps for the first time in human history, vast numbers of young adults, blessed with an expectation of a long disease-free and war-free future, are living childlessly through their most fertile years, pursuing their own fulfillment now, but with the (often mistaken) expectation that there will always be time enough later to start a family.

One important reason for the apparent experiential link between longevity and childbearing seems readily intelligible: without some presentiment of our mortality, there might be less desire for renewal. And so a world of men and women who do not hear the biological clock ticking or do not feel the approach of their own decline might have far less interest in bearing—and, more important, caring for—children. Children are one answer to mortality. But people in search of other more direct and immediate answers, or, more to the point, people whose longer lease on life leaves them relatively heedless of its finitude, might very well be far less welcoming of children, and far less interested in making the sacrifices needed to promote human renewal through the coming of new generations. Whether this would in fact occur is an empirical question, and not all Council Members are convinced of this connection between awareness of finitude and devotion to perpetuation. But we all believe these are possibilities well worth contemplating.

---

* The great "baby boom" of the 1950s and '60s in the United States was not, as one might imagine, a result of substantially increased birth rates. In 1900, the birth rate was just above 30 births per thousand population; in 1950 (roughly the beginning of the period called the "baby boom") it was 24.1, and in 1965 (the end of that period) it was 18.4. It is not increased rates of childbearing but rather extraordinary reductions in infant mortality (allowing many more children to live to adulthood) that explain the relative size of the generation born in those years. The birthrate has since continued to decline, reaching approximately 15 births per thousand population in 2001, bringing it closer to the death rate, and therefore bringing population growth roughly into line with figures from the early twentieth century.

Related to the subject of the effects of longevity on procreation is the subject of the effects of longevity on marriage and the resulting family connections. These topics are too large—and perhaps too speculative—to explore here. Yet two questions may suffice to point to what may be at stake. Would people in a world affected by age-retardation be more or less inclined to swear lifelong fidelity "until death do us part," if their life expectancy at the time of marriage were eighty or a hundred more years, rather than, as today, fifty? And would intergenerational family ties be stronger or weaker if there were five or more generations alive at any one time?

5. Attitudes Toward Death and Mortality

How a greatly increased lifespan lived in good health would affect attitudes toward death is another important matter. Certainly, the removal of the numerous causes of premature death has diminished through much of life the fear of *untimely* death, though its overall effects on our views of mortality are less easy to discern. Yet it is possible that an individual committed to the technological struggle against aging and decline would be less prepared for and less accepting of death, and the least willing to acknowledge its inevitability. Given that these technologies would not in fact achieve immortality, but only lengthen life, they could in effect make death even less bearable, and make their beneficiaries even more terrified of it and obsessed with it. The fact that we might die at any time could sting more if we were less attuned to the fact that we must die at some (more-or-less known) time. In an era of age-retardation, we might in practice therefore live under an even more powerful preoccupation with death, but one that leads us not to commitment, engagement, urgency, and renewal, but rather to anxiety, self-absorption, and preoccupation with any bodily mishap or every new anti-senescence measure.

Much may depend on how people actually grow old and die in a new world of increased longevity. Should the end come swiftly, with little premonitory illness (the third of the possibilities discussed above), death might always be regarded as untimely, unprepared for, shocking, and anxiety about accidents or other health hazards might rise.* But what if, in

---

* Montaigne puts it this way: "I notice that in proportion as I sink into sickness, I naturally enter into a certain disdain for life. I find that I have much more trouble digesting this resolution when

the "stretched rubber band" sort of life cycle, the period of debility became even more protracted and difficult than it now is? We have already seen how, thanks to antibiotics, techniques of life-support, and medicine's general success in preventing quick deaths from infectious diseases, heart attacks, and strokes, many more people are now spending prolonged periods in decay, or subject to Alzheimer disease and other age-related degenerative disorders. One of the costs we are already paying for the gift of longevity is the placement of elderly citizens and their families in degrading and difficult situations that simply were not possible in earlier times. Even a cure for Alzheimer disease, welcome as it most surely would be, would very likely leave some other chronic debilitating illness in command of those declining years. Under such circumstances, death might come to seem a blessing. And in the absence of fatal illnesses to end the misery, pressures for euthanasia and assisted suicide might mount.

6. The Meaning of the Life Cycle

There is also more to the question of aging than the place of death and mortality in our lives. Not just the specter of mortality, but also the process of aging itself affects our lives in profound ways. Aging, after all, is a process that mediates our passage through life, and that gives shape to our sense of the passage of time and our own maturity and relations with others. Age-retardation technologies make aging both more manipulable and more controllable as explicitly a human project, and partially sever age from the moorings of nature, time, and maturity. They put it in our hands, but make it a less intelligible component of our full human life. Having many long, productive years, with the knowledge of many more

I am in health than when I have a fever. Inasmuch as I no longer cling so hard to the good things of life when I begin to lose the use and pleasure of them, I come to view death with much less frightened eyes. This makes me hope that the farther I get from life and the nearer to death, the more easily I shall accept the exchange. . . . If we fell into such a change [decrepitude] suddenly, I don't think we could endure it. But when we are led by Nature's hand down a gentle and virtually imperceptible slope, bit by bit, one step at a time, she rolls us into this wretched state and makes us familiar with it; so that we find no shock when youth dies within us, which in essence and in truth is a harder death than the complete death of a languishing life or the death of old age; inasmuch as the leap is not so cruel from a painful life as from a sweet and flourishing life to a grievous and painful one." (Montaigne, M., "That to Philosophize Is to Learn to Die," *The Complete Essays of Michel Montaigne*, trans. Donald M. Frame, Stanford: Stanford University Press, 1965, p. 63.)

to come, would surely bring joy to many of us. But in the end, these techniques could also leave the individual somewhat unhinged from the life cycle. Without the guidance of our biological life cycle, we would be hard-pressed to give form to our experiential life cycle, and to make sense of what time, age, and change should mean to us.

Any of the foregoing effects of course would most likely be subtle, and it would be exceedingly difficult to hold them up against the promise of longer and longer life and to expect any of us simply to reject the offer. But in considering the offer, we must take into account the value inherent in the human life cycle, in the process of aging, and in the knowledge we have of our mortality as we experience it. We should recognize that age-retardation may irreparably distort these and leave us living lives that, whatever else they might become, are in fundamental ways different from—and perhaps less serious or rich than—what we have to this point understood to be truly human.

Powerful as some of these concerns are, however, from the point of view of the individual considered in isolation, the advantages of age-retardation may well be deemed to outweigh the dangers. But individuals should not be considered in isolation, and the full potential meaning of age-retardation cannot come into view until we take in the possible consequences for society as a whole. When we do so, some of these individual concerns become far more stark and apparent, and new concerns emerge as well.

B. Effects on Society

To begin to grasp the full implications of significant age-retardation, we must imagine what our world would look like if the use of such techniques became the norm. This is both a reasonable expectation and a useful premise for analysis. If effective age-retardation technologies became available and relatively painless and inexpensive,* the vast

---

* Other sorts of problems, involving aggravated social stratification based on the gift of lengthened life, might emerge if the lifespan-extending technologies were very expensive and available only to the privileged few, as they well might be, at least initially. Such difficulties, already anticipated in the current inequities in health care, could be much exacerbated even short of technolo-

majority of us would surely opt to use them, and they would quickly become popular and widely employed. Moreover, viewing the effects of these technologies in the aggregate both highlights the consequences they would have for individuals by drawing them out and showing what they would mean on a large scale, and allows us to see certain consequences that affect the society and its institutions directly, and that are not just individual effects writ large. Individual changes in attitude and outlook toward children or mortality would have far more profound effects if they were widely shared throughout society. And at the same time, some changes, like age distributions in the population, only become apparent at all when we take in a view of entire communities or societies all at once.

The full social effects of age-retardation probably would not be evident until the first cohort to benefit from treatment began to cross the barrier of the present maximum lifespan, but lesser consequences would become evident much sooner, as more and more of the population survived to older ages, and lived with the plausible expectation of doing so.

Consequences will likely be apparent at every level of society, and in almost every institution. Among the more obvious may be effects on work opportunities, new hires, promotions and retirement plans; housing patterns; social and cultural attitudes and beliefs; the status of traditions; the rate and acceptability of social change; the structure of family life and relations between the generations; and political priorities and choices, and the locus of rule and authority in government. The experiences of the past century offer us some clues in this regard, though the effects of significant increases in lifespan would likely be more radical than those we have seen as a result of twentieth-century advances.

To paint a fuller picture, we consider the potential social implications of age-retardation in three areas: generations and families; innovation, change, and renewal; and the aging of society.

gies to retard senescence. The projected opportunities for "regenerative medicine"—featuring stem-cell-based tissue transplantation or more extensive organ replacement—may turn out to be very expensive and available mainly to the wealthy.

1. Generations and Families

Family life and the relations between the generations are, quite obviously, built around the shape of the life cycle. A new generation enters the world when its parents are in their prime. With time, as parents pass the peak of their years and begin to make way and assist their children in taking on new responsibilities and powers, the children begin to enter their own age of maturity, slowly taking over and learning the ropes. In their own season, the children bring yet another generation into the world, and stand between their parents and their children, helped by the former in helping the latter. The cycle of succession proceeds, and the world is made fresh with a new generation, but is kept firmly rooted by the experience and hard-earned wisdom of the old. The neediness of the very young and the very old puts roughly one generation at a time at the helm, and charges it with caring for those who are coming and those who are going. They are given the power to command the institutions of society, but with it the responsibility for the health and continuity of those institutions.

A society reshaped by age-retardation could certainly benefit from the wisdom and experience of more generations of older people, and from the peace, patience, and crucial encouragement that is often a wonderful gift of those who are no longer forging their identity or caught up in economic or social competition. But at the same time, generation after generation would reach and remain in their prime for many decades.* Sons might no longer surpass their fathers in vigor just as they prepared to become fathers themselves. The mature generation would have no obvious reason to make way for the next as the years passed, if its peak became a plateau. The succession of generations could be obstructed by a glut of the able. The old might think less of preparing their replacements, and

---

* Combined with patterns of decreasing family size in the West, this might create a peculiar reorienting of the generational makeup of families, with fewer children and far more and older adults, layered in succeeding generations—the opposite of a branching family tree. A lifespan of approximately 150 years could reasonably be expected to allow one to see his or her great-great-great-great-grandchild. But this child would have as many as 63 other such great-great-great-great-grandparents, along with 32 great-great-great-grandparents, 16 great-great-grandparents, eight great-grandparents, four grandparents and two parents—and, if certain demographic trends continue, few if any siblings, uncles and aunts, or cousins.

the young could see before them only layers of their elders blocking the path, and no great reason to hurry in building families or careers—remaining functionally immature "young adults" for decades, neither willing nor able to step into the shoes of their mothers and fathers. Families and generational institutions would surely reshape themselves to suit the new demographic form of society, but would that new shape be good for the young, the old, the familial ties that bind them, the society as a whole, or the cause of well-lived human lives?

2. Innovation, Change, and Renewal

The same glut might also affect other institutions, private and public. From the small business to the city council, from the military to the Fortune 500 corporation, generational succession might be disrupted, as the rationale for retirement diminished. Again, these institutions would benefit from greater experience at the top, but they might find it far more difficult to adjust to change. With the slowing of the cycles of succession might also come the slowing of the cycles of innovation and adaptation in these institutions.

Cultural time is not chronological time. Beliefs and attitudes tend to be formed early in life, and few of us can really change our fundamental outlook once we have reached our intellectual maturity. Serious innovation, and even just successful adaptation to change, is therefore often the function of a new generation of leaders, with new ideas to try and a different sense of the institution's mission and environment. Waiting decades for upper management to retire would surely stifle this renewing energy and slow the pace of innovation—with costs for the institutions in question and society as a whole.

A society's openness and freshness might be diminished not only because large layers of elders block paths to youthful advancement. They might also be jeopardized more fundamentally by the psychological and existential changes that the mere passing of time and "learning how things are" bring to many, perhaps most, people. After a while, no matter how healthy we are or how well placed we are socially, most of us cease to look upon the world with fresh eyes. Familiarity and routine blunt awareness. Fewer things shock or surprise. Disappointed hopes and broken dreams, accumulated mistakes and misfortunes, and the struggle to meet the economic and emotional demands of daily life can take their toll in diminished ambition, insensitivity, fatigue, and cynicism—not in everyone, to be sure, but in many people growing older.* As a general matter, a society's aspiration, hope, freshness, boldness, and openness depend for their continual renewal on the spirit of youth, of those to whom the world itself is new and full of promise.

3. The Aging of Society
Even as the ravages of aging on the lives of individuals were diminished, society as a whole would age. The average age of the population would, of course, increase, and, as we have seen, the birthrate and the inflow of the young would likely decrease. The consequences of these trends are very difficult to forecast, and would depend to a great extent on the character of the technique employed to retard aging. If the delay of senescence made it more acute when it did come, then the costs of caring for the aged would not be reduced but only put off, and perhaps increased. The trend we have already seen in our society, whereby a greater share of private and public resources goes to pay for the needs of the aged and a lesser share for the needs of the young, would continue and grow. But society's institutions could likely adapt themselves to this new dynamic (though of course the fact that we can adjust to something does not in itself settle the question of whether that something is good or bad). More important is the change in societal attitudes, and in the culture's view of itself. Even if age-retardation actually decreased the overall cost of caring for the old, which is not unimaginable, it would still increase the age of society, affecting its views and priorities. The nation might commit less of its intellectual energy and social resources to the cause of initiating the young, and more to the cause of accommodating the old.

---

* As Aristotle noted in his remarkable portrait of the old, the young, and those in their prime, the old often "aspire to nothing great and exalted and crave the mere necessities and comforts of existence." (Aristotle, *Rhetoric*, Book II, Ch. 13, 1389b22, trans. L. Cooper, Englewood Cliffs, N.J.: Prentice-Hall, 1960, p. 135.)

A society is greatly strengthened by the constant task of introducing itself to new generations of members, and might perhaps be weakened by the relative attenuation of that mission. A world that truly belonged to the living—who expected to exercise their ownership into an ever-expanding future—would be a very different, and perhaps a much diminished, world, focused too narrowly on maintaining life and not sufficiently broadly on building a good life. If individuals did not age, if their functions did not decline and their horizons did not narrow, it might just be that societies would age far more acutely, and would experience their own sort of senescence—a hardening of the vital social pathways, a stiffening and loss of flexibility, a setting of the ways and views, a corroding of the muscles and the sinews. This sort of decline would be far less amenable to technological solutions.

A society reshaped in these and related ways would be a very different place to live than any we have known before. It could offer exciting new possibilities for personal fulfillment, and for the edifying accumulation of individual and societal experience and wisdom. But it might also be less accommodating of full human lives, less welcoming of new and uninitiated members, and less focused on the purposes that reach beyond survival. If so, retardation of aging—like sex selection, as discussed in an earlier chapter—might turn out to be a Tragedy of the Commons, in which the sought-for gains to individuals are undone or worse, owing to the social consequences of granting them to everyone. Contemplating these concerns in advance forces us to consider carefully the sort of world we wish to build, or to avert.

V. CONCLUSION

The prospect of effective and significant retardation of aging—a goal we are all at first strongly inclined to welcome—is rife with barely foreseeable consequences. We have tried to gesture toward some possible effects, both positive and negative, though no one can claim to know what a world remade by unprecedented longevity on a mass scale would really look like.

On its face, our effort to propose some possible concerns about such a world is open to the charge that we have taken the present to be "the best of all possible worlds." Indeed, simply by raising any doubts, some may accuse us—wrongly—of believing that the present is no longer the best of the worlds we have known. Some questions we have raised about the social implications of future increases in maximum lifespan might well have been raised a century ago, were someone then to have proposed—no one, of course, did—to increase the average life expectancy at birth by the amount in fact realized since 1900 (thirty years, from 48 to 78). Empirical studies of the consequences of that large increase are lacking, for obvious reasons, and it would be virtually impossible to try to assess now the full social costs of this widely welcomed change. Yet if there is merit in the suggestion that too long a life, with its end out of sight and mind, might diminish its worth, one might wonder whether we have already gone too far in increasing longevity. If so, one might further suggest that we should, if we could, roll back at least some of the increases made in the average human lifespan over the past century.

These remarks prompt some large questions: Is there an optimal human lifespan and an ideal contour of a human life? If so, does it resemble our historical lifespan (as framed and constrained by natural limits)?* Or does the optimal human lifespan lie in the future, to be achieved by some yet-to-be-developed life-extending technology? Whatever the answers to these intriguing and important questions, nothing in our inquiry ought to suggest that the present average lifespan is itself ideal. We do not take the present (or any specific time past) to be "the best of all possible worlds," and we would not favor rolling back the average lifespan even if it were doable. Although we suggest some possible problems with substantially longer lifespans, we have not expressed, and would not

---

* The natural history of longevity might after all teach us something about the value of extended life. Lifespans have increased dramatically through evolution, and apparently to great advantage. Contemporary species are the products of evolutionary changes that have likely included something on the order of 1,000-fold increases of lifespan since the very short-lived earliest living forms. If increased longevity were inherently detrimental, we humans would not have evolved to have both great abilities and long lifespans. This result of natural and enormously gradual evolutionary change, however, cannot in itself be taken as a reassuring precedent for any humanly engineered change, especially if produced rapidly without the opportunity for evolutionary testing of the resulting changes in fitness.

express, a wish for shorter lifespans than are now the norm. To the contrary, all of us surely want more people to be able to enjoy the increased longevity that the last century produced. Those previous efforts that have increased *average* lifespans have done so by reducing the risks and removing the causes of *premature* death, allowing many more people to live out their biblical three-score (today, four-score) and ten. Yet during that time, there has been relatively little increase in the *maximum* human lifespan, and not many people are living longer than the longest-lived people ever did. Although we may learn about the future by studying somewhat similar changes in the past, the effects of changes of the past are not an adequate guide for the radically new possibilities that age-retardation may bring into being. Thus, to be committed, as we are, to trying to help everyone make it through the natural human lifespan (surely a better world than the present) does not require our being committed to altering or increasing that lifespan. Conversely, to be concerned about the implications of departing from a three-to-four-generational lifespan does not necessitate a reactionary embrace of any putative virtues of premature death.

The past century's advances in average lifespan, now approaching eighty years for the majority of our fellow citizens, have come about through largely intelligible operations within a natural world shaped by human understanding and human powers. It is a conceptually manageable lifespan, with individuals living not only through childhood and parenthood but long enough to see their own grandchildren, and permitted a taste of each sort of relationship. It is a world in which one's direct family lineage is connected by both genetics and personal experience, not so attenuated by time that relatives feel unrelated. Generation and nurture, dependency and reciprocated generosity, are in some harmony of proportion, and there is a pace of journey, a coordinated coherence of meter and rhyme within the repeating cycles of birth, ascendancy, and decline—a balance and beauty of love and renewal giving answer to death that, however poignant, bespeaks the possibility of meaning and goodness in the human experience. All this might be overthrown or forgotten in the rush to fashion a technological project only along the gradient of our open-ended desires and ambitions.

Contemplating the speculative prospect of altering the human life cycle brings us to the crucial question: Is there a goodness and meaning in life so fundamental that it is too wide to be grasped by our scientific vision and too deep to be plumbed by the imperious exigencies of our natural desire? If we go with the grain of our desires and pursue indefinite prolongation and ageless bodies for ourselves, will we improve the parts and heighten the present, but only at the cost of losing the coherence of an ordered and integrated whole? Might we be cheating ourselves by departing from the contour and constraint of natural life (our frailty and finitude), which serve as a lens for a larger vision that might give all of life coherence and sustaining significance? Conversely, in affirming the unfolding of birth and growth, aging and death, might we not find access to something permanent, something beyond this "drama of time," something that at once transcends and gives purpose to the processes of the earth, lifting us to a dignity beyond all disorder, decay, and death? To raise these questions is not to answer them, but simply to indicate the enormous matters that are at stake.

Without some connection between change and permanence, time and the eternal, it is at best an open question whether life could be anything but a process without purpose, a circumscribed project of purely private significance. Our natural desires, focused on ourselves, would lead us either to attempt to extend time as far as technologically possible or to dissolve it in the involution of a ceaseless series of self-indulgent distractions. In Aldous Huxley's *Brave New World*, Bernard and Lenina are hovering in a helicopter over the city, wondering how to best spend their evening together. Lenina (typically jejune) suggests a game of electromagnetic golf. Bernard demurs and replies, "No, that would be a waste of time." Lenina answers back, "What's time for?" Only aging and death remind us that time is of the essence. They invite us to notice that the evolution of life on earth has produced souls with longings for the eternal and, if recognized, a chance to participate in matters of enduring significance that ultimately could transcend time itself.

The broader issue has to do with the meaning of certain elements of our human experience that medical science may now allow us to alter and manipulate. The ability to retard aging puts into question the meaning of aging in our lives, and the way we ought best to regard it: Is aging a disease? Is it a condition to be treated or cured? Does that mean that all the generations that have come before us have lived a life of suffering, either waiting for a cure that never came or foolishly convincing themselves that their curse was just a blessing in disguise? Is the finitude of human life, as our ancestors experienced it and as our faiths and our philosophies have taught us to understand it, really just a problem waiting to be solved? The anti-aging medicine of the not-so-distant future would treat what we have usually thought of as the whole, the healthy, human life as a condition to be healed. It therefore presents us with a questionable notion both of full humanity and of the proper ends of medicine.

The attempt to overcome aging puts in stark terms the question that defines much of our larger investigation of the uses of biotechnology that go beyond the treatment of the sick and wounded: Is the purpose of medicine to make us perfect, or to make us whole? And, medicine's purpose aside, would we really be better off as individuals (happier and more fulfilled) and as a society (more cultivated, more accomplished, more just) if we had more perfect and more ageless bodies? The human being in his or her natural wholeness is not a perfect being, and it is that very imperfection, that never fully satisfactory relation with the world, that gives rise to our deepest longings and our greatest accomplishments. It is what reminds us that we are more than mere chemical machines or collections of parts, and yet that we are less than flawless beings, seamlessly a part of and perfectly content in a world fully under our control and direction. It is the source of some of what we most appreciate about ourselves.

Some foreseeable biotechnologies, like those of effective age-retardation, hold out the prospect of perfecting some among our imperfections, and must lead us to ask just what sort of project this is that we have set upon. Is the purpose of medicine and biotechnology, in principle, to let us live endless, painless lives of perfect bliss? Or is their purpose rather to let us live out the humanly full span of life within the edifying limits and constraints of humanity's grasp and power? As that grasp expands, and that power increases, these fundamental questions of human purposes and ends become more and more important, and finding the proper ways to think about them becomes more vital but more difficult. The techniques themselves will not answer these questions for us, and ignoring the questions will not make them go away, even if we lived forever.

ENDNOTES

[1] Olshansky, S., et al., "No truth to the Fountain of Youth," *Scientific American*, June 2002, pp. 92-95.

[2] Shakespeare, W., *King Henry the Fourth, Part 2*, Act II, Scene 4, 259-260.

[3] Owino, V., et al., "Age-related loss of skeletal muscle function and the ability to express the autocrine form of insulin-like growth factor-1 (MGF) in response to mechanical overload," *FEBS Letters*, 505: 259-263, 2001.

[4] Brown, W., "A method for estimating the number of motor units in thenar muscles and the changes in motor unit count with aging," *Journal of Neurology, Neurosurgery, and Psychiatry* 35: 845-852, 1972.

[5] Roubenoff, R., et al., "Sarcopenia: Current concepts," *The Journal of Gerontology, Biological and Medical Sciences*, Series A, 55A, M716-M724, 2000.

[6] Rose, S., "'Smart drugs': do they work, are they ethical, will they be legal?," *Nature Reviews, Neuroscience* 3: 975-979, 2002. This discussion also draws on James McGaugh's presentation before the President's Council on Bioethics, October 17, 2002 (available at www.bioethics.gov).

[7] Rose, *ibid*.

[8] Yesavage, J., et al., "Donepezil and flight simulator performance: effects on retention of complex skills," *Neurology* 59: 123-125, 9 July 2002.

[9] McGaugh, J., "Significance and Remembrance: The Role of Neuromodulatory Systems," *Psychological Science* 1: 15-25, 1990.

[10] Langreth, R., "Viagra for the Brain," *Forbes*, 4 February 2002.

[11] Ibid.

[12] Wade, N., "Of Smart Mice and an Even Smarter Man," *New York Times*, September 7, 1999. See also Tsien, J., et al., "Genetic enhancement of learning and memory in mice," *Nature* 401: 63-69, 2 September 1999.

[13] A useful review of caloric restriction work in animals is Weindruch, R., et al., *The Retardation of Aging and Disease by Dietary Restriction*. Springfield, IL: Charles Thomas Publishers, 1998.

[14] The study of caloric restriction in dogs, conducted by researchers at the University of Pennsylvania, the University of Illinois, Cornell University, and Michigan State University, is expected to be published in an upcoming issue of the *Journal of the American Veterinary Medical Association*. Preliminary results were announced by the University of Pennsylvania in September 2002.

[15] Ramsey, J., et al., "Dietary restriction and aging in rhesus monkeys: the University of Wisconsin study," *Experimental Gerontology* 35 (9-10): 1131-1149, 2000.

[16] These results refer to a yet-unpublished study brought to the Council's attention by Steven Austad in his presentation at its December 2002 meeting. (Available on the Council's website at www.bioethics.gov.)

[17] Dillin, A., et al., "Timing requirements for insulin/IGF-1 signaling in C. elegans," *Science* 298(5594): 830-834, 2002.

[18] See the NIH News Release, "Researchers Identify Gene for Premature Aging," April 16, 2003, available on the NHGRI website at http://genome.gov/11006962; Eriksson, M., et al., "Recurrent de novo point mutations in lamin A cause Hutchinson-Gilford progeria syndrome," *Nature* 423: 293-298, 2003; and Vastag, B., "Cause of progeria's premature aging found: expected to provide insight into normal aging process," *Journal of the American Medical Association* 289: 2481-2482, 2003.

[19] Rudman, D., et al., "Effects of human growth hormone in men over sixty years old," *The New England Journal of Medicine* 323:1-5, 1990.

[20] Olshansky, S., *op. cit.*

[21] An overview of the subject by Council Member Elizabeth Blackburn in the journal *Nature* from November 2000 sheds light on this controversial question (Blackburn, E., "Telomere states and cell fates," *Nature* 408(6808): 53-56, 2000).

[22] Cawthon, R., et al., "Association between telomere length in blood and mortality in people aged 60 years or older," *Lancet* 361(9355): 393-395, 2003.

[23] Shakespeare, *op. cit.*, Act I, Scene 2, 179-183.

5

Happy Souls

Who has not wanted to escape the clutches of oppressive and punishing memories? Or to calm the burdensome feelings of anxiety, disappointment, and regret? Or to achieve a psychic state of pure and undivided pleasure and joy? The satisfaction of such desires seems inseparable from our happiness, which we pursue by right and with passion.

According to the Declaration of Independence, the right to pursue happiness is one of the unalienable rights that belong equally to all human beings. Indeed, the American Founders held that governments exist mainly to safeguard this right—along with the rights to life and liberty—against those who would seek to deny or suppress it. Life, the foundational good, is good also because it makes liberty possible. And liberty is good both in itself and as the prerequisite for pursuing happiness in ways that each of us may freely choose for ourselves.* Our interest in happiness is not, however, merely one interest among many. It is an overarching interest in our complete and comprehensive well-being.

For this reason, the pursuit of happy souls is not simply, in this report, just another case study. At the same time it implicates or points to something final and all-embracing. For it is ultimately our desire for happiness—for the fulfillment of our aspirations and the flourishing of our lives—that leads us to seek, among other things, better children, superior performance, and ageless bodies (and minds). Yet the contribution of those proximate and

---

* "Pursuit" is here properly ambiguous, encompassing both the quest to find happiness and the enjoyment of happiness once found (as in "my favorite pursuits").

subordinate ends to the ultimate and supreme end of happiness* is partial and indirect. Having better and more accomplished children or a more vigorous and well-working body surely can contribute to our happiness, but they are not the thing itself: there are people with splendid children and perfectly toned bodies who are nonetheless miserable. Superior performance, though perhaps more integral to our own flourishing, is likewise not the whole story: everything depends on how it fits into the larger psychic, moral, and spiritual economy of our lives—what we long for and how well we attain it, and whether we are satisfied with ourselves in relation to our ideals, aspirations, and actual achievements and experiences.

Such self-satisfaction and sense of fulfillment are, needless to say, not easily attained. On the contrary, obstacles to human happiness abound, ranging from overt illnesses of brain and psyche, through grief and guilt, shame and sorrow, to simple frustrations of hopes and plans. Dementia, depression, disappointment, and despair are, alas, all too common, and many—perhaps most—people are more often bent on overcoming these and other impediments to happiness than on seeking it in its positive fullness.** In these efforts at peace of mind, human beings have from time immemorial sought help from doctors and drugs. In a famous literary instance, Shakespeare's Macbeth entreats his doctor to free Lady Macbeth from the haunting memory of her own guilty acts:

MACBETH: Canst thou not minister to a mind diseas'd,
Pluck from the memory a rooted sorrow,
Raze out the written troubles of the brain,
And with some sweet oblivious antidote
Cleanse the stuff'd bosom of that perilous stuff
Which weighs upon the heart?

---

* We note at the outset of this discussion that some people do not regard happiness as the supreme goal, preferring instead to place righteousness, duty, virtuous and creative activity, or holiness and serving God at the peak of human aspiration. Whether or not this remains a disagreement depends finally on whether happiness, if understood as human fulfillment, embraces these other goals as well, or whether it is distinct from them.

** John Locke, one source of our present views of happiness, wrote that the quest for happiness is, in fact, nothing more than an effort to alleviate "the uneasiness a man is at present under." (*Essay Concerning Human Understanding* [1690], Chapter XXI, "Of Power," §31.)

DOCTOR: Therein the patient
                Must minister to himself.

Ministering to oneself, however, is easier said than done, and many people have found themselves unequal to the task without some outside assistance. For centuries, they have made use of external agents to drown their sorrows or lift their spirits. Alcohol, in different measures, can accomplish both. So, too, certain naturally occurring psychotropic agents, from the mythical lotus flower described in Homer's *Odyssey* to the very real euphoriants derived from the opium poppy. Yet until recently, biotechnological aids to psychic flourishing have been relatively feeble and non-specific. Drugs for soothing bad memories have been utterly lacking. And drugs to brighten mood or raise self-esteem have been imperfect: unsafe, inadequately effective, transient, liable to side effects, and frequently illegal or stigmatized. Thanks to recent breakthroughs, however, the situation is changing rapidly. The burgeoning field of neuroscience is providing new, more specific, and safer agents to help us combat all sorts of psychic distress. Soon, doctors may have just the "sweet oblivious antidote" that Macbeth so desired: drugs (such as beta-adrenergic blockers) that numb the emotional sting typically associated with our intensely bad memories, and "mood brighteners" (such as serotonin reuptake inhibitors) that lift and stabilize our general disposition and make us feel good (or better) about ourselves.

To be sure, these agents—and their better versions, yet to come—are, for now at least, being developed not as means for drug-induced happiness but rather as agents for combating major depression or preventing posttraumatic stress disorder (PTSD). Yet once available for those purposes, they could also be used to ease the soul and enhance the mood of nearly anyone. Should this occur, further research and development of drugs helpful to the direct pursuit of happier souls—surely a profitable business venture—would very likely take place. As a result, our pursuit of happiness and our sense of self-satisfaction will become increasingly open to *direct* biotechnical intervention. Such possibilities raise many large questions.

By directly inducing changes in our subjective experience, the new psychotropic drugs create the possibility of severing the link between feelings of happiness and our actions and experiences in the world. Who would need better children, superior performance, or more youthful bodies if medication could provide the pleasure and sense of well-being that is the goal of so many of our aspirations? Indeed, why would one need to discipline one's passions, refine one's sentiments, and cultivate one's virtues, in short, to organize one's soul for action in the world, when one's aspiration to happiness could be satisfied by drugs in a quick, consistent, and cost-effective manner?

Yet it is far from clear that feelings of contentment severed from action in the world or from relationships with other people could make us truly happy. Would a happiness that did not flow from what we do and say, usually in association with others, be more than a simulacrum of that happiness for which our souls fit us? More generally, would the pharmacological management of our mental lives draw us toward or estrange us from the true happiness that we seek? It is hard to answer in the abstract. In some cases, it might bring us nearer, by restoring our natural ability to take satisfaction in joyous events and satisfying deeds. In other cases, it might estrange us, by substituting the mere feelings divorced from their natural and proper ground.

The currently available drugs to alter memory and mood, and the new drugs and their uses that may be just around the corner, invite other large questions about the character of human life. By using drugs to satisfy more easily the enduring aspirations to forget what torments us and approach the world with greater peace of mind, what deeper human aspirations might we occlude or frustrate? What qualities of character may become less necessary and, with diminished use, atrophy or become extinct, as we increasingly depend on drugs to cope with misfortune? How will we experience our incompleteness or understand our mortality as our ability grows to medically dissolve all sorts of anxiety? Will the availability of drug-induced conditions of ecstatic pleasure estrange us from the forms of pleasure that depend upon discipline and devotion? And, going beyond the implications for individuals, what kind of a society are we likely to have when the powers to control memory, mood, and mental life through drugs reach their full maturity and are widely used?

On one level, as observed above, these questions are already with us, and have been for centuries. Alcohol, marijuana, cocaine, and other consciousness-affecting drugs offer temporary pleasures and escapes, and they can surely alter behavior and sense of self. But the difference (or potential difference) with the biotechnical interventions explored in this chapter is their capacity for more *precise, long-term,* and *sought-after* alterations in the human psyche. While current drugs may have more-or-less predictable effects, psyche-altering agents of the future, devised unlike those of the past on the basis of exact knowledge of the brain, will permit more refined and effective interventions. While current drugs used in moderation may give those who use them the feeling states they desire, these feeling states quickly wear off and the psyche returns to normal. And while current drugs used in excess may have long-term effects on the trajectory of one's life, these effects are typically destructive—*not* the effects we seek. Thus, while some of the ethical questions explored in this chapter surely apply to current drugs—which is not, of course, a reason to dismiss them—the core issues involved with recreational drugs and new psychotropic biotechnologies are, in important respects, psychologically and ethically distinct.

To be sure, the answers to the important questions raised above must in some measure be speculative, at least for now. They will depend on many factors: the pace of biotechnological developments; the range of physiological and psychological effects of the new drugs; debatable opinions about the hierarchy of human aspirations or the happiness most appropriate to the human soul; and the actual consequences, individual and social, of the drugs used and the purposes served. In due course, the answers about consequences can be found only by careful empirical social and psychological research. Yet figuring out which effects social scientists should investigate requires prior reflection and thoughtful analysis of the *possible* results and their likely human significance. And, despite lack of foreknowledge, we are obliged now to address these questions to the best of our abilities, if we wish to act responsibly regarding the biotechnical future that we might be, willy-nilly, in the midst of creating for ourselves and our descendants.

This chapter explores some of the questions connected with possibilities for directly altering our psychic state of well-being, using technologies that affect our memories (section II) or our moods and dispositions (section III). But before turning to these prospects, we begin with questions about the goal itself: What is a "happy soul"? As with the goals discussed in the previous three chapters, the goal here too is fraught with rich ambiguity.

I. WHAT ARE "HAPPY SOULS"?

The nature or meaning of happiness has always been a contested matter. Near the start of his inquiry into the supreme human good, Aristotle remarks that everyone agrees regarding its *name*—"happiness" or "flourishing"—but regarding *what it is*, most people do not give the same account as the wisest.[1] Some equate it with pleasure, others with honor or recognition, wealth or power, while still others locate it in virtuous deeds, love, or understanding. Adjudicating these competing claims is, of course, beyond the scope of this report. But a few pertinent questions about the character of happiness may prove useful for what is to come. Is happiness a feeling, sensation, or mood, or is it rather an activity? Is it a state of restful contentment or of focused and energetic striving? Some people, especially those who are troubled by the obstacles to happiness, equate it with peace of mind or an untroubled soul. Others demand something more: not just the absence of distress or discomfort, but a fullness or richness or flourishing of being. What, then, is the relation between being happy and being (merely) satisfied? Between being satisfied and being (merely) content? Between being content and being not discontent, or between the latter and being not dissatisfied? And in the face of all the obstacles to human happiness, isn't it happiness enough not to be genuinely miserable, not to be "uneasy"? Formally speaking, one might suggest that happiness consists in a coincidence between one's desires and one's power to satisfy them. But, as the well-known rejoinder has it, desires come in all sizes: Is it better to be a pig satisfied or Socrates dissatisfied? If the content matters as well as the form, how is happiness materially related to the activities of love and friendship, work and play, song and worship? Are social ties and activities important, or is happiness a purely solitary endeavor?

Whatever answers one might give to those questions, there are two further questions especially pertinent to the present inquiry: Is happiness a momentary matter or is it something experienced only over time, or even only over a complete life? And how can one tell the difference between true and false happiness, between the real thing and the mere likeness?

The first question introduces us to perplexities about the subject or bearer of happiness, here called, for lack of a better term, "soul"—a term no less problematic than "happiness." By "soul" we mean something *psychological* rather than theological: indeed, "soul" is the exact English translation of the Greek *psyche*, a term we sometimes use directly as its equivalent, as well as in the compounds "psychology" ("the account or science of the soul") and "psychiatry" ("the doctoring of the soul"). We mean here by "soul" or "psyche" the interacting powers of "mind and heart"— powers of reason, speech, understanding, intuition, memory, and imagination, as well as of desire, passion, and feeling—powers that make us human, powers that we know from the inside that we enjoy (and that dead or inanimate bodies lack). We mean also not just these generically human powers, but our particular and unique constellation of them, shaped by our own experiences, aspirations, attachments, achievements, disappointments, and feelings. We mean at once that which makes all of us human and that which makes each of us individually who we are. Because the happiness we seek we seek for *ourselves*—for *our* self, not for someone else's, and for our *self* or embodied soul, not for our bodies as material stuff—our happiness is bound up with our personhood and our identity. We would not want to attain happiness (or any other object of our desires) if the condition for attaining it required that we become someone else, that we lose our identity in the process.

The importance of identity for happiness implies necessarily the importance of memory. If experiencing our happiness depends upon experiencing a stable identity, then our happiness depends also on our memory, on knowing who we are in relation to who we have been. A person with Alzheimer disease, no matter how cheerful his mood, we hesitate to call happy precisely because, in some important sense, he is no longer altogether there as himself. His actions in the present are severed, through the loss of memory, from the actions and experiences that made him who and what he was and is. Indeed, much of the dread of this disease is connected with the erosion of personal identity that the loss of memory brings with it.

But if enfeebled memory can cripple identity, selectively altered memory can distort it. Changing the content of our memories or altering their emotional tonalities, however desirable to alleviate guilty or painful consciousness, could subtly reshape who we are, at least to ourselves. With altered memories we might feel better about ourselves, but it is not clear that the better-feeling "we" remains the same as before. Lady Macbeth, cured of her guilty torment, would remain the murderess she was, but not the conscience-stricken being even she could not help but be.

The second question takes us directly to mood, and to its link with the truth of things. In the pursuit of happiness, human beings have always worried about falling for the appearance of happiness and missing its reality. We are all too familiar with desires that lead astray, pleasures that cause serious harm, temporary satisfactions that leave us depleted and diminished. Yet however routinely we may mistake a fleeting sense of happiness for the real thing, we regard distinguishing between the two as crucial to our happiness. And for good reason. We don't really believe that ignorance is bliss; we say it ruefully to bolster spirits in the face of a sudden encounter with a painful truth. We may manage to convince ourselves that cheating is better than losing or that love based on a lie is better than no love at all. But seldom do those who win by cheating or who love by deceiving cease to long for the joy and fulfillment that come from winning fair and square or being loved for who one truly is. Many stoop to fraud to obtain happiness, but none want their feeling of flourishing itself to be fraudulent. Yet a fraudulent happiness is just what the pharmacological management of our mental lives threatens to confer upon us.

Anticipating the ethical analyses that come later in this chapter, we identify a two-fold threat of fraudulent happiness. First, an unchecked power to erase memories, brighten moods, and alter our emotional dispositions could imperil our capacity to form a strong and coherent personal identity. To the extent that our inner life ceases to reflect the ups and downs of daily existence and instead operates independently of them, we dissipate our identity, which is formed through engagement with others and through immersion in the mix of routine and unpredictable events that constitute our lives. Second, by disconnecting our mood and memory from what we do and experience, the new drugs could jeopardize the fitness and truthfulness of how we live and what we feel, as well as our ability to confront responsibly and with dignity the imperfections and limits of our lives and those of others. Instead of recognizing distress, anxiety, and sorrow as appropriate reflections of the fragility of human life and inseparable from the setbacks and heartbreaks that accompany the pursuit of happiness and the love of fellow mortals, we are invited to treat them as diseases to be cured, perhaps one day eradicated. Instead of recognizing contentment, pleasure, and joy as appropriate reflections of the richness of human life and inseparable from the fulfilling activities and attachments that are the heart of human happiness, we are invited to treat them as ends in themselves, perhaps one day inducible at will.*

To be sure, our emotions can play cruel tricks on us and fail us in myriad ways. They often wax and wane without reason, and they are not in themselves given to maintaining proper measure. And for those afflicted by debilitating memories of traumatic events, or who chronically suffer depression, despair, or a sense of deep unworthiness, the new drugs are likely to prove a great boon, by repairing crucial capacities for a normal and fitting emotional life. Nevertheless, it behooves us to explore the potential uses and misuses of these new drugs carefully, for drugs that erase memories or alter our temperaments and emotional outlooks deal with that which is most us, our hearts and minds. If we, as individuals and as a society, fail to proceed responsibly, the pharmacological management of our mental lives could seriously impair our ability to pursue that happiness for which our hearts long and to which our minds guide us.

---

* Once again, whether we in fact accept these invitations to change our self-understanding and whether, if we do, the baneful consequences (for the fitness and truthfulness of our emotional lives) will in fact follow are empirical questions, to be investigated in future research, but not therefore to be banished from current reflection.

II. MEMORY AND HAPPINESS

At first glance, the pursuit of happiness—a forward-looking activity—might seem to have little to do with memory—the remembrance of things past. Yet a closer look reveals some deep connections. Could we be happy if we were unable to remember our own past, if we lived only day-to-day, one moment to the next? Could we be happy if we were unable to assimilate present experience into the remembered narrative of previous experience? Could we be happy in the absence of happy memories? Conversely, could we be happy in the presence of terrible memories, memories so traumatic and so life-altering that they cast a deep shadow over all that we do, today and tomorrow? As these questions imply, both our capacity to remember—our ability to recall and recollect—and the content of what we remember—the banked "traces" of specific past experiences—may well be crucial to our prospects for happiness.*

A good memory is necessary even to do the little things that contribute to our happiness: preparing the foods we like, riding a bicycle, finding our way home or to the home of friends. Guiding us with little conscious effort, such memories are silently yet deeply part of who we are. Memory is also indispensable for our ability to learn new things: the name of a new acquaintance, the title of a new book, the contours of a new place. This forward-looking but memory-dependent readiness to capture and incorporate the not-yet-known and the not-yet-lived makes possible new pursuits, new associations, and new ways of getting along in the world—in a word, new ways of becoming happy.

Memory is important not only for retaining knowledge of what we can do. It is important also for allowing and enabling us to "know"—virtually without any deliberate effort on our part—*who we are*. Our memory, by its own activity, preserves for us the complex web of lived experiences that furnish our sense of self: the shared memories of living side-by-side with loved ones; the class long ago that changed our lives; the

---

* At the same time, it is important to note that "stored memories" do not remain static. Every time we recall a memory, what gets stored after such acts of recollection is a different memory, altered on account of how we, in recollecting it, have "received" and reacted to it. Once encoded, memories can be altered by recall.

days we spent in sickness and celebration; our finest moments and most shameful acts. The memories and the "self" they shape are acquired over time. At each moment, our then-existing web of memories shapes the way we face and understand our everyday lives. But this web of memories is, paradoxically, not permanently fixed, unlike an image recorded on a photograph. As we give new meaning to old happenings and try to fit them within the larger narrative of our unfolding existence, it changes over the course of life. Our experiences at age sixteen will have a different meaning to us when remembered at age eighteen, and a very different meaning yet again when remembered at age fifty. As we grow older, memories become less vivid, but perhaps their significance becomes more clear; although they are less immediate, they are now part of the larger story of who we are. We can consciously re-examine the meaning of remembered events and, as a result, change *how* they are remembered. Yet the memories themselves set limits on how much can be re-written, and much of the "re-construction" or "re-membering" of our remembered lives results from *undirected* "editorial" work. Astonishingly, memory itself selectively retains and deletes, reconfigures and reintegrates, the experiences that comprise who we have been and, therefore, *are*. Our identity or sense of self emerges, grows, and changes. Yet, despite all the changes, thanks to the integrating powers of memory, our identity also, remarkably, persists *as ours*.

If the capacities of remembering are crucial for preserving the "my-ness" of any happiness that comes our way, the *content* of the memories are crucial for our happiness itself. We do not wish merely to remember having had satisfying experiences; we wish to remember them with satisfaction. We desire not only even-keeled memories, but also memories with feeling and with sense: we relish the memory of devoted parents, of first love, the birth of a child; we delight in recalling beautiful sights seen, good deeds done, worthy efforts rewarded. We especially want our memories to be not simply a sequence of disconnected experiences, but a narrative that seems to contain some unfolding purpose, some larger point from beginning to end, some aspiration discovered, pursued, and at least partially fulfilled.

Memory is central to human flourishing, in other words, precisely because we pursue happiness in time, as time-bound beings. We have a past and a future as well as a present, and being happy through time requires that these be connected in a meaningful way. If we are to flourish *as ourselves*, we must do so without abandoning or forgetting who we are or once were. Yet because our lives are time-bound, our happiness is always incomplete—always not-yet and on-the-way, always here but slipping away, but also always possible again and in the future. Our happiest experiences can be revivified. And, as we reminisce from greater distance and with more experience, even our painful experiences can often acquire for us a meaning not in evidence when they occurred.

The place of memory in the pursuit of happiness also suggests something essential about human identity, a theme raised in various places and in different ways throughout this report: namely, our identities are formed both by what we do and by what we undergo or suffer. We actively choose paths and do deeds fit to be remembered. But we also live through memorable experiences that we would never have chosen—experiences we often wish never happened at all. To some extent, these unchosen memories constrain us; though we may regret the shadows they cast over our pursuit of happiness, we cannot simply escape them while remaining who we really are. And yet, through the act of remembering—the act of discerning and giving meaning to the past as it really was—we can shape, to some degree, the meaning of our memories, both good and bad.

The contribution of good memories to happiness, presented in this overly rosy account, makes clear how bad memories can undermine happiness, indeed, can cause misery. We can lose our memory through injury or illness; we can be plagued by terrifying, shameful, or guilty memories. Even for the fortunate and virtuous, life is not a bowl of cherries. To live, as we emphasized in the last chapter, is to age and decline, in memory as well as in muscle. To aspire is to risk disappointment. To love is to risk loss, and eventually to lose what one loves altogether in death. Bad memories, present inevitably to all of us, can not only mar present happiness; if sufficiently grave, they can overwhelm us and crush the prospect of seeking happiness any time in the future. Memory is not *always* a friend to happiness.

For this reason, people interested in happiness are interested, among other things, in better memories. Precisely because, in order to be happy, we need to be able to remember, we would like to find ways to keep our memory capacity intact, against the dangers of senility. Precisely because we desire happier memories, we might be tempted to "edit out," if we could, those memories that most disturb us or even to seek a new life history entirely.* For understandable reasons, we might seek to restore the innocence or peace of mind that our actions or our sufferings have disrupted.

Until recently, the prospect of altering our remembrance of things past—and doing so with precision, getting the better memories we desire without compromising memory as a whole—was a mere fantasy. But in the near future that may not be so. Much memory research over the past decades has focused on finding the causes and then the remedies for forgetfulness, in the first instance to forestall or treat the senile dementias, but, in the second place, to prevent also the annoying lapses of memory in the elderly and middle-aged, who have trouble remembering, for example, where they left the house keys. Although the field is full of promise,** there is little of practical value to report at the present time. Should such remedies for failing memories be found, their use would be welcomed by most people as a great boon. Assuming that there were no physical or mental side effects—a large assumption—there is little obvious reason to be concerned about the ethical or social implications.†

Scientists have also sought ways to alter the *content* and *feeling tone* of specific memories, with the goal of helping people whose lives are

---

* We also know that individuals "naturally" edit their memory of traumatic or significant events— both giving new meaning to the past in light of new experiences and in some cases distorting the past to make it more bearable. The question before us is how or whether new biotechnical interventions alter this inborn capacity to refine, reshape, and edit the way we remember the past.

** A few recent findings were noted in Chapter Four, "Ageless Bodies."

† Of course, this is not to say that the use of "memory-enhancers" would be a simple matter, ethically or socially. Such drugs, if they became available, would likely have many "beyond therapy" uses; they would raise questions about the meaning of enhancing cognitive performance pharmacologically and the meaning of "normal" memory decline that accompanies aging, both matters we discuss or at least touch on in other parts of this report.

crushed by remembered trauma. This research has yielded some novel pharmacological interventions, still rather limited in their effect but perhaps a harbinger of things to come, that change the way we remember the most emotionally affecting experiences of life, specifically by "numbing" the discomfort connected with the memory of our most painful experiences. The capacity to alter or numb our remembrance of things past cuts to the heart of what it means to remember in a human way, and it is this biotechnical possibility that we focus on here. Deciding when or whether to use such biotechnical power will require that we think long and hard about what it means to remember truthfully, to live in time, and to seek happiness without losing or abandoning our identity. The rest of this discussion of "memory and happiness" is an invitation to such reflection.

A. Good Memories and Bad

If happiness requires better memories, how would we improve them if we could? What would be an excellent or perfect memory?

The most obvious answer is "perfect recall." An individual with a perfect memory, forgetting nothing, would remember every fact, face, and encounter, every mistake he ever made, every injury suffered at the hands of others. But even a little reflection shows that indiscriminate and total recall is not a blessing but a curse. Those who have it suffer like the Jorge Luis Borges character, "Funes, the Memorious," who describes his "all-too-perfect" memory as "a garbage disposal"; or like the famous memory patient Shereshevskii, whose photographic memory prevented him from forming normal human relationships.[2] "Perfect memory" makes those who possess it miserable and dysfunctional.

An excellent memory might instead mean the ability to *remember things as they really are* or *as they actually happen*. Yet mere accuracy of recall without guidance about what is worth remembering would burden us with an inability to separate the important from the trivial. Perhaps, then, an excellent memory would recall accurately only those things that are meaningful, important, or worth remembering. Yet the significance of past events often becomes clear to us only after much rumination in light of later experience, and what seems trivial at one time may appear crucial at another. Neither can an excellent memory be one that remembers only what we *want* to remember: sometimes our most valuable memories are of events that were painful when they occurred, but that on reflection teach us vital lessons.

Speaking loosely, one might suggest that remembering well is *remembering at the right pitch:* neither too much, engulfing us in trivia or imprisoning us in the past, nor too little, losing track of life's defining moments or of knowledge needed for everyday life; neither with too much emotion, allowing past misfortunes to haunt or consume us, nor with too little emotion, recalling what is joyful, or horrible, or inconsequential, all with the same monotone affect.

The difficulty of describing an "excellent memory" makes this a problematic target for those seeking to improve human memory. They will find more likely targets in the various forms of "bad" memories, which are more easily described.

Curiously, some apparent weaknesses of memory are in fact integral to its sound functioning; some of memory's "vices" are inextricably linked to its "virtues." "Sometimes we forget the past and at other times we distort it; some disturbing memories haunt us for years," writes psychologist Daniel Schacter. But these failings of memory, he suggests, are "by-products of otherwise desirable and adaptive features of the human mind."* Put differently, to isolate and seek to "cure" each of memory's individual failures would risk distorting the way memory works as a whole, weaving past, present, and future together in a meaningful way.

Yet many defects of memory are not adaptive but destructive, diminishing life, not facilitating it. Some people just have *weak memories;* owing to

---

* Schacter finds that our memory commits the following "seven sins": transience, absent-mindedness, blocking, misattribution, suggestibility, bias, and persistence. While each of these failings can sometimes be a nuisance, they are also, he argues, necessary for our survival. See Schacter, D., Presentation at the October 2002 meeting of the President's Council on Bioethics, Washington, D.C. Transcript available on the Council's website at www.bioethics.gov; also Schacter, D., *The Seven Sins of Memory: How the Mind Forgets and Remembers,* New York: Houghton Mifflin, 2001, pp. 4 ff.

inborn or acquired defects, they fail to develop normal powers of memory. There is, for the foreseeable future, little anyone can do to help these people.

A far more common problem is *memory loss*. Indeed, most people gradually lose their capacity to remember (especially recent events) as they age, but some do so much more severely. Patients with Alzheimer disease sense early on that memory is beginning to slip away. As the disease progresses, they suffer loss of self-consciousness itself—of life lived, people loved, and the world once known—and cease to live as the persons they once were. The amnesias, caused by trauma and much rarer than dementia, produce some similar results.*

Finally, there are *terrible memories*, a class of destructive memory problems most relevant to the present inquiry concerning happy souls. These troubles result from the lived experience of dreadful events (for example, violent crime or war) or one's own awful deeds (for example, betrayal of a friend or abuse of spouse or child), amplified by the harrowing ways those events or deeds are remembered by especially vulnerable individuals. In certain cases, traumatic memories grossly distort and disfigure the individual's psyche: such people are diagnosed with PTSD. In the most severe cases, the traumatic memories cast a shadow over one's whole life, making the pursuit of happiness impossible.

Whereas weak memory (and weak cognition generally) limits one's ability to become the person one might wish to be, and lost memory destroys one's ability to know who one is, these traumatic memories can make it extremely difficult to live with oneself and with one's life as remembered. All these "bad memories" jeopardize happiness, and, in principle, all offer potentially worthy targets for biotechnological efforts to improve memory. But only the last—the use of drugs to erase or blunt

---

* An individual with "retrograde amnesia" suffers from a sudden loss, either partial or total, of his own memory of the past. His personal past is inaccessible to him; it remains known and remembered only (and necessarily only in part) by others. Though he can learn new things, he remains a stranger to his world, thrown into a life and human relationships that he has no memory of forming. In contrast, an individual with "anterograde amnesia" suffers from the inability to remember new things, new events, or new experiences. The past remains intact as memory, but he is unable to move beyond it. Although the sufferer remains himself, he remains psychically fixed in time, with mind and body, self-consciousness and reality, alienated from one another.

the emotional content of our memories—would give rise to the most serious ethical and social questions. We therefore confine our attention, for the remainder of this analysis, to the emerging pharmacological means for altering our memory of traumatic events.

B. Biotechnology and Memory Alteration

It is a commonplace observation that, while some events fade quickly from the mind, emotionally intense experiences form memories that are peculiarly vivid and long-lasting. Not only do we recall such events long after they happened, but the recollection is often accompanied, in some measure, by a recurrence of the emotions aroused during the original experience. The usefulness—but also the danger—of this natural strengthening of emotionally charged memories was observed already by Descartes more than 350 years ago.* But it is only in our time that scientists have begun to understand the mechanisms by which emotion and memory are linked.

A body of recent research on the formation of long-term memory has established two crucial facts about this phenomenon. First, immediately following a new experience there occurs a period of *memory consolidation,* during which some memories are encoded in the brain with more lasting impact than others. Second, strong emotional arousal is attended by the release of certain *stress hormones* (such as epinephrine, also known as adrenaline), and the presence or absence of these hormones in the brain during the period of memory consolidation greatly affects how strong and durable a memory is formed.

By the early 1990s, research on animals had shown that these stress hormones enhance the encoding of memories by activating the amygdala, a small almond-shaped region of the brain deep inside the temporal

---

* "The utility of all the passions consists only in their fortifying and prolonging in the soul those thoughts which it is good for it to conserve and which otherwise may be easily effaced; as also all the harm they can cause consists in their fortifying and conserving these thoughts more than is needed, or in fortifying and conserving others which ought not to be fixed there." (Descartes, *The Passions of the Soul* [1649], § 74.)

lobe.* Experiments on rats showed that the memory of an experience can be strengthened if epinephrine (which produces high arousal) is injected into the amygdala immediately afterwards; conversely, such memory can be weakened by injecting into the amygdala drugs (called beta-blockers)** that suppress the action of epinephrine.[3]

Research with human subjects broadened these results and shed further light on the neuromodulatory processes that regulate the encoding of memories in the brain. Studies of patients with amnesia confirmed the crucial role of the amygdala in the consolidation of emotionally charged memories. People who have suffered damage to the amygdala typically have no difficulty remembering recent mundane events, but they do not exhibit the enhanced long-term memory normally produced by emotionally arousing experiences. Furthermore, a person with a damaged amygdala will typically recall emotional experiences *without* the normal repetition of the original emotion. In healthy subjects, fearful experiences are encoded with fearful memories, but subjects with amygdala damage often exhibit "abnormal fear response": they have difficulty learning to fear (and hence avoid) dangerous situations because they do not recall fearful events with the appropriate emotion. Evidently, the activation of the amygdala by stress hormones during highly emotional experiences leads to the encoding of memories that are not only more persistent but also more apt to return with the appropriate emotional accompaniment.

The results described above may help to explain what happens when, after living through particularly horrifying experiences, some people experience symptoms of PTSD. When a person experiences especially shocking or violent events (such as a plane crash or bloody combat), the release of stress

---

* As crucial as animal research is to providing insight about the workings of human memory, we must also keep in mind the limits of the comparison. The character of human memory is so distinct, involving experiences so foreign to other animals, that shared systems of the brain may have very different functional and experiential meanings, and crucial subtleties may be lost in seeing only the broad neurological similarities. The hazard of extrapolating too much from other animals to human beings is always present in research—but perhaps especially in the case of memory and other psychological-moral experiences that are singularly human.

** Beta-blockers—more precisely, beta-adrenergic receptor antagonists—such as propranolol were originally developed in the 1960s (and today are still chiefly used) for the prevention and treatment of heart disease and hypertension.

hormones may be so intense that the memory-encoding system is over-activated. The result is a consolidation of memories both far stronger and more persistent than normal and also more apt, upon recollection, to call forth the intense emotional response of the original experience. In such cases, each time the person relives the traumatic memory, a new flood of stress hormones is released, and the experience may be so emotionally intense as to be encoded as a new experience. With time, the memories grow more recurrent and intrusive, and the response—fear, helplessness, horror—more incapacitating. As we shall see, drugs that might prevent or alleviate the symptoms of PTSD are among the chief medical benefits that scientists expect from recent research in the neurochemistry of memory formation.

In fact, the discovery of hormonal regulation of memory formation was quickly followed up by clinical studies on human subjects demonstrating that memory of emotional experiences can be altered pharmacologically. In one particularly interesting series of experiments, Larry Cahill and his colleagues showed that injections of beta-blockers can, by inhibiting the action of stress hormones, suppress the memory-enhancing effects of strong emotional arousal. The researchers showed their subjects a series of slides and told them one of two stories to explain the events depicted; one story was mundane and emotionally neutral, the other was tragic and emotionally gripping. Two weeks later, the participants were asked to recall the story, and those who had heard the emotionally arousing story were found—as expected—to recall what was depicted in the slides in far greater detail than those who had heard the mundane version. The experiment was then repeated, except that half the participants were given an injection of the beta-blocker propranolol and half were injected with a saline placebo one hour before the slide show. What they found was that, after two weeks, those who had heard the more mundane version of the story had the same level of recollection regardless of whether they had received the beta-blocker or the placebo. But of the subjects who had heard the more arousing version of the story, only those receiving the placebo showed an enhanced level of recollection. Those who heard the arousing story after receiving the beta-blocker found it extremely sad and emotional at the time, but two weeks later they remembered it at the same emotional level as the group that had heard the neutral story.[4]

Thus, taking propranolol appears to have little or no effect on how we remember everyday or emotionally neutral information. But when taken at the time of highly emotional experiences, propranolol appears to suppress the normal memory-enhancing effects of emotional arousal—while leaving the immediate emotional response unaffected. These results suggested the possibility of using beta-blockers to help survivors of traumatic events to reduce their intrusive—and in some cases crippling—memories of those events. In 2002 Roger K. Pitman and his colleagues published a pilot study reporting the use of propranolol administered to emergency room patients within six hours after a traumatic experience (mostly car accidents) and for an additional ten days thereafter. The patients—both those taking the drug and those taking placebos—were tested for their psychological and physiological response to a re-telling (with related images) of the traumatic event. One month after the event, those taking propranolol showed measurably lower incidence of PTSD symptoms than the control group. And three months later, while the PTSD symptoms of both groups had returned to comparable levels, the propranolol group showed measurably lower psycho-physiological response to "internal cues (that is, mental imagery) that symbolized or resembled the initial traumatic event."[5]

This study, while very preliminary, suggests that drugs may become available that will enable us not only to soften certain powerful memories but to detach them from the strong emotions evoked by the original experience. Propranolol and other currently available beta-blockers may not be able to do the whole job,* and, until more evidence is acquired, we do well to regard them as weak precursors of subsequent drugs that might be more powerful and effective. Yet the prospect of such "memory numbing" drugs has already elicited considerable public interest in and concern about their potential uses in non-clinical settings: to prepare a soldier to kill (or kill again) on the battlefield; to dull the sting of one's own shameful acts; to allow a criminal to numb the memory of his or her victims.[6]

---

* Long-time and sizable clinical experience with beta-blockers in treatment of heart disease and hypertension has not revealed memory defects or personality change to be major side effects. Yet one might not expect to see their memory-blunting power except in the face of the huge adrenaline outpourings associated with frightening and horrifying experiences.

Some of these scenarios are perhaps far-fetched. But although the pharmacology of memory alteration is a science still in its infancy, the significance of this potential new power—to separate the subjective experience of memory from the truth of the experience that is remembered—should not be underestimated. It surely returns us to the large ethical and anthropological questions with which we began—about memory's role in shaping personal identity and the character of human life, and about the meaning of remembering things that we would rather forget and of forgetting things that we perhaps ought to remember.

C. Memory-Blunting: Ethical Analysis

If we had the power, by promptly taking a memory-altering drug, to dull the emotional impact of what could become very painful memories, when might we be tempted to use it? And for what reasons should we yield to or resist the temptation?

At first glance, such a drug would seem ideally suited for the prevention of PTSD, the complex of debilitating symptoms that sometimes afflict those who have experienced severe trauma. These symptoms— which include persistent re-experiencing of the traumatic event and avoidance of every person, place, or thing that might stimulate the horrid memory's return[7]—can so burden mental life as to make normal everyday living extremely difficult, if not impossible.* For those suffering these disturbing symptoms, a drug that could separate a painful memory from its powerful emotional component would appear very welcome indeed.

Yet the prospect of preventing (even) PTSD with beta-blockers or other memory-blunting agents seems to be, for several reasons, problematic. First

---

* These symptoms are observed especially among combat veterans; indeed, PTSD is the modern name for what used to be called "shell shock" or "combat neurosis." Among veterans, PTSD is frequently associated with recurrent nightmares, substance abuse, and delusional outbursts of violence. There is controversy about the prevalence of PTSD, with some studies finding that up to 8 percent of adult Americans have suffered the disorder, as well as a third of all veterans of the Vietnam War. See Kessler, R. C., et al., "Post-Traumatic Stress Disorder in the National Comorbidity Survey," *Archives of General Psychiatry* 52(12): 1048-1060, 1995; Kulka, R. A., et al., *Trauma and the Vietnam War Generation: Report of Findings from the National Vietnam Veterans Readjustment Study*, New York: Brunner/Mazel, 1990.

of all, the drugs in question appear to be effective only when administered during or shortly after a traumatic event—and thus well before any symptoms of PTSD would be manifested. How then could we make, and make on the spot, the *prospective* judgment that a particular event is sufficiently terrible to warrant preemptive memory-blunting? Second, how shall we judge *which* participants in the event merit such treatment? After all, not everyone who suffers through painful experiences is destined to have pathological memory effects. Should the drugs in question be given to everyone or only to those with an observed susceptibility to PTSD, and, if the latter, how will we know who these are? Finally, in some cases merely witnessing a disturbing event (for example, a murder, rape, or terrorist attack) is sufficient to cause PTSD-like symptoms long afterwards. Should we then, as soon as disaster strikes, consider giving memory-altering drugs to all the witnesses, in addition to those directly involved?

These questions point to other troubling implications. Use of memory-blunters at the time of traumatic events could interfere with the normal psychic work and adaptive value of emotionally charged memory. A primary function of the brain's special way of encoding memories for emotional experiences would seem to be to make us remember important events longer and more vividly than trivial events. Thus, by blunting their emotional impact, beta-blockers or their successors would concomitantly weaken our recollection of the traumatic events we have just experienced. Yet often it is important, in the aftermath of such events, that at least someone remembers them clearly. For legal reasons, to say nothing of deeper social and personal ones, the wisdom of routinely interfering with the memories of trauma survivors and witnesses is highly questionable.

If the apparent powers of memory-blunting drugs are confirmed, some might be inclined to prescribe them liberally to all who are involved in a sufficiently terrible event. After all, even those not destined to come down with full-blown PTSD are likely to suffer painful recurrent memories of an airplane crash, an incident of terrorism, or a violent combat operation. In the aftermath of such shocking incidents, why not give everyone the chance to remember these events without the added burden of painful emotions? This line of reasoning might, in fact, tempt us to give beta-blockers liberally to soldiers on the eve of combat, to emergency

workers en route to a disaster site, or even to individuals requesting pro-
phylaxis against the shame or guilt they might incur from future mis-
deeds—in general, to anyone facing an experience that is likely to leave
lasting intrusive memories.

Yet on further reflection it seems clear that not every intrusive memory is a suitable candidate for prospective pharmacological blunting. As
Daniel Schacter has observed, "attempts to avoid traumatic memories
often backfire":

> Intrusive memories need to be acknowledged, confronted, and
> worked through, in order to set them to rest for the long term.
> Unwelcome memories of trauma are symptoms of a disrupted psy-
> che that requires attention before it can resume healthy functioning.
> Beta-blockers might make it easier for trauma survivors to face and
> incorporate traumatic recollections, and in that sense could facilitate
> long-term adaptation. Yet it is also possible that beta-blockers would
> work against the normal process of recovery: traumatic memories
> would not spring to mind with the kind of psychological force that
> demands attention and perhaps intervention. Prescription of beta-
> blockers could bring about an effective trade-off between short-term
> reductions in the sting of traumatic memories and long-term
> increases in persistence of related symptoms of a trauma that has not
> been adequately confronted.[8]

The point can be generalized: in the immediate aftermath of a painful
experience, we simply cannot know either the full meaning of the experience in question or the ultimate character and future prospects of the
individual who experiences it. We cannot know how this experience will
change this person at this time and over time. Will he be cursed forever by
unbearable memories that, in retrospect, clearly should have been blunted
medically? Or will he succeed, over time, in "redeeming" those painful
memories by actively integrating them into the narrative of his life? By
"rewriting" memories pharmacologically we might succeed in easing real
suffering at the risk of falsifying our perception of the world and under-
mining our true identity.

Finally, the decision whether or not to use memory-blunting drugs must be made in the absence of clearly diagnosable disease. The drug must be taken right after a traumatic experience has occurred, and thus before the different ways that different individuals handle the same experience has become clear. In some cases, these interventions will turn out to have been preventive medicine, intervening to ward off the onset of PTSD before it arrives—though it is worth noting that we would lack even post hoc knowledge of whether any particular now-unaffected individual, in the absence of using the drug, would have become symptomatic.* In other cases, the interventions would not be medicine at all: altering the memory of individuals who could have lived well, even with severely painful memories, without pharmacologically dulling the pain. Worse, in still other cases, the use of such drugs would inoculate individuals in advance against the psychic pain that *should* accompany their commission of cruel, brutal, or shameful deeds. But in all cases, from the defensible to the dubious, the use of such powers changes the character of human memory, by intervening directly in the way individuals "encode," and thus the way they understand, the happenings of their own lives and the realities of the world around them. Sorting out how and why this matters, and especially what it means for our idea of human happiness, is the focus of the more particular—albeit brief—ethical reflections that follow.

1. Remembering Fitly and Truly

Altering the formation of emotionally powerful memories risks severing what we remember from how we remember it and distorting the link between our perception of significant human events and the significance of the events themselves. It risks, in a word, falsifying our perception and understanding of the world. It risks making shameful acts seem less shameful, or terrible acts less terrible, than they really are.

---

* There is already ongoing controversy about excessive diagnosis of PTSD. Many psychotherapists believe that a patient's psychic troubles are generally based on some earlier (now repressed) traumatic experience which must be unearthed and dealt with if relief is to be found. True PTSD is, however, generally transient, and the search for treatment is directed against the symptoms of its initial (worst) phase—the sleeplessness, the nightmares, the excessive jitteriness.

Imagine the experience of a person who witnesses a shocking murder. Fearing that he will be haunted by images of this event, he immediately takes propranolol (or its more potent successor) to render his memory of the murder less painful and intrusive. Thanks to the drug, his memory of the murder gets encoded as a garden-variety, emotionally neutral experience. But in manipulating his memory in this way, he risks coming to think about the murder as more tolerable than it really is, as an event that should not sting those who witness it. For our opinions about the meaning of our experiences are shaped partly by the feelings evoked when we remember them. If, psychologically, the murder is transformed into an event our witness can recall without pain—or without *any* particular emotion—perhaps its moral significance will also fade from consciousness. If so, he would in a sense have ceased to be a genuine witness of the murder. When asked about it, he might say, "Yes, I was there. But it wasn't so terrible."

This points us to a deeper set of questions about bad memories: Would dulling our memory of terrible things make us too comfortable with the world, unmoved by suffering, wrongdoing, or cruelty? Does not the experience of hard truths—of the unchosen, the inexplicable, the tragic—remind us that we can never be fully at home in the world, especially if we are to take seriously the reality of human evil? Further, by blunting our experience and awareness of shameful, fearful, and hateful things, might we not also risk deadening our response to what is admirable, inspiring, and lovable? Can we become numb to life's sharpest sorrows without also becoming numb to its greatest joys?

These questions point to what might be the highest cost of making our memory of intolerable things more tolerable: Armed with new powers to ease the suffering of bad memories, we might come to see all psychic pain as unnecessary and in the process come to pursue a happiness that is less than human: an unmindful happiness, unchanged by time and events, unmoved by life's vicissitudes. More precisely, we might come to pursue such happiness by willingly abandoning or compromising our own truthful identities: instead of integrating, as best we can, the troubling events of our lives into a more coherent whole, we might just prefer to edit them out or make them less difficult to live with than they really are.

There seems to be little doubt that some bitter memories are so painful and intrusive as to ruin the possibility for normal experience of much of life and the world. In such cases the impulse to relieve a crushing burden and restore lost innocence is fully understandable: If there are some things that it is better never to have experienced at all—things we would avoid if we possibly could—why not erase them from the memory of those unfortunate enough to have suffered them? If there are some things it is better never to have known or seen, why not use our power over memory to restore a witness's shattered peace of mind? There is great force in this argument, perhaps especially in cases where children lose prematurely that innocence that is rightfully theirs.

And yet, there may be a great cost to acting compassionately for those who suffer bad memories, if we do so by compromising the truthfulness of how they remember. We risk having them live falsely in order simply to cope, to survive by whatever means possible. Among the larger falsehoods to which such practices could lead us, few are more problematic than the extreme beliefs regarding the possibility—and impossibility—of human control. Erring on the one side, we might come to imagine ourselves as having more control over our memories and identities than we really do, believing that we can be authors and editors of our memories while still remaining truly—and true to—ourselves. Erring on the other side, we might come to imagine that we are impotently in the grip of the past as we look to the future, believing that we can never learn to live with this particular memory or give it new meaning. And so we ease today's pain, but only by foreclosing, in a certain way, the possibility of being the kind of person who can live well with the whole truth—both chosen and unchosen—and the kind of person who can live well as himself.

2. The Obligation to Remember

Having truthful memories is not simply a personal matter. Strange to say, our own memory is not merely our own; it is part of the fabric of the society in which we live. Consider the case of a person who has suffered or witnessed atrocities that occasion unbearable memories: for example, those with firsthand experience of the Holocaust. The life of that individual might well be served by dulling such bitter memories,* but such a humanitarian intervention, if widely practiced, would seem deeply troubling: Would the community as a whole—would the human race—be served by such a mass numbing of this terrible but indispensable memory? Do those who suffer evil have a duty to remember and bear witness, lest we all forget the very horrors that haunt them? (The examples of this dilemma need not be quite so stark: the memory of being embarrassed is a source of empathy for others who suffer embarrassment; the memory of losing a loved one is a source of empathy for those who experience a similar loss.) Surely, we cannot and should not force those who live through great trauma to endure its painful memory *for the benefit of the rest of us.* But as a community, there are certain events that we have an obligation to remember—an obligation that falls disproportionately, one might even say unfairly, on those who experience such events most directly.[9] What kind of people would we be if we did not "want" to remember the Holocaust, if we sought to make the anguish it caused simply go away? And yet, what kind of people are we, especially those who face such horrors firsthand, that we can endure such awful memories?

The answer, in part, is that those who suffer terrible things cannot or should not have to endure their own bad memories alone. If, as a people, we have an obligation to remember certain terrible events truthfully, surely we ought to help those who suffered through those events to come to terms with their worst memories. Of course, one might see the new biotechnical powers, developed precisely to ease the psychic pain of bad memories, as the mark of such solidarity: perhaps it is our new way of meeting the obligation to aid those who remember the hardest things, those who bear witness to us and for us. But such solidarity may, in the end, prove false: for it exempts us from the duty to suffer-with (literally, to feel *com*-passion for) those who remember; it does not

---

* Of course, many Holocaust survivors managed, without pharmacological assistance, to live fulfilling lives while never forgetting what they lived through. At the same time, many survivors would almost certainly have benefited from pharmacological treatment.

demand that we preserve the truth of their memories; it attempts instead to make the problem go away, and with it the truth of the experience in question.

3. Memory and Moral Responsibility

The question of how responsible we are or should be held for our memories, especially our memory failures, is a complicated one: Are remembering and forgetting voluntary or involuntary acts? To what extent should a man who forgets his child in a car, by mistake, be held "morally accountable" for his forgetting? Is remembering "something we do" or "something that happens to us"?

Hard as these questions are, this much seems clear: Without memory, both our own and that of others, the notion of moral responsibility would largely unravel. In particular, the power to numb or eliminate the psychic sting of certain memories risks eroding the responsibility we take for our own actions—since we would never have to face the harsh judgment of our own conscience (Lady Macbeth) or the memory of others. The risk applies both to self-serving uses of such a power (for example, drugs taken after a criminal act and before the next one) and to more ambiguous "social" uses (for example, drugs taken after killing in war and before killing again). Without truthful memory, we could not hold others or ourselves to account for what we do and who we are. Without truthful memory, there could be no justice or even the possibility of justice; without memory, there could be no forgiveness or the possibility of forgiveness—all would simply be *forgotten*.

The desire for powers that numb our most painful memories is largely a personal desire: to have such drugs for myself, in the service of my own peace of mind and happiness. Yet we cannot be blind to the potentially coercive and immoral uses—by other individuals and by the state—of biotechnical interventions that alter how we remember and what we forget, and that indirectly affect our well-being. Just as drugs that dull the emotional sting of certain memories might be desired by the victim to ease his trauma, so they might be useful to the assailant to dull his victim's sense of being wronged. Perhaps no one has a greater interest in blocking the painful memory of evil than the evildoer. We also cannot ignore the potentially coercive nature of normalizing the use of such drugs in certain occupations: that is, by making chemically aided desensitization part of the "job description" (augmenting or replacing existing non-chemical means of desensitization). Nor can we forget the central place of manipulating memory in totalitarian societies, both real and imagined, and the way such manipulation made living truthfully—and living happily—impossible.

4. The Soul of Memory, The Remembering Soul

Perhaps more than any other subject in this report, memory is puzzling. It is both central to who we are as individuals and as a society, yet very hard to pin down—so variable in its many meanings and many manifestations. Jane Austen may have captured this complexity best:

> If any one faculty of our nature may be called more wonderful than the rest, I do think it is memory. There seems something more speakingly incomprehensible in the powers, the failures, the inequalities of memory, than in any other of our intelligences. The memory is sometimes so retentive, so serviceable, so obedient—at others, so bewildered and so weak—and at others again, so tyrannical, so beyond control!—We are to be sure a miracle every way—but our powers of recollecting and of forgetting, do seem peculiarly past finding out.[10]

On the one hand, when considering the meaning of human memory, we need to face the fact that there are limits to our control over who we are and what we become. We are not free to decide everything that happens to us; some experiences, both great joys and terrible misfortunes, simply befall us. These experiences become part of who we are, part of our own life as truthfully lived. And yet, we do have some measure of freedom in *how* we live with such memories—the meaning we assign them, the place we give them in the larger narrative of our lives. But this meaning is not simply arbitrary; it must connect the truth or significance of the events themselves, as they really were and really are, with our own continuing pursuit of a full and happy life. In doing so, we might often be tempted to sacrifice the accuracy of our memories for the sake of easing our pain or expanding our control over our own psychic lives. But doing so means, ultimately, severing ourselves from reality and leaving our own identity behind; it risks making us false, small, or capable of great illusions, and thus capable of great decadence or great evil, or perhaps simply willing to accept a phony contentment. We might be tempted to alter our memories to preserve an open future—to live the life we wanted to live before a particular experience happened to us. But in another sense, such interventions assume that our own future is not open—that we cannot and could never redeem the unwanted memory over time, that we cannot and could never integrate the remembered experience with our own truthful pursuit of happiness.

In the end, we must wonder what life would be like—and what kind of a people we would become—with only happy memories, with everything difficult, uncertain, and hard edited out of our lives as we remembered and understood them. We would suffer no loss, but perhaps only because we loved feebly and cared little for what we had. We would never shudder at life's injustices, but perhaps only because we had little interest in justice. We would little relish our own achievements, since we would achieve them without any memory of hardship along the way and with no recollection of achieving in spite of the odds. To have only happy memories would be a blessing—and a curse. Nothing would trouble us, but we would probably be shallow people, never falling to the depths of despair because we have little interest in the heights of human happiness or in the complicated lives of those around us. In the end, to have only happy memories is not to be happy in a truly human way. It is simply to be free of misery—an understandable desire given the many troubles of life, but a low aspiration for those who seek a truly human happiness.

III. MOOD AND HAPPINESS

Even more than memory, mood conditions and is conditioned by our happiness. Thoughtful reflection reveals that memory is crucial to human happiness because it links our present identity with our past deeds and experiences; but the connection between mood and happiness (and also unhappiness) is self-evident to all. Indeed, the content of our happiness seems at first glance to be largely a function of our present mood: the word "happy" is normally taken as the opposite of "sad," and the question, "Are you happy?" is typically understood as an inquiry about one's mood. Yet although many people, if asked, might say that being happy and being in a good mood are one and the same, the truth of the matter is not so simple. If happiness were nothing other than "good mood," it would seem to follow that anything that elevates one's mood automatically increases one's happiness. And if that were the case, the development of safe and effective mood-elevating drugs—not only for the clinically depressed but also for the merely sad or discontented—would seem to herald a future blessed by ever-greater numbers of ever-happier people. But, as we shall see, closer examination reveals that the connection between mood and happiness is much more subtle, and the prospects for making people happy through pharmacology are much more ambiguous.

The first complication concerns "mood" itself: what it is, and how to think about it. Narrowly understood, "mood" refers to a frame of mind or state of feeling: "I am feeling blue," "I am in a grumpy mood," or "I am in the mood for dancing." These more or less transient feeling states come and go, shifting or persisting in ways over which we have only limited control. Although they rise and fall as we prosper or fail in the things we try to do from day to day, our moods are also at the mercy of fortune. They may be soured by hunger, fatigue, or illness; they may be sweetened by a call from an old friend, a kindness shown to a stranger, or a simply beautiful day; they may soar into ecstasy at the birth of a child, they may sink into despair at the death of a spouse.

Yet beneath our shifting moods are more pervasive and persistent dispositions of feeling, commonly called "temperaments."* Temperament is the general orientation of "feeling," "mood," and "outlook" that we bring

---

* The term harkens back to the time when these dispositions were thought to be the result of the temper, or balance, of the body's so-called "four humors": blood, phlegm, bile, and black bile. As a result of insufficiently tempered mixtures, so the theory had it, persons with an unbalanced excess of one or another of the humors would be of sanguine, phlegmatic, choleric, or melancholic temperaments. It has been noted that current scientific efforts to tie temperaments to various imbalances in neurotransmitter levels in the brain may be regarded as a modern scientific "revival" of the idea that "humoral tempering" is central to determining our emotional outlooks.

to all experience and on which particular experiences work to produce the various and shifting states of emotion. It is our temperament that inclines us toward being generally upbeat or gloomy, hopeful or fearful, extroverted or introverted, emotionally quick and mercurial or emotionally slow and phlegmatic. Seen through the wider lens of temperament, "mood" means more than cheerful or sad, "good mood" or "bad." It covers the ranges between—and combinations among—being confident and reticent, outgoing and shy, bold and timid, engaged and apathetic, excitable and calm, irascible and easygoing, ambitious and lazy, proud and humble. Although rooted in some combination of inborn natural gifts and altered by nurture and experience, temperament is also somewhat shapable through habituation into more or less stable traits of character: depending on how we recurrently react to fearful situations, we become more courageous, cowardly, or rash; depending on how we recurrently react to other people, we become more amiable, unfriendly, or obsequious. Although temperaments are centrally matters of feeling or emotion, they are also related to awareness and thought. They will both color and be colored by opinions and beliefs we have about the world and about ourselves. People with unduly high expectations are probably more easily disappointed and discouraged; people who believe that "selfish genes" govern behavior may be less troubled by their own moral failings; people who trust in a loving and forgiving God may be less susceptible to despair.

As these last comments indicate, mood and temperament are not only outward-looking and responsive to worldly happenings. They are also much connected with our inner sense of self. Animals no doubt experience feelings of pleasure and pain, fear and calm, frustration and satisfaction, and something that looks from the outside like spiritedness, anger, and even pride. But it is unlikely that they harbor humankind's explicitly judgmental feelings of self-love, self-esteem, self-worth, self-doubt, and self-loathing, especially as these are tied in human beings *to some explicit or tacit idea of who one thinks one is, judged in relation to who one thinks one should be and (especially) in relation to others.* Some of us are very hard on ourselves, filled with self-criticism and doubt about self-worth at even the smallest falling short; others of us are very self-content or even self-indulgent, able to brush aside even large failures with what looks like blithe indifference. Like the other temperaments, the self-regarding dispositions are, of course, not simply inborn and fixed; cumulative life experience, including our history of genuine successes and failures, no doubt contributes much. But self-demanding perfectionists are unlikely to turn into laid-back "accommodationists," especially from life experience alone. Accordingly, these self-regarding feelings and dispositions—no less than our basic temperaments and supervening moods—play a major role in whether we find satisfaction in life, or the opposite.

A second difficulty concerns the range and "spectral" character of moods, however narrowly or broadly defined. Human moods, temperaments, and attitudes of self-regard vary enormously in character, intensity, and persistence, as well as in their effects on the way each of us lives our lives. The possible combinations of particular dispositional traits seem virtually limitless, and they defy the capacity of ordinary language to describe them accurately and fully, *even for any one individual.* One feeling or mood blends into another, and all of them admit of degree. When we analytically separate out any one dimension for description—say, for example, the range from cheerful to gloomy—we notice that people distribute themselves along a full and continuous spectrum of "normal" mood states and dispositions, and this seems true across the board.

Yet it is clear that there are many individuals who are not emotionally normal, whose psyches are "taken over" for long periods of time by a dominant and debilitating mood or outlook. They live in the grip of profound sadness, hopelessness, or despair, or of panic and terror regarding social situations, or unrelieved guilt, shame, or feelings of abject unworthiness. Not liking the way they feel and are, sometimes suicidal and often desperate for help, these people bring themselves (or are brought by others) to the doctor's door, where, fortunately, in many cases real help is increasingly available. Indeed, vast numbers of people suffering persisting and disabling disorders of mood and temperament are today diagnosed and treated by psychiatrists and other physicians for numerous affective disorders, including major depression, bipolar disorder, social anxiety disorder, obsessive-compulsive disorder, oppositional disorder, and the like. Scientists increasingly believe that most of these psychic disorders are—like schizophrenia—partly the product of, or at least correlated with, certain underlying abnormalities and (partially heritable) disorders in the brain. Yet there are at present no specific diagnostic tests to prove the point. For this reason, it is often hard to determine whether any given individual suffering the symptoms that define these disorders belongs simply to the extreme end of a spectral distribution of "normal" temperaments or rather to a separate "class" of people with a specific brain disorder. What is, however, easy to recognize is the enormous misery these symptoms and conditions cause, and the further fact that such patients often respond well to so-called "mood-altering" or "mood-brightening" drugs.

The different meanings of "mood" and the wide range of their character, both negative and positive, give rise to a third complication regarding the relation of mood and happiness, this one regarding human aspiration: What mood or moods, what states of feeling, what emotional outlook on life and self do we aspire to? As one would expect, our aspirations in this realm are many and varied. Some of us, depressed or despairing, crave merely a cessation of pain, our troubles lifted. Some of us, bored or listless, would like spikes of bliss—to get "high"—and some would even want that bliss perpetually, if that were possible. Some would prefer simply peace or contentment, never to be sad again. Some would have their dispositions brightened and stabilized, inhibitions eased, optimism and resilience gained or restored. Some strive for the best experiences—falling in love, attaining some honor, performing at one's best—in order to enjoy the good feelings and self-esteem that accompany those experiences, whereas others would be satisfied by the feelings alone, without actually having to endure the work, hardship, and risk of failure. As this variety suggests, while the desire for happiness is universal, the content of happiness is elusive, opinions and wishes varying from person to person depending in part on "where we start," "who we are," and what we desire as the things most needful. Increasingly, however, both our culture's preoccupation with "how we feel about ourselves," and especially the availability of mood-altering drugs that can change those feelings, have encouraged us to treat "states of mind"—mood, feeling, disposition—as goals and targets that can be separated and pursued apart from the actions and experiences they normally accompany.

In the remainder of this discussion, and very mindful of all the ambiguities and uncertainties involved in doing so, we will use "mood" in the very broadest sense, to embrace the transient and supervening states of feeling, the basic underlying temperaments, and the emotionally charged outlooks we have on ourselves and the world. Any of them, if negative and severe enough, mars the chance for happiness. Any of them, if sufficiently enduring and disabling, deserves to be classified as illness or disease. All of them are in principle subject to pharmacological intervention, if not today, very likely sometime soon. Given the wide variety of mood-altering agents, present and projected, and given our ignorance of the precise effect any particular drug will bring about in any given person, we are somewhat at a loss about what to call these chemicals: "antidepressants" seems too narrow, "mood-altering-agents" too non-specific, "mood-elevators" or "mood-brighteners" too specialized, "euphoriants" inaccurate.* Moreover, no single name describes a drug that, in different people, can alleviate depression, calm panic, moderate compulsions, boost confidence, or improve self-esteem. Somewhat arbitrarily, we will use "mood-brighteners," despite the inaccuracy, so as to keep before us their ability not only to lift mood but also to improve the outlook of the person, including about himself.

A. Mood-Improvement Through Drugs

Whereas drugs designed to alter memory are new, mood-altering agents are not. Alcohol and opiates have been with us for centuries. Doctors first used lithium for its mood-stabilizing effects in the early twentieth century. Since the 1950s, psychiatrists have used tricyclics and monoamine-oxidase inhibitors (or their precursors) to treat depression. The desire to use these

---

* The difficulty in describing the effects of psychotropic agents is very likely inherent in the difficulty in describing the psychic phenomena themselves. Regarding our "inner experience," we are often stuck with metaphors—"higher," "brighter," "depressed"—including the spatial metaphor of "inwardness" itself. We return to this topic when we treat the effects of some of the drugs now most commonly in use.

and other technological means to take control of our mood abides and likely will abide so long as there are human beings who wish for happiness and do not have it. The desire being so strong and the technologies so familiar, we have developed a network of laws, social taboos, professional standards, and understandings of risks, both physical and moral, through which we more or less manage the technologies' use—though there continue to be many casualties along the way, and alcoholism and drug abuse remain massive social problems. Now, as rapid advances in scientific and medical research are producing new technologies of feeling—safer, more powerful, and more specific than any that came before—there is reason to suspect that our laws, knowledge, and ethical practice are lagging behind our technology. So we must ask anew what to think of the powers over mood we are in the midst of developing. The question, if more familiar, is also more pressing than any connected with powers over memory, for the technologies of mood-control are not only coming but already here.

1. Mood-Brightening Agents: An Overview

We already have at our disposal a wide range of newer psychotropic agents useful in altering mood, some named above. But selective serotonin reuptake inhibitors (SSRIs), such as Prozac, Paxil, Zoloft, Celexa, Lexapro, and Effexor, stand out.* SSRIs are the newest and most advanced mood-brighteners available. There is nothing futuristic about them—a recent poll suggests one in eight adult Americans use them today, mostly as treatment for diagnosed illness[11]—yet they give some sense of what mood-brightening technologies are to come, at least in the near future. Their effects appear to be far-reaching, touching not only those with obvious mental illness but also those in the penumbra of depression, those with merely melancholy or inhibited temperaments, and possibly those who are emotionally or temperamentally balanced or normal.[12] But their effects and the reason for their effects are not understood with any precision.

---

* Effexor also inhibits norepinephrine and is sometimes referred to as an SNRI (serotonin-norepinephrine reuptake inhibitor). In this chapter, for convenience, it can be assumed under the heading of SSRI. Some other agents, such as the aminoketone Wellbutrin, are used in ways similar to SSRIs; the analysis that follows may also apply or apply partially to them.

They are fairly safe and non-addictive, and they are legal, yet there is no consensus in America about the limits of their appropriate use. A public conversation has begun, but only begun.[13] While we will focus much of our discussion on SSRIs—with occasional turns to other mood-elevating drugs, such as MDMA (methylenedioxy-n-methylamphetamine, or "Ecstasy")—we also keep in mind the prospect of more advanced pharmacological means for altering mood in the not-too-distant future. We are interested not in the SSRIs as such, but in the insights we might gain from their current uses regarding the ethical and social implications of mood-brightening pharmacology in general, today and especially tomorrow.

As we noted at the start of this chapter, medical researchers developed SSRIs, and doctors by and large prescribe them, not to stave off ordinary unhappiness, but to treat major depression and other emotional problems so disabling as to indicate the presence of mental illness. For these conditions, the drugs are true medicines of great benefit. In efforts to help those afflicted with the worst anxieties and depressions, those sliding into similar afflictions, and those suffering psychic pain severe enough—diagnosable illness or not—to make claims on a doctor's duty to save (that is, those at risk of suicide), SSRIs are often indispensable, and patients and doctors have every reason to use them.[14] As far as we know, most prescription and use of SSRIs are of this therapeutic character.

Yet some doctors are prescribing mood-brighteners for people whose troubles are not so severe and whose neurochemistry may not be abnormal. This should not be surprising or shocking, given that the boundaries between mental illness and misery or between mental health and happiness are not easily drawn. Physicians are prescribing for patients with lesser and lesser forms of depression, psychiatrist Peter Kramer has argued, precisely because Prozac and similar drugs can give them relief, a classic case in which the availability of a technology of cure drives, and expands, the definition of illness.[15] But whether or not diagnostic categories are being expanded, and properly or not, two separate human enterprises—curing mental illness and pursuing happiness—appear to be converging, because of the development of medicines so effective that their use overshoots the illness for which they were developed and because they aid or seem to aid the realization of ordinary human desires for happier souls.

Also worth noting at the outset is the astonishing variety of individual situations for which people use these drugs and the diverse effects they have on users' minds and lives. No single ethical inquiry can hope to discuss, much less resolve, the questions attending every particular case of use. Moreover, much hard-to-design empirical research would be needed to verify whether the troubling consequences that ethical reflection identifies as possible are in fact coming to pass. The subject is too subtle, the emotional lives of human beings too diverse and elusively complex. Yet many of our ethical and social questions cannot on those grounds be set aside.

The millions of Americans now taking SSRIs are probably only the beginning. Epidemiologists widely consider depression to be *under*treated in America: according to recent studies, between 9.5 percent and 20 percent of Americans suffer from some form of depression.[16] If all were treated with mood-brighteners, one out of every five to ten people would use them. Moreover, the rate of diagnosed depression appears to be climbing in the United States, as in all developed countries—probably due not just to greater reporting, but to real increase.[17] At the same time, the diagnosis of depression seems to be expanding to include lesser and lesser forms of sadness,[18] while more and more conditions besides depression (social phobia, obsessive-compulsive disorder, and many others) are being treated with mood-brighteners.[19] Although data is hard to come by, according to some reports as many as 20 percent of students on elite college campuses now take or have taken prescription mood-brighteners.[20] As these trends dovetail with new drugs still to come, whose risk and side-effect profiles may well be increasingly gentle, use of mood-brighteners will almost certainly expand.

In light, then, of both present actualities and future possibilities, we need now to deepen our understanding of mood-brighteners, and to evaluate their human costs as well as their benefits, as we strive to reach sensible judgments about how they should be used. At stake are not only questions of private health and happiness, but also, as we shall see, questions regarding the character of American society.

2. Biological and Experiential Effects of SSRIs

Assessment begins with trying to understand the effects of SSRIs, both on the brain and on felt human experience. In both cases, we know only a little of what we seek to know, and still less about the connection between the biological and experiential effects.

Neurologically, what SSRIs do is alter the brain's handling of serotonin. Like other neurotransmitters, serotonin is released from one neuron to bind with and thereby activate another. The brain recycles serotonin after each release, gathering it up again by means of a "reuptake system." SSRIs inhibit the serotonin reuptake system, thus increasing the concentration of serotonin available to the receiving neurons—hence the name, "serotonin reuptake inhibitor." (Since SSRIs inhibit serotonin reuptake without interfering with reuptake of other neurotransmitters, we get the full name, "selective serotonin reuptake inhibitor.") When given to patients diagnosed with mood disorders, SSRIs brighten or stabilize moods in most of them, presumably as a result of the increased availability of serotonin in certain crucial places in the brain.

Scientists do not yet know how inhibiting the reuptake of serotonin alters the mental state. What serotonin does, how it functions, and even whether it is a serotonin problem that causes depression in the first place, remain largely unknown.[21] Serotonin does not alter mood directly, such that more of it produces more pleasure or confidence and less of it the opposite; that much is clear. Serotonin is not an opiate or a euphoriant. But just what does happen when more or less serotonin is available— whether mood is eventually reoriented by some plastic development in the brain, or by some other downstream effect, some subtle influence over feeling, perceiving, and thinking, or something else entirely—is at present a mystery.* Neuroscience is a young field; many of the powers it is yield-

---

* There is some evidence that major depression may be associated with reduced volume in the hippocampus, perhaps reflecting a loss of neurons in that part of the brain; furthermore, very recent studies suggest that treatment with SSRIs (as well as other antidepressants) leads to significant neurogenesis (new growth of neuron cells) in the hippocampus. It is, however, far too early to say whether hippocampal atrophy is a major cause of depression, or whether the antidepressant efficacy of SSRIs and other drugs is in fact mediated by stimulation of neurogenesis. See Sheline, Y. I., et al., "Hippocampal atrophy in recurrent major depression," *Proceedings of the National*

ing arrive in advance of its capacity to understand them. And even if we knew more about brain chemistry and its functional significance, it is not clear that such knowledge would be of a sort to help ethical inquiry. How to characterize and assess what someone's mood becomes when it is serotonin-enabled—whether "happy" or "calm" or "confident" or "insensible" or something else again—is outside of strictly biological inquiry. Brain science is and likely will remain silent on the nature and significance, in *human* terms, of the experienced changes in mood that the SSRIs produce.

One effect of SSRIs is clear: they relieve a number of disorders of mood, particularly depression. Yet the nature of these disorders is complicated and their causes remain largely unknown. In DSM-IV* the lengthy discussion of depression (like the discussions of other psychiatric disorders) is essentially a compendium of symptoms, with no attempt at a coherent account of the nature or causes of the illness.[22] Although studies of patients' family histories suggest an important role for genetic predispositions and inherited susceptibilities, no underlying biological counterpart to major depression, let alone its specific variants, has so far been found, no broken part identified—not even a disorder in the serotonin system.[23] There is as yet no genetic or blood test, brain scan, or electroencephalogram for diagnosing depression. The very term "depression" seems to refer not to one thing, but to a heterogeneous collection of conditions with different symptoms, causes, courses of illness—and responses to SSRIs.[24] This last point is especially important: how serotonin affects a person appears to depend—though few studies address the matter directly—on what the person's starting point is. The mentally ill and the more-or-less-healthy-but-unhappy experience, it seems, different effects from the drugs. Those with the type of depression seen in bipolar disorder often make a full recovery, becoming steady in mood and capable of fit-

---

Academy of Sciences, 93: 3908-3913, 1996; Santarelli, L., et al., "Requirement of Hippocampal Neurogenesis for the Behavioral Effects of Antidepressants," *Science,* 301: 805-809, 2003.

* *The Diagnostic and Statistical Manual of Mental Disorders, Fourth Edition* (DSM-IV) is the psychiatric community's authoritative guide to diagnosis. Its chief and stated purpose is to "provide a helpful guide to clinical practice" (p. xxiii).

ting emotional responses to all the highs, lows, and "middles" of life. Those with something closer to ordinary sadness or grief, or those with a melancholy or inhibited temperament, seem to have subtler responses, though ones they still welcome. And some individuals respond to one medication but not another, while others have no response at all.

Our attention here is mainly on the latter group, "normal" people who want to feel "better than normal," or at least better than *they* normally do. People who take SSRIs in the absence of definite mental illness, and the physicians who observe them, commonly report that negative feelings such as sadness and anger do not disappear but diminish, as does the inclination to brood over them. Loss, disappointment, and rejection still sting, but not as much or as long, and one can cope with them with less disturbance of mind. Sensitivity also declines, along with obsession, compulsion, and anxiety, while self-esteem and confidence rise. Fear, too, is reduced, and one is more easily able to experience pleasure and accept risk. Mental agility, energy, sleep, and appetite become more regular, typically increasing. And mood brightens—though not to the point of perpetual bliss or anywhere near it.[25] People *do* indeed feel better.

Still, it is hard to know what to make of this bundle of reported effects. Speaking abstractly, one can see a certain unity to them, a reduction of various negative feelings, an increase in positive ones, a general moderation prevailing where once there was excess or deadness. Also, it seems that only the "positive/negative axis" of feeling is touched: SSRIs do not directly affect other aspects of feeling—do not impart or remove empathy, have no direct effect on moral conscience, neither increase nor lessen one's ability to appreciate beauty. Might there be some way of understanding and characterizing these effects as a whole?

One suggestion is that SSRIs alter a person's native temperament or affective disposition—an individual's tendency to respond to the circumstances and events of life in a particular emotional fashion. Temperaments vary, for example, in characteristic intensity of emotions and moods, from strong (or intense) to weak (or mild). While a severely stressful event will of course provoke a strong reaction from almost anyone, some people react more strongly (and some more mildly) to equivalent stresses, and—

important for our purposes—their tendencies to react at such a pitch are long-lasting.* SSRIs affect this dimension of temperament: they tend to reduce the intensity of emotional responsiveness.[26] One might say that SSRIs, at base, make people calmer.**

Yet "calmness" is not the only way to understand the effects of SSRIs on mood and psychic experience. For one thing, the calmness explanation stumbles on the example of MDMA (Ecstasy), which also makes more serotonin available and which induces not calm but bliss, social and sensory openness, and feelings of intense affection.[127] A second view of serotonin function is that it deals with something more basic than emotion and mood: a nondescript measure of well-being. This idea takes off from findings in animal research, indicating that serotonin systems are active in brains of lower organisms, organisms that almost certainly do not experience conscious moods or emotions.[††] One could easily imagine how it might be useful for any organism to have an internal gauge of its well-being—satisfaction of its needs and desires, its social status, and the like—that would prod it to undertake actions that foster survival and reproduction. Perhaps serotonin is part of such a gauge, a mechanism by which organisms set their background level of felt well-being.[28]

---

* This line of variation has been differently described as the neuroticism-stability dimension, the unstable-stable dimension, or the strong-weak dimension, of human temperament. But as the names suggest, part of the model's clinical importance is in explaining emotional vulnerability: the more intense one's moods and emotions, the more likely one is to fall into a variety of behaviors and states of mind that are troubling.

** A calmer disposition might then permit more fitting emotional responses to particular experiences. Arguably, SSRIs might also shrink the range of emotional responses, raising the floor but lowering the ceiling.

† MDMA functions differently from SSRIs: rather than inhibiting serotonin reuptake, it increases serotonin production, causing massive dumps of serotonin into the synapses. Yet to the receiving neuron, more serotonin is available either way. Whether the difference between SSRIs and MDMA is one of degree or of kind, and what the example of one means for the other, is not clear.

†† For example, lobsters show increased serotonin production when nearing food sources. Primates' levels of serotonin correlate with their position in the social hierarchy. (Peter Kramer, presentation at the September 2002 meeting of the President's Council on Bioethics, Washington, D.C. Transcript available on the Council's web site at www.bioethics.gov.) The examples are both suggestive and perplexing. Lobsters seem unlikely to have emotions or moods of a fine-grained sort. Yet primates of high social status show a wide range of emotions and moods (presumably while enjoying high serotonin levels). Perhaps serotonin is involved with something more basic than emotion and mood, something less specific yet still registering the difference between positive and negative.

A variety of human observations support the "background level of felt well-being" thesis. With humans, as with primates, SSRIs do not directly introduce or block emotions and moods; one can experience a variety of emotions and moods—including negative ones—while taking them, and presumably while enjoying elevated levels of serotonin. Also, while SSRIs change a user's serotonin levels within hours, they produce no experienced psychic effect for weeks. Something subtler than direct control of emotion and mood is taking place, something that would create tendencies toward, and shape the intensity of, certain emotions and moods, but not simply implant them.

In this regard, it is striking that SSRIs are effective in relieving symptoms for so many conditions: social phobia, obsessive-compulsive disorder, post-traumatic stress disorder, generalized anxiety disorder, premenstrual dysphoric disorder, a variety of eating disorders and sexual compulsions, and the whole range of conditions clustered around major depression, possibly ranging all the way from melancholic dispositions to ordinary sadness. The emotions and moods, not to mention the causes, symptoms, and courses of illness of these conditions, are very different. How is it that SSRIs address them all? This broad efficacy makes sense if SSRIs establish a background sense of well-being, for in the presence of such a sense those many conditions could not persist; each disorder is an instance of feeling unwell, and so each is inconsistent with a general sense of being well. It is as if SSRIs erect the kind of healthy dispositional foundation that those blessed with fortunate genetics and favorable environments tend to have (without the need for drugs), below which, apart from the most crushing circumstances, one's despair will not fall.

A third hypothesis suggests that SSRIs can sometimes transform personality. Consider, for example, the story of "Sally," a patient of psychiatrist Peter Kramer, who describes her case in *Listening to Prozac*. Shy by nature, raised by depressed and inhibited parents, sexually abused by an uncle, Sally developed an "entrenched timidity and social discomfort," which led to "a sameness to her life, a terrible monotony . . . a life of intolerable bleakness."[29] It had few pleasures, no lovers or close friends, little to look forward to or to relish, and—though she did not think of herself as depressed until midlife—she became then not just depressed but "openly desperate." As she wrote to Kramer before seeing him:

> I am forty-one years old. I feel angry and hurt most of the time. I feel like my spirit has been shattered and fragmented with each piece having been trampled on and bruised. I am very, very anxious. I am afraid of everything, even centipedes and roaches. I keep thinking something very, very bad is going to happen to me, some great misfortune, or that I'll become handicapped and have to depend on people to take care of me. I don't know who I am, because that person stopped growing at the age of four, and it makes me very sad.[30]

Sally's touching story is, in outline, widely shared: a difficult environment amplifies a troubled or troublesome predisposition and sets in motion a great unhappiness. Prozac had a dramatic effect on her. She felt that the drug cleared her head, made her more calm and confident. With her new assertiveness, she negotiated a promotion at work, where she had been locked into one job for eighteen years. The changes in her social life were positively stunning. More easygoing, more cheerful, and—most of all—unafraid at last, she dated several men, came to love one, and married him: "an extraordinary achievement, a sign of victory over a crippling aspect of the self." Sally said the Prozac had let her true personality finally emerge, the personality deflected by hardship and inborn fear; it let her truly live for the first time. When her doctor expressed some concerns and suggested suspending the use of it temporarily, Sally flatly refused.

Trying to understand the nature of Sally's transformation, Kramer suggests that it was social inhibition, not depression or anxiety, that led to her unhappiness and stagnation, and concludes as follows:

> The vast majority of these [naturally shy] people, including those who are outright inhibited socially, will be "normal" in psychological terms. Most of them will be highly functional in their careers and private lives. No one has ever called people with inhibited personality mentally ill. The brief conclusion to this line of reasoning is that in patients like Sally, and in many others with less dramatic

stories and perhaps with no history of depression at all, what we are changing with medication is the infrastructure of personality. That is, Sally is able to marry on Prozac because she has achieved chemically the interior milieu of someone born with a different genome and exposed to a more benign world in childhood.[31]

Yet SSRIs do not transform personality utterly: Prozac only changed the easily measured, gross traits of Sally's temperament, Kramer explains, not the "many small and consequential features that make each person unique . . . [their] opinions, aspirations, bêtes noires, mannerisms, and memories."[32] Sally acquired the states of feeling not of anyone, but of Sally, had Sally been born and raised to be well.*

Many psychiatrists disagree with Kramer's conclusion, arguing that people like Sally are chronically depressed or otherwise disordered, and what appears to be personality change is actually just the liberation of their true self.[33] Yet, be this as it may, we may still share Kramer's wonder at "the capacity of modern medication to allow a person to experience, on a stable and continuous basis, the feelings of someone with a different temperament and history." Indeed, in response to his critics, Kramer presents a sharp challenge to the view that SSRIs cannot alter personality, in the process clearly articulating this Council's concern regarding the "beyond therapy" uses of these drugs. Arguing that SSRIs clearly can produce dramatic improvements in people who were once not considered ill, he insightfully suggests that this fact presents doctors, along with society more generally, with the choice either to expand the notion of mental illness or to see SSRIs as medicating personality.**

---

* We are not unaware of the strangeness of the claim that such a hypothetical identity, previously hidden but newly released, would be identical to one that would have been formed *in a life differently lived.*

** "This research is pushing psychiatry toward the treatment of ever more minor levels of mood disruption; there is, in other words, an empirical rationale for expanding the range of psychiatric diagnosis. It may be appropriate to medicate patients whose level of depression is "subsyndromal"—certainly a melancholic person may be a fit candidate for that other mental health technology, psychotherapy—but I would say that an honest labeling of this use of antidepressants would deem it an attempt, through pharmacology, to replace a normal if unrewarded personality style with another normal style that is more comfortable or better socially rewarded." (Kramer, P., *Listening to Prozac*, Second Edition, New York: Penguin, 1997, p. 322.)

These three accounts of what SSRIs fundamentally do—induce calmness, provide a background sense of well-being, change personality—probably ought not to be looked at as mutually exclusive competitors. Inducing a background sense of well-being could be the cause of greater calm, and greater calm in turn the cause of a transformed personality. The three could also be identical: the difference between a background sense of well-being and a greater sense of calm may be, at least in part, one of description, and each of those could be understood as personality changes. The three accounts double back, overlap, and imply one another at many points, and we can perhaps see them as three ways of making the same change, whose results can, in summary, be called a "brighter mood."

This very confusion, however—the uncertainty regarding what SSRIs do, the unclear relationship between the various accounts—is instructive for thinking about the future of mood-brighteners, and we have dwelt on it for this reason. Our technological powers often arrive far ahead of our capacity to understand them. This is only partly due to the fact that researchers often first come across a new and effective mood-altering drug by accident, and only later learn the mechanism of its action. It is also due to the enormous complexity of the brain and the still greater complexity of mental life. And it is due especially to the deep and unbridgeable divide between the language of inner experience and the language of neurochemistry, a fact that will always bedevil efforts to understand the humanly felt import of molecular events in the brain. The outcome: We acquire drugs that satisfy our aspirations, yet we know not how or why. As the example of SSRIs shows, even though we are ignorant, even though we suspect that the unknown effects of the drugs are subtle and deep, we make substantial use of them nonetheless. The generalizable lesson seems clear: in the years to come, SSRIs will in all likelihood become more effective in accomplishing what they accomplish; they will be modified to produce fewer and gentler side effects and they will be utilized more and more. When some discovery leads to an altogether new drug with even greater powers to satisfy our aspirations for a happier soul, it will also be used despite much ignorance and uncertainty. Where deep human desires are present, and where the effects of technology are so attractive, most people will prefer benefits despite ignorance to knowledge without benefits.

B. Ethical Analysis

From an ethical perspective that gives primacy to personal freedom and an individual's right to pursue happiness as he or she defines it, the use of mood-brighteners in search of a happier soul might seem at first glance to be largely unproblematic. If we have available to us a drug that induces a background sense of well-being, why shouldn't we use it when we feel unfulfilled or steadily "blue"? What could be wrong with, or even just disquieting about, wanting to feel better about ourselves and our lives, and availing ourselves of the necessary assistance in doing so? If we may embrace psychotherapy for the same purpose, why should we not embrace mood-brighteners, especially if they are not only safe but also cheaper and more effective than "talk therapy"? Only a person utterly at peace with the world and content with himself would be beyond temptation at the prospect of having his troubles effortlessly eased. And even were we to resist the temptation for ourselves, we might seek it for our unhappy children, whose sorrows are for most of us much more painful than our own.

Yet further reflection gives rise to questions—about both ends and means—that ought, at the very least, to give pause to anyone tempted by the pharmacological road to happiness. For we care that our children—and that we ourselves—have not only the sense or feeling of well-being, but well-being itself. We desire not simply to be satisfied with ourselves and the world, but to have this satisfaction as a result of deeds and loves and lives worthy of such self-satisfaction. We do not want to kill our aspiration for a better life by drowning in a self-absorbed contentment those experiences of lack and self-discontent that serve as aspiration's source, or those engagements with the world and other people that serve as aspiration's vehicle.*

---

* Consider the analogy of "treating" the anxiety and disproportionate urgency (and associated danger) of adolescent sexuality by extinguishing it at its biochemical source (note that in some patients Prozac will diminish libido). This fundamental biological drive, and its attendant discontent, is inextricably related to the larger longings of romantic love and in turn to some of life's highest aspirations and achievements.

Here, then, lie several potential grounds of our unease about—not rejection of—mood-elevating drugs: the prospect of mistaking some lesser substitute for real happiness; the danger of seeking happiness at the cost of confounding our own identity or losing our longings for the real thing; and the price to be paid—in personal aspiration, interpersonal relations, and communal character—should a large fraction of our society (successfully) pursue happier souls by this inward-turning means.

1. Living Truly

Most people seek some form of the well-being that Sally came to experience, in her case only with the help of medication: We seek to be confident in everyday life, to form lasting and meaningful relationships with others, to pursue worthy goals and take pleasure in their achievement. But what is the significance in relying on mood-brightening drugs to achieve such happiness? To what extent is the happiness of the happy person attributable to the drug and to what extent is it "her own"? To what extent are drug-induced psychic states connected with or disconnected from life as really lived? Surely, for Sally and others who benefit greatly from mood-brightening drugs, the drugs are not the direct cause of their happiness. Sally's happiness has much to do with her new husband and new job, her new attachments and new achievements, though she would likely not have sought or found them without taking Prozac. The drug itself did not make her happy; it merely enabled her *to do and experience* the many things that make her happy. But now imagine being Sally's husband: Just *to whom* am I married? Would I love Sally if she stopped taking Prozac and relapsed into timidity and hopelessness? Would Sally love me? Would Sally be Sally?

With a drug like Ecstasy, the answers to such strange and difficult questions—about the identity of the person taking such drugs and the status of the positive feelings they induce—are more obvious, if no less disquieting. People high on Ecstasy routinely profess their love for perfect strangers. Imagine that a young party-goer, under the influence of the drug, tells a young woman that he loves her and wants to marry her. Imagine also that he means it, insofar as the feeling he now has is indistinguishable from what he might one day feel when he truly falls in love with a woman. Should the fact that his feelings are produced by the drug, rather than inspired by the woman, matter? It should of course matter to *her*. His drug-based professions of love cannot be taken seriously. Neither should a marriage proposal that owes everything to his being "high." But it should also matter to *him*, once he awakens from the "alternative reality" induced by taking Ecstasy and recovers the real identity that the drug temporarily erased.

The young man's drug-induced "love" is not just incomplete—an emotion unconnected with knowledge of and care for the beloved. It is also unfounded, not based on anything—not even visible beauty—from which such emotions normally grow. The young woman, were she to learn about his use of Ecstasy, might readily agree: "He doesn't really love me. It's just the drugs talking." She might even say that the man is *not really himself*: "This isn't the real him; he isn't in his right mind." Insofar as his feelings are attributable to Ecstasy, the young man's feelings and words are, to speak plainly, fake, indeed, doubly fake: they are neither *true* nor truly *his*.* The drugs deceive him and induce him to behave in ways that could deceive another.

In human affairs, we care a great deal about the difference between "the real" and "the merely appearing." We care about "living truly." To be sure, people for centuries have produced spurious feelings of all types with alcohol and other agents. Yet although our society is generally tolerant of the practice—alcohol, if not "harder" drugs—we do recognize the risks, limits, and costs, not to mention the heightened possibilities of wrongdoing, connected with "not being in one's own right mind." In fact, much of the disquiet often voiced about mood-brightening drugs—*even when appropriately used to treat serious mental illness*—clusters around this concern. Some patients fear personality change, fear losing the "real me." Some also worry about using artificial means to change their psyches, a concern that springs ultimately from their desire that feelings and personalities not be artificial and false but genuine and true. Their worry, also

---

* The subject of true love and love potions is, of course, a familiar theme of great literature, from the myth of Tristan and Isolde to Shakespeare's *A Midsummer Night's Dream*. These writings are interested in the degree to which eros itself is like divine, demonic, or "magical" possession. Are people who fall in love in their own "right minds"?

widely shared, about having one's experiences of the world mediated by a drug is, at least in part, a worry about having one's real experience distorted. Even the expressed concern over "taking the easy way out" may involve not so much an opposition to ease, but a concern about distortion and self-deception.

With mood-brightening drugs like SSRIs, questions of truthfulness and identity are indeed complicated. Unlike Ecstasy (a drug regarded on multiple grounds as dangerous and declared illegal), SSRIs cannot implant a groundless emotion, and they cannot instantly transform a soul. Especially for the mentally ill, these drugs, far from distorting reality, may enable patients to "*get into* their right mind" and to experience the richness of life more fully and truthfully, sometimes for the first time. It would thus be wrong and unfair to say that people whose lives are improved by mood-brightening drugs live falsely or untruthfully, or that people taking Prozac do not really love the husbands or wives they fell in love with while taking their medication.

But while they do not live falsely, many of them do live different lives than they would otherwise have lived, lives first made possible because of the drug and often requiring its continued use to be sustained. Though SSRIs do not instantly change the psyche, they can, gradually and over time, induce a persisting background sense of well-being, even where well-being itself is lacking. As a result, they can significantly change a person's temperament and therewith his personality, often markedly. According to the striking testimony of some users, SSRIs allow them to "become themselves" again or—strangely—to gain their true identity for the "first time." This matter of changed or transformed identity is, on its face, perplexing, with individuals living lives and doing deeds they never did or could have done before taking the drugs. And it remains for many a source of persisting disquiet.

Many people—perhaps all people, at some point—desire a happier life than the one they have now. Dissatisfied with themselves, they want to do better or feel better. In some cases, they opt for sharp and sudden highs, for a brief "holiday from reality" made possible by drugs like alcohol, heroin, or Ecstasy. In other cases, discontent spurs changed habits, new pursuits, and better ways of living and behaving.

In yet other cases, people are and will be tempted to turn to mood-brightening drugs—SSRIs today, perhaps more advanced drugs in the future—that might enable them more easily to do for themselves the things they wish to do but cannot, or to feel the things they wish to feel but do not, or to feel the things they once felt but can feel no longer. While such drugs often make things better—they often help individuals achieve some measure of the happiness they desire—taking such drugs may also leave many of the same individuals wondering whether their newfound happiness is fully *their own*—and in this sense, fully real. This concern persists even when one becomes happy about genuinely happy things—like a new spouse or new job. It is even more pertinent, and more disquieting, should one come to feel happy for no good reason at all, or happy even when there remains much in one's life to be truly unhappy about.

2. Fitting Sensibilities and Human Attachments

A central concern with mood-brightening drugs is that they will estrange us emotionally from life as it really is, preventing us from responding to events and experiences, whether good or bad, in a fitting way. Of course, changing the way we respond to life's happenings is a prime motive for developing such drugs in the first place: to help individuals feel more joyful about joyful things or less overwhelmed by their troubles and sorrows. And many people, their neurobiological "equipment" defective, surely need psychopharmacological assistance if they are to become able to respond fittingly to life's many ups and downs. But there is a danger that our new pharmacological remedies will keep us "bright" or impassive in the face of things that ought to trouble, sadden, outrage, or inspire us—that our medicated souls will stay flat no matter what happens to us or around us.

Writing in his *Confessions* about the death of his mother, St. Augustine provides a moving account of what it means to respond to real life in a fitting way:

> I closed her eyes; and there flowed a great sadness into my heart, and
> it was passing into tears, when mine eyes at the same time, by the

violent control of my mind, sucked back the fountain dry, and woe was me in such a struggle! . . . [I]n Thine ears, where none of them heard, did I blame the softness of my feelings, and restrained the flow of my grief, which yielded a little unto me; but the paroxysm returned again, though not so as to burst forth into tears, nor to a change of countenance, though I knew what I repressed in my heart. And as I was exceedingly annoyed that these human things had such power over me, which in the due order and destiny of our natural condition must of necessity come to pass, with a new sorrow I sorrowed for my sorrow, and was wasted by a twofold sadness.[34]

At first blush, St. Augustine's comments may strike a modern reader as strange. He regarded his own grief, at least partially, as a failing, believing that it betrayed too much concern for earthly things. But such grief was, by his own admission, a "human thing," a fitting response to the death of the mother he loved dearly. What he felt was deep sadness at a deeply sad event. If his response to his mother's death had been hysterical unremitting sorrow, we might think it excessive. And if he had been coldly indifferent, we would wonder at his lack of humanity. The sadness he actually felt was the humanly fitting response, the emotion called for and appropriate to the circumstances. And yet, his sorrow, while fitting, also troubled him greatly.

Permit a somewhat outrageous thought experiment: might St. Augustine's physician, were such a drug available, have offered him a mood-brightener? With it, St. Augustine might still have mourned, but with less misery. He might have had to struggle less to "suck back the fountain dry," or to sorrow less for his own sorrowing. He might even have been less deflected from his primary aspiration to attend to matters divine—if, that is, the drug did not also flatten his longings. Would he, should he, have accepted such pharmacological assistance?

If St. Augustine's grief bothered him for theological reasons, because of its excessive worldliness, the prospect of such grief troubles many of our contemporaries for psychological reasons, either because we want no such psychic burdens interfering with our worldly doings or because we think we cannot endure them on our own. A desire for pharmacologic relief is understandable. Some things, we fear, will simply hurt too much, if faced in their unvarnished reality without somehow dulling the pain.* Yet especially in matters of love and death, such psychic relief may also estrange us from the attachments that matter most. Seeking to "make the pain go away," or simply to ease it in the moment of its greatest sting, we risk giving our departed loved one less significance than he or she deserves. Suffering "less than we should," we risk diminishing our appreciation of the depth of our love and of the one whose absence now causes our pain.

This dilemma holds not only in matters of mourning. It applies also to the pain of failing to achieve our goals or uphold our highest principles, the pain of betraying or being betrayed by a friend, the pain of no longer being able to do the things we once did with great ability and great joy. Nothing hurts only if nothing matters. And while we rightly seek to reduce the causes of gratuitous suffering, both physical and psychic, we do not want to remove the *capacity* to suffer when suffering is called for.**

It is true that in order to function in everyday life, one needs some measure of detachment from the things that touch us most deeply. We cannot and should not be filled to the emotional brim at every moment or wear all our feelings on our sleeves. To feel things deeply and fittingly does not require living without reticence or self-restraint. Yet by seeking psychic detachment by means that pharmacologically insulate or remove us from the highs and lows of real life, we may risk coming to love feebly or to care shallowly, losing the fine texture of emotional and psychic life and weakening our appreciation for the very human attachments that make life most meaningful.

---

* Many a person has drowned his sorrows in alcohol, though it should be added that—unlike with the use of mood-brighteners—sorrow returns the morning after, often made worse by a hangover. And chronic drunkenness brings its own miseries and sorrows.

** This point about psychic pain and psychic fitness exactly parallels the situation regarding bodily pain and fitness. We try to prevent or treat gratuitous pain, but we recognize the life-saving and fitness-preserving virtues of the capacity to feel pain. Full analgesia is deadly.

3. What Sorrow Teaches, What Discontent Provokes

The previous reflection casts a small doubt on the unqualified goodness of the goal of a "happy soul." "Feeling good" may not always be good or good for us. Never to suffer loss may mean never to love deeply; never to feel ashamed may mean that our standards for ourselves are too low; never to be dissatisfied with ourselves may mean that we aspire to too little. Even as we seek happiness, in other words, we must not overlook what sorrow teaches and what discontent provokes—the intuitions, longings, and hunger for improvement and understanding that make for a fuller and more flourishing life.

There is, despite what the Romantics thought, no nobility in having consumption (tuberculosis)—though there may be in how one copes with it. So, too, there is no nobility in suffering from major depression or crippling despair or even protracted grief following the death of a spouse or child. In some cases, the very possibility of doing and living nobly and finely may be crushed in ways that only mood-brightening drugs, properly used, can help restore or repair. And clearly, one should not actively seek misery for the lessons it might teach us, any more than one should seek to gain a fatal disease in order to face it with courage or to relate better to those who suffer from it.

But we cannot ignore the truth that life's hardships often make us better—more attuned to the hardships of others, more appreciative of life's everyday blessings, more aware of the things and the people that matter most in our lives. Sadness in the recollection of a loss or a national tragedy (for example, September 11) keeps alive and pays tribute to the blessings we once enjoyed or still enjoy, gratuitously and vulnerably. Anxiety in the face of a crucial meeting or big decision registers the importance of the undertaking and prods us to rise to the occasion. Shame at our own irresponsible or duplicitous conduct exhibits knowledge of proper conduct and provides a spur to achieving it. These emotional stings not only reflect the truth. If they do not crush us, they may make us better.

It seems paradoxical: sane people would never choose or pray for sorrow, yet it is common to hear people say, after the fact, that their darkest times were in some respects their finest hours and the source of a better future. True, sorrows can often cripple or destroy. But sometimes, as the philosopher Nicholas Wolterstorff writes in his *Lament for a Son*:

> there emerges a radiance which elsewhere seldom appears: a glow of courage, of love, of insight, of selflessness, of faith. In that radiance we see best what humanity was meant to be. . . . In the valley of suffering, despair and bitterness are brewed. But there also character is made.[35]

Sorrow, courageously confronted, can make us stronger, wiser, and more compassionate.

To what extent might SSRIs, when used to reduce our troubles and sorrows, endanger this aspect of affective life? Although they do not prevent psychic pain, SSRIs may generally dull our capacity to feel it, rendering us less capable of experiencing and learning from misfortune or tragedy or empathizing with the miseries of others. If some virtues can only be taught through very trying circumstances, those virtues might be lost or at least less developed.

But it is not only the discontent thrust upon us by external events or great misfortunes that can help to make us better. We can benefit too from the discontent with our own deeds, actions, and character that comes from honest self-examination. To be sure, many forms of self-loathing are destructive or excessive, ranging from joyless perfectionism to suicidal despair. But without some proper measure of self-discontent, there would be no spur to self-improvement. If we never felt the emotional pangs of our own shortcomings and limitations, we would never aspire to become better or wiser. Just as physical pain prods us, say, to remove our hand from the hot stove, psychic pain prods us, when it functions well, to improve those aspects of our daily life (at work, at home, in the community) that are not "working well." Just as the pangs of hunger push us to nourish the body, so the pangs of psychic hunger spur us to nourish the soul.

The motive force of passion is not confined to the negative emotions. Positive emotions, too, when they are fitting and function well, reinforce our attachment to what is good in our lives, encouraging us to continue in the activities and human relationships that are fulfilling and to preserve and enlarge the good things we seek and cherish. In a word, healthy affect, negative as well as positive, is efficacious. It guides us to overall well-being. Undermine that function—by means, say, of a drug that induces a sense of well-being-no-matter-what in a person whose ordinary emotions are functioning properly—and the cost is a life in which fitting feeling can no longer guide or spur us toward living well.

In sum, a mood-brightening drug that always made us pleased with ourselves no matter what we did—a drug that guaranteed our self-esteem, even when such esteem is not warranted—might shrink our capacity for true human flourishing.* Possessed of full self-satisfaction, why would we be spurred to seek improvement? Possessed of full peace of mind, why would we risk loss by giving our heart to another or hazard disappointment by aspiring to something difficult and noble? The example of "soma," the drug in Aldous Huxley's fictional *Brave New World*, illustrates the debased value of a spurious, drug-induced contentment.[36] Soma—like cocaine, only without side effects or addiction—completely severs feeling from living, inner sensation from all external relations, the feeling of happiness from leading a good life. Rendered impotent in their aspirations, the denizens of Huxley's dystopia do not loathe their condition and do not yearn for another, largely because they cannot loathe and cannot yearn. They imagine themselves to be happy as they are, and thus never pursue a life that would be more fully human, with the ups and downs that come from having aspirations self-consciously chosen and ardently pursued.

SSRIs do not completely sever how one feels from how one lives. On the contrary, in many therapeutic uses, they probably re-link feeling and living, permitting passionate experience its proper role in fostering further growth. But in certain uses and in certain people, these drugs may fracture the relationship between passion and action, inducing calm, apathy, and easy self-satisfaction where energy, engagement, and the desire for self-improvement might be called for.

---

* The cultivation and corruptions of a spurious self-esteem are, of course, possible without using drugs. Examples abound in our current cultural climate.

4. Medicalization of Self-Understanding

Welcome though they are for those who really need them, even the proper use of mood-brighteners to treat emotional disorders is not without hazard. Precisely because of the effectiveness of the medication to alter mood and self-esteem, there may well be a tendency to redefine, in medical and biological terms, what are currently considered normal emotions, moods, and temperaments. Because the psychic pains of mental illness are akin or sufficiently similar to the psychic pains of ordinary life, there will be a natural tendency to regard ordinary affective life through the lens first polished for viewing mental disorders.* Such medicalized understanding might well make suffering easier to cope with. For example, a person who attributes his discontent or sadness to sickness may spare himself difficult self-examination and self-recrimination, as well as arduous attempts to change the way he lives. He can take mood-brighteners without guilt or without any sense that he is missing something. But this benefit, if it is that, may well come at considerable cost. For one reconceives sadness as sickness only by emptying it of psychic or spiritual significance and turning it into a mere thing of the body. Not only is the soul seen as dissolved into the body, but the body itself is seen as dissolved into genes and neurochemicals. Ardent desire is reduced to an elevated peptide concentration in the hypothalamus, righteous indignation is reduced to an elevated serotonin level in the temporal lobe. In the limit, happiness itself, along with misery, can be reconceived as a matter of neurons and neurotransmitter levels. No longer a spiritual achievement or the fruit of a life well-lived, it can come to be seen as the gift of either natural good fortune or biotechnical manipulation. The medicalization of psychic pain, however necessary as a path to providing much needed relief for the sick, indicates (whether intended or not) a great advance for biological reductionism against the citadel of mind and soul, a march that knows no natural stopping place, and that at each point along the

---

* The same thing happened with psychoanalysis, where a theory devised to explain neurosis became the ruling explanation of all psychic life, abnormal and normal.

advance threatens to reduce further the dignity of our inner life—or at least our self-understanding of it.

Our concern regarding such a transformation is not merely of theoretic or conceptual importance. It is also practical, affecting how doctors treat patients and the problems they bring to the doctor's door. Thanks to the efficacy of mood brightening agents, and of psychotropic drugs more generally, there may well be a temptation to redefine and *to treat* what are currently considered normal emotions, moods, and temperaments on the model of mental illness, and mental illness as a matter purely of bodily—ultimately, of molecular—character and causation. Should this occur, there will be large difficulties in assigning moral responsibility for any improper (or, for that matter, admirable) behavior, not only in matters criminal but in all interpersonal relations.

Are normal emotions or normal problems of living today being "diagnosed" or regarded in the way we regard mental illness? Is medicalization actually taking place, in practice as well as in thought? It is hard to say, and careful social science research would be needed before an answer could be hazarded with confidence. And a positive answer, *in some cases,* need not be cause for concern. It is possible that temperaments we once saw as typically human—habitual mild melancholy, for example, or shyness, or alienation, or inhibition—will be shown indisputably to result from definite neurochemical abnormalities. Epilepsy was once thought to show demonic possession ("The Sacred Disease"), and manic depression was thought to reveal bad character. Both diseases were stigmatized and treated ineffectively. Now, thankfully, both epilepsy and bipolar disorder have been entirely medicalized, both in idea and in practice. Medicalizing the problems of living, and using drugs to brighten a healthy mood, may have serious human costs, but so does refusing to use beneficial medication when one is sick and treating problems of health as problems of character. Good medicine and sound ethics thus have the same interest: effectively treating the sick in light of a sound conception of human health, without treating as illness every troubled state of soul.

Many psychiatrists, keenly aware of the problem, already understand their mission in these terms. A leading book in the field introduces the subject of depression by explaining that, of the patients who turn to a doctor because they are feeling downhearted, "the majority . . . will be facing a serious life situation," while some "will be suffering not from some responsive mood but from a fixed depressive state," which then "must be recognized for what it is, major depression."[37] The DSM-IV requires for a diagnosis of major depression or dysthymia that "[t]he symptoms cause clinically significant distress or impairment in social, occupational, or other important areas of functioning."[38] If doctors maintain high diagnostic standards, treating with mood-brightening drugs only those patients who have an illness, are sliding into one, or whose emotional troubles are so urgent as to make claims on the duty to save, the worst excesses of using mood-brighteners can perhaps be avoided or reduced.

Yet we should not be complacent. Many forces and incentives are pushing us in the opposite direction. As already noted, the arrival of efficacious mood-brightening (and other psychotropic) drugs invites enlargement of the domain of illness and further reductionist thinking about its cause. Doctors are the gatekeepers to drugs, drugs are prescribed (and their costs reimbursed) only for diagnosed illnesses, and the growing demand for drugs—a demand in part deliberately created by their manufacturers in direct advertising to consumers—exerts great pressure for the expansion of diagnostic categories. Even were the medical profession interested in developing a sound and limited concept of health, a workable account is hard to come by, and, truth to tell, the search for it is rarely undertaken. Especially as health comes to be regarded less as the absence of disease but as some positive state of well-being, ever open-ended and unlimited in its boundaries, the incentive increases to medicalize not only health but all human activities, psychic and social.* One need not philosophically embrace the World Health Organization's notorious definition of health—as "complete physical, mental, and social well-being"—to contribute in practice to making human happiness a growing part of the doctor's business, ever more open to pharmacological assistance.

---

* Proposals are now circulating among psychiatrists to define a new "relational disorder" to cover people with serious marital difficulties, including spousal abuse.

5. The Roots of Human Flourishing

As we noted at the start of this chapter, the nature of human happiness is a contested matter, not only between different cultures but within any one culture. Western thought boasts many distinguished accounts of how emotions and feelings are, and should be, involved with human flourishing or human happiness. An important issue in dispute is the connection between "feeling pleasure" and "being happy," a question advertised in the ambiguities of the word "happiness," perched as it is between "pleasure" and "flourishing," between "feeling good" and "living well." A most prominent ethical outlook, utilitarianism, seeks the greatest happiness for the greatest number, with happiness often measured solely by self-reported pleasure or contentment. On such a view, mood-brightening technology might be regarded as an unequivocal good, a direct contribution to greater human happiness, whose only cost would be any pleasure it might prevent or obstruct, say, through side effects or addiction.

A very different picture of what it means to flourish emotionally emerges from the ethical analysis presented above. Perpetual bliss would not be the emotional ideal (at least in the world we inhabit), because emotional flourishing of human beings in this world requires that feelings jibe with the truth of things, both as effect and as cause. As response, affect is at its best when it exhibits certain cognitive and aesthetic virtues like measure and proportion; the criterion is that it be fitting. As motive, affect should lead a person to seek out a good life or to preserve the one he has; the criterion is that it be efficacious in service to the good to which the emotion points, whether positively or negatively. When affect is a healthy part of a psychic whole, it serves not the limited purpose of pleasure alone, but serves and helps constitute overall human flourishing.

Taking an additional step, we suggest that, under conditions of psychic health, the moods of the mind and the experienced pleasures, both of soul and body, are neither primary nor independent aspects of our lives. They are rather derived from and tied to the things we do and encounter: the people we meet, love, and lose, and the children we rear; the activities we pursue and the successes and failures that we encounter; the thoughts we have and the judgments we make; the beauty we admire and the evils we abhor. Moreover, because human activities and experiences differ greatly among themselves, so, too, do the attendant pleasures and pains differ in kind and in quality. Whatever we may assert in speech about the supremacy and homogeneity of pleasure or satisfaction, we care in fact primarily about activity and experience, and we care also about the quality of the pleasure and satisfaction. We do not really want the pleasure without the activity: we do not want the pleasure of playing baseball without playing baseball, the pleasure of listening to music without the music, the satisfaction of having learned something without knowing anything. Pleasure follows in the wake of the activity and, as it were, lights it up into consciousness. But without the activity there is and can be no happiness. We embrace neither suffering nor self-denial by suggesting that disconnected pleasure (or contentment or self-esteem or brightness of mood) produced from out of a bottle is but a poor substitute for happiness.

Where does this leave us regarding the relation between mood-brighteners and happy souls? We human beings share with all higher animals a predilection for feelings of comfort and pleasure. But our uniquely human capacity is to recognize that all the pokings, proddings, and temptings of feeling are like arrows that point us to lives of meaning and purpose. And recognizing the direction of our aspiration, we also find in ourselves the eminently human capacity to desire and direct its aim. There have always been those who, seeing how intense and how woven into our various enterprises is the desire for pleasure, think its satisfaction the whole point of human life. If that were true, the potential appeal of mood-brightening drugs would appear limitless.

But if, as we have suggested, it is not true, then to put mood-brightening technology to its best human use is to use it sparingly, medically, to help those who cannot do so unassisted to attain the capacity for securing fitting relationships between their feelings, their causes, and their effects. It is to help them achieve an appropriate relationship between their circumstances, inner life, and possibilities for action, so that they are able to feel joy at joyous events and sadness at sad ones, to marvel at the world's wonders, resist cruelties, and all the while strive to develop their talents, honor their obligations, and cherish their friendships and loves. For none of us lives humanly by the feeling of untroubled ease alone.

6. The Happy Self and the Good Society

So far, we have focused largely on the meaning of using mood-brightening drugs for the individual, and the danger of gaining peace of mind at the cost of living less truly or not being oneself. But individuals do not pursue happiness alone as solitary beings, nor is the search for individual well-being, narrowly understood, the sole or even central purpose of our lives. The individual depends on others to live a full and flourishing human life—on farmers to feed him, teachers to guide him, soldiers to protect him, family and friends to stand with him. His very identity is embedded in a web of overlapping communities—family, neighborhood, institutions of work and worship, nation. And these communities often need individuals to put the good of the whole before their own inner (or inward-looking) search for happiness. If human beings were merely self-absorbed, all good and lasting things would wither.

At the same time, we also cannot ignore the great achievement of liberal society in its concern for the dignity of the individual person—for seeing individuals not simply as useful and expendable means to society's ends, but as ends in themselves. Their individual well-being must be regarded and protected, not only against oppressive government or religious authority, but also against the tyranny of the majority and the ruling opinions and conventions of society.

The availability and use of mood-brightening drugs creates (and reflects) potential dangers in these two corresponding directions. The first danger is that individuals will become so preoccupied with their own state of mind that they remove themselves increasingly from active participation in civic life, discarding those attachments without which they cannot achieve the happiness they seek and without which the community cannot survive and flourish. The second danger is that social goals or expectations—the external pressure to be productive, to gain status and recognition, to get ahead—will produce a "mood-brightened society," where pharmacological interventions in our psyches become normal or expected for students, employees, and ultimately everyone. Put simply, the first danger involves the solipsistic self, worried only about the state of his feelings, who uses psychopharmacology to ensure a flat and shallow self-regarding psychic pleasure. The second danger involves the slavish self, whose worth is measured only in the eyes of others or according to his success in the rat race, and who takes mood-brightening (or other) drugs to assert himself or to increase his chances of meeting society's demands. Neither alternative bodes well for a free society.

Needless to say, one is hesitant to fault doctors and individuals who use mood-brightening drugs in search of relief from melancholy or malaise in cases where indications of serious depression are unclear. The decision to medicate in such cases, often difficult and full of ambivalence, is usually best made by patients and physicians in private. But we also cannot ignore the potential social consequences if self-medication of the soul, freely and individually chosen, were to become the social norm. Nor can we ignore the present culture in which these individual choices are made: a culture that prizes self-esteem, self-fulfillment, and self-advancement, and that increasingly looks to modern medicine to heal the troubled self. Indeed, new drugs for the psyche, new direct-to-consumer advertisements promising greater happiness through pharmacology, an expanding number of mental illnesses with ever broader criteria of diagnosis—this potent brew may already be creating new anxieties about mental health and new desires for mood-brightening drugs where neither existed before. These newly created desires, and the self-understanding that accompanies them, can transform the souls of a society even more profoundly than the drugs themselves.

Perhaps a remedy for our psychic troubles lies in the rediscovery of obligations and purposes outside the self—a turn outward rather than inward, a turn from the healthy mind to the good society. And perhaps the most promising route to real happiness is to live a fully engaged life, as teachers and parents, soldiers and statesmen, doctors and volunteers—in short, to follow the vocations of life that involve not the self alone, but the ties that bind and that ultimately give the individual's identity its true shape. To be sure, there are many people whose deep psychic distress precludes meeting obligations and forming close relationships, and for whom the proper use of mood-brighteners is the blessed gift that can restore to them the chance for a full and flourishing life. But there is also a danger that such drugs, suitably improved and refined, may one day offer us peace of mind not only without side effects but also without exertion or interest in human attachments—a peace of mind that might rival friends, family, and country for our deepest devotion.

IV. CONCLUSION

The promise and the peril of memory-blunting and mood-brightening drugs may prove to be quite profound. The awesome powers modern science has placed in our hands to control the external world increasingly enable us to control our inner experience, indeed to sever the link between subjective experience and our actions in the world. Not only can we produce an enormous range of things that make us happy—including stronger bodies, smarter minds, and stronger and smarter children—but increasingly we can produce through drugs the subjective experience of contentment and well-being in the absence of the goods that normally engender them. In some cases—as with traumatic memories or a pervasive and crippling sense of anxiety and despair—the new drugs can help return a person to the world and enable him to take responsibility for his life. But in many other cases, the growing power to manage our mental lives pharmacologically threatens our happiness by estranging us not only from the world but also from the sentiments, passions, and qualities of mind and character that enable us to live in it well.

Living well in the world has always meant striving for physical pleasure, wealth, honor, recognition, friendship, love, understanding, and spiritual fulfillment. And no small part of the challenge has been to reconcile the conflicting demands of these abiding human goods. In responding to the challenge, it has always been advantageous to be strong of body and sound of mind, and it has always been a pleasure to move freely under one's own power and to understand accurately the ways of the world.

Nearly all the goods we seek involve living well with others, so some knowledge of the human heart is indispensable to our happiness. Since friendship and love, the goods for which we often long most, indissolubly link the happiness of others to our happiness, we also have a keen interest in that sympathetic understanding that allows us to figure out both our own wants, needs, and desires and those of our friends and family members. In other words, happiness today, as always, consists in the activity of the well-functioning and self-aware soul.

Memory- and mood-altering drugs pose a fundamental danger to our pursuit of happiness. In the process of satisfying our genuine desires for peace of mind, a cheerful outlook, unclouded self-esteem, and intense pleasure, they may impair our capacity to satisfy the desires that by nature make us happiest. The fashioning of a memory that does not reflect how we have shaped and been shaped by experience threatens to bestow upon us satisfactions that are not truly our own. And the creating of calmer moods and moments of heightened pleasure or self-satisfaction that bear no relation to our actual undertakings threatens to erode our sentiments, passions, and virtues. What is to be particularly feared about the increasingly common and casual use of mind-altering drugs, then, is not that they will induce us to dwell on happiness at the expense of other human goods, but that they will seduce us into resting content with a shallow and factitious happiness.

It is no great surprise that it is our freedom-loving, technology-fancying, and happiness-chasing society that is bringing these wares to market. Yet these drugs also pose a fundamental danger to a society based on the individual's right to the pursuit of happiness. A society whose citizens can obtain tranquility on demand and enjoy no-fault ecstasy is a society whose citizens are bound to be less prepared to perform the responsibilities incident to citizenship in a free country. Wise policy is not derived from a formula. Laws are not self-enacting. Emergencies, resulting both from acts of nature and from acts of human recklessness and cruelty, will happen. But who will judge wisely, who will act honorably, who will rise to the occasion should drugs increasingly estrange us from the satisfactions connected to acting wisely and well? Who will take seriously even the everyday duties to kith and kin in a world that esteems—and uses medicine to produce—self-satisfied egos, looking out only for Number One?

The remedy for the new individual and social dangers to which our freedom exposes us must be consistent with our right to "the pursuit of happiness." And so it is. For the remedy consists in organizing our lives around happiness rightly understood, and our freedom gives us the opportunity to acquire that understanding and act upon it. In the end, it is happiness understood as complete and comprehensive well-being, or happiness of the soul, that we seek. And the happiness of the soul is inseparable from the pleasure that comes from perfecting our natures and living fruitfully with our families, friends, and fellow citizens.

No doubt the amazing new world of biotechnology has an enormous role to play in our soul's aspiration for happiness. Whether it will further or frustrate that aspiration depends in no small measure on our ability to clarify happiness's character and content. It depends especially on our willingness, both as individuals and as a society, not to settle for a shallow and shrunken imitation.

ENDNOTES

[1] Aristotle, *Nicomachean Ethics,* 1095a17-20.

[2] Borges, J. L., "Funes the Memorious," in *Ficciones,* John Sturrock, ed. (original publication 1942; English transl., Grove Press, 1962; rpt. by Alfred A. Knopf/Everyman, 1993), pp. 83-91; Luria, A. R., *The Mind of a Mnemonist: A little book about a vast memory* (Solotaroff, L., trans.), New York: Basic Books, 1968.

[3] On this research see LeDoux, J. E., "Emotion, Memory, and the Brain," *Scientific American,* 270: 32-39, 1994; McGaugh, J., "Emotional Activation, Neuromodulatory Systems and Memory," in *Memory Distortion: How Minds, Brains, and Societies Reconstruct the Past,* edited by D. Schacter, et al., pp. 255-273, 1995; and McGaugh, J., "Memory consolidation and the amygdala: a system perspective," *Trends in Neuroscience,* 25(9): 456-461, 2002.

[4] Cahill, L., et al., "Beta-Adrenergic activation and memory for emotional events," *Nature,* 371: 702-704, 1994.

[5] Pitman, R. K., et al., "Pilot Study of Secondary Prevention of Posttraumatic Stress Disorder with Propranolol," *Biological Psychiatry,* 51: 189-192, 2002.

[6] See, for example, Goodman, E., "Matter Over Mind?," *Washington Post,* November 16, 2002, and Baard, E., "The Guilt-Free Soldier," *Village Voice,* 28 January 2003. It is interesting to note the dual appeal of such drugs to both the traumatized victim seeking escape from the horror of his or her experience and the traumatizing assailant looking to escape the inconvenience of his guilty memory.

[7] There is no definitive diagnostic criterion for PTSD, but the core symptoms are thought to include persistent re-experiencing of the traumatic event, avoidance of associated stimuli, and hyperarousal. See *Diagnostic and Statistical Manual of Mental Disorders, Fourth Edition, text revision,* Washington, D.C.: American Psychiatric Association, 2000, pp. 463-486.

[8] Schacter, D., *The Seven Sins of Memory: How the Mind Forgets and Remembers,* New York: Houghton Mifflin, 2001, p. 183.

[9] For a discussion of memory-altering drugs and the meaning of "bearing witness," see the essay by Cohen, E., "Our Psychotropic Memory," *SEED,* no. 8, Fall 2003, p.42.

[10] Austen, Jane, *Mansfield Park* (1814), Ch. 22.

[11] See http://abcnews.go.com/onair/WorldNewsTonight/poll000410.html.

[12] Kramer, P., *Listening to Prozac,* New York: Penguin, 1997, p. 66. The point is thematic throughout the book; see also, for example, pp. 46, 89, 125-127, and 320-322. See also Braun, S., *The Science of Happiness: Unlocking the Mysteries of Mood,* New York: John Wiley & Sons, 2000, pp. 8-9 and 161-181, and Barondes, S., *Better Than Prozac: The Future of Psychiatric Drugs,* Oxford:

Oxford University Press, 2003. Relatively little academic research, as opposed to clinical observation, has been done on this issue. What has been done supports the idea that SSRIs affect the mood of people without severe illness, ranging from mild depression to normalcy. See Dunlop, S. R., et al., "Pattern Analysis Shows Beneficial Effect of Fluoxetine Treatment in Mild Depression," *Psychopharmacology Bulletin*, 26: 173-180, 1990; Knutson, B., et al., "Selective Alteration of Personality and Social Behavior by Serotonergic Intervention," *American Journal of Psychiatry* 155: 373-379, 1998; Liotti, M., et al., "Differential Limbic-Cortical Correlates of Sadness and Anxiety in Healthy Subjects: Implications for Affective Disorders," *Biological Psychiatry*, 48: 30-42, 2000.

[13] Dozens of books aimed at a general audience about mood-brighteners, in particular the SSRI Prozac, have been published in the last decade alone (some are listed in endnote 12). Popular articles abound in publications ranging from the *New York Times* to *Newsweek* to *Glamour* (Slater, L., "Prozac Mother and Child," *New York Times Magazine*, 17 October 1999, pp. 15-17; Gates, D., "The Case of Dr. Strangedrug," *Newsweek*, 19 June 1993; Fried, S., "Addicted to Antidepressants? The Controversy Over a Pill Millions of Us Are Taking," *Glamour*, April 2003, pp. 178-180, 262). Television programs have also covered the matter, including "Nightline," "Geraldo," the "Today" show, "60 Minutes," "Donahue," "Larry King," "Eye on America," and "Prime Time Live." The tremendous coverage, while highly varied in quality, indicates the degree to which drugs that touch on such deep and universal human aspirations provoke interest.

[14] For one, among many, moving accounts of major depressive illness and its associated risks, including risk of suicide, see Rosenberg, L., "Brainsick: A Physician's Journey to the Brink," *Cerebrum*, 4: 43-60, 2002.

[15] Kramer, P., *Listening to Prozac*, pp. 15-16, 44-46, 321-322. This point is one of Kramer's principal themes. See also Barondes, S., *Better Than Prozac, op. cit.*

[16] The National Institute of Mental Health, *The Numbers Count: Mental Disorders in America*, Washington, D.C.: NIH Publication No. 01-4584, 2003, p. 1; Sapolsky, R., "Will We Still Be Sad Fifty Years from Now?" in Brockman, J., *The Next Fifty Years: Science in the First Half of the Twenty-First Century*, New York: Vintage, 2002, p. 106; Nestler, E.J., et al., "Neurobiology of Depression," *Neuron*, 34: 13-25, p. 13, 2002.

[17] Klerman, G., et al., "Increasing rates of depression," *Journal of the American Medical Association*, 261(15): 2229-2235, 1989; see also Sapolsky, R., "Will We Still Be Sad Fifty Years from Now?" *op. cit.*, pp. 106-107.

[18] See the references cited in endnotes 12 and 16.

[19] The National Institute of Mental Health, *Medications*, Washington, DC: NIH Publication No. 02-3929, 2002, p. 20; Nestler, "Neurobiology of Depression," *op. cit.*, p. 15.

[20] Glader, P., "From the Maker of Effexor: Campus Forums on Depression," *Wall Street Journal*, 10 October 2002, p. B1. Very little definitive information on the prevalence of mood-brighteners among college students is available. One survey suggests that only slightly over 4 percent of students are currently taking mood-brighteners (American College Health Association, *National College Health Assessment: Reference Group Executive Summary Spring 2002*, Baltimore: American College Health Association, 2002). But this assessment does not speak to how many have taken them, and it contradicts the impressions of many college officials.

[21] Nestler, "Neurobiology of Depression," *op. cit.*

[22] *Diagnostic and Statistical Manual of Mental Disorders, op. cit.*, pp. 345-428.

[23] Nestler, *op. cit.*; Healy, D., *The Antidepressant Era*, Cambridge: Harvard 1997, p. 174.

[24] Nestler, "Neurobiology of Depression," *op. cit.*, p. 13. Braun, *The Science of Happiness, op. cit.*, pp. 17-18.

[25] See *Listening to Prozac, op. cit.*; *The Science of Happiness, op. cit.*, p. 12 and pp. 161-181; *Better Than Prozac, op. cit.*

[26] For a discussion of both this aspect of temperament and the capacity of SSRIs to affect it, see McHugh, P., et al., *The Perspectives of Psychiatry*, Baltimore: Johns Hopkins, 1998, pp. 132-135.

[27] For a report of the experience of taking MDMA, see Klam, M., "Experiencing Ecstasy," *The New York Times Magazine*, 21 January 2001.

[28] A related line of thought has been developed by Michael McGuire. See Kramer, *Listening to Prozac*, 169.

[29] *Listening to Prozac*, pp. 144-148, 162, 177, and 195.

[30] *Listening to Prozac*, pp. 145-146.

[31] *Listening to Prozac*, p. 177.

[32] *Listening to Prozac*, p. 195.

[33] Healy, *The Antidepressant Era, op. cit.*, p. 173.

[34] *The Confessions of St. Augustine*, trans. J. G. Pilkington, Norwalk: Easton Press, 1979, ch. 9, pp. 160-162.

[35] Wolterstorff, N., *Lament for a Son*, Grand Rapids: Eerdman's, 1987, pp. 96-97.

[36] Huxley, A., *Brave New World*, Norwalk: Easton Press, 1978.

[37] McHugh, P., et al., *The Perspectives of Psychiatry*, p. 71.

[38] *Diagnostic and Statistical Manual of Mental Disorders, op. cit.*

"Beyond Therapy": General Reflections

The four preceding chapters have examined how several prominent and (generally) salutary human pursuits may be aided or altered using a wide variety of biotechnologies that lend themselves to purposes "beyond therapy." In each case, we have discussed the character of the end, considered the novel means, and explored some possible implications, ethical and social. In surveying the pertinent technologies, we have taken a somewhat long-range view, looking at humanly significant technical possibilities that may soon—or not so soon—be available for general use, yet at the same time trying to separate fact from science fiction. In offering ethical analysis, we have tried to identify key issues pertinent to the case under discussion, asking questions about both ends and means, and looking always for the special significance of pursuing the old human ends by these new technological means. In this concluding chapter, we step back from the particular "case studies" to pull together some common threads and to offer some generalizations and conclusions to which the overall inquiry has led.

I. THE BIG PICTURE

The first generalization concerns the wide array of biotechnologies that are, or may conceivably be, useful in pursuing goals beyond therapy. Although not originally developed for such uses, the available and possible techniques we have considered—techniques for screening genes and testing embryos, choosing sex of children, modifying the behavior of children, augmenting muscle size and strength, enhancing athletic performance, slowing senescence, blunting painful memories, and brightening mood—do indeed promise us new powers that can serve age-old human desires. True, in some cases, the likelihood that the new technologies will be successfully applied to those purposes seems, at least for the foreseeable future, far-fetched: genetically engineered "designer babies" are not in the offing. In other cases, as with psychotropic drugs affecting memory, mood, and behavior, some uses beyond therapy are already with us. In still other cases, such as research aimed at retarding senescence, only time will tell what sort of powers may become available for increasing the maximum human lifespan, and by how much. Yet the array of biotechnologies potentially useful in these ventures should not be underestimated, especially when we consider how little we yet know about the human body and mind and how much our knowledge and technique will surely grow in the coming years. Once we acquire technical tools and the potential for their use based on fuller knowledge, we will likely be able to intervene much more knowingly, competently, and comprehensively.

Second, despite the heterogeneity of the techniques, the variety of purposes they may serve, and the different issues raised by pursuing these differing purposes by diverse means, we believe that all of these matters deserve to be considered together, just as we have done in this report. Notwithstanding the multiplicity of ends, means, and consequences that we have considered, this report offers less a list of many things to think about than a picture of *one big thing* to think about: the dawning age of biotechnology and the greatly augmented power it is providing us, not only for gaining better health but also for improving our natural capacities and pursuing our own happiness. The ambitious project for the mastery of nature, the project first envisioned by Francis Bacon and René Descartes in the early seventeenth century, is finally yielding its promised abilities to relieve man's estate—and then some. Though our society will, as a matter of public practice, be required to deal with each of these techniques and possibilities as they arrive, piecemeal and independently of one another, we should, as a matter of public understanding, try to see what they might all add up to, taken together. The Council's experience of considering these disparate subjects under this one big idea—"beyond therapy, for the pursuit of happiness"—and our discovery of overlapping ethical implications would seem to vindicate the starting assumption that led us to undertake this project in the first place: *biotechnology beyond therapy deserves to be examined not in fragments, but as a whole.*

Yet, third, the "whole" that offers us the most revealing insights into this subject is not itself technological. For the age of biotechnology is not so much about technology itself as it is about *human beings empowered by biotechnology.* Thus, to understand the human and social meaning of the new age, we must begin not from our tools and products but from where human beings begin, namely, with the very human desires that we have here identified in order to give shape to this report: desires for better children, superior performance, younger and more beautiful bodies, abler minds, happier souls. Looking at the big picture through this lens keeps one crucial fact always in focus: how people exploit the relatively unlimited uses of biotechnical power will be decisively determined by the perhaps still more unlimited desires of human beings, especially—and this is a vital point—as these desires themselves become transformed and inflated by the new technological powers they are all the while acquiring. Our desires to alter our consciousness or preserve our youthful strength, perhaps but modest to begin with, could swell considerably if and when we become more technically able to satisfy them. And as they grow, what would have been last year's satisfaction will only fuel this year's greater hunger for more.

Fourth, as the ubiquitous human desires are shaped and colored not only reactively by the tools that might serve them but also directly by surrounding cultural and social ideas and practices, the "one big picture" will be colored by the (albeit changeable) ruling opinions, mores, and institutions of the society in which we live and into which the technologies are being introduced. For example, the desire for performance-enhancing drugs will be affected by the social climate regarding competition; the eagerness to gain an edge for one's children will be affected by whether many other parents are doing so; and the willingness to use or forego medication for various sorts of psychic distress will be affected by the poverty or richness of private life, and the degree to which strong family or community support is (or is not) available for coping with that distress directly. Moreover, in a free and pluralistic society, we may expect a very diverse popular reaction to the invitation of the new technologies, ranging from exuberant enthusiasm to outright rejection, and the overall public response cannot be judged in advance. Yet because the choices made by some can, in their consequences, alter the shared life lived by all, it behooves all of us to consider the meaning of these developments, whether we are privately tempted by them or not. It is in part to contribute to a more thoughtful public appraisal of these possibilities that we have undertaken this report.

By beginning with the common human desires, we have sought to place what may be new and strange into a context provided by what is old and familiar. We recognize the temptation to add biotechnological means to our "tool kits" for pursuing happiness and self-improvement, and it is not difficult to appreciate, at least at first glance, the attractiveness of the goods being contemplated. We want to give our children the best start in life and every chance to succeed. We want to perform at our best, and better than we did before. We want to remain youthful and vigorous for as long as we can. We want to face life optimistically and with proper self-regard. And since we now avail ourselves of all sorts of means toward these ends, we will certainly not want to neglect the added advantages that biotechnologies may offer us, today and tomorrow.

At the same time, however, we have identified, in each of the previous four chapters, several reasonable sources of concern, ethical and social. And, in each case, we have called attention to some of the possible hidden costs of success, achieved by employing these means. The chapter on better children raised questions about the meaning and limits of parental control and about the character and rearing of children. The chapter on superior performance raised questions about the meaning of excellence and the "humanity" of human activity. The chapter on ageless bodies raised questions about the significance of the "natural" life cycle and life-span, and their connection to the dynamic character of society and the prospects for its invigorating renewal. And the chapter on happy souls raised questions about the connections between experienced mood or self-esteem and the deeds or experiences that ordinarily are their foundation, as well as the connections between remembering truly and personal identity. Looking again at these subjects, now seen as part of "one big picture," we think it useful here to collect and organize the various issues into a semi-complete account, so that the reader may see in outline the most important and likely sources of concern.

Before proceeding, we wish to reiterate our intention in this inquiry, so as to avoid misunderstanding. In offering our synopsis of concerns, we are not making predictions; we are merely pointing to possible hazards, hazards that become visible only when one looks at "the big picture." More important, we are not condemning either biotechnological power or the pursuit of happiness, excellence, or self-perfection. Far from it. We eagerly embrace biotechnologies as aids for preventing or correcting bodily or mental ills and for restoring health and fitness. We even more eagerly embrace the pursuits of happiness, excellence, and self-improvement, for ourselves, our children, and our society. Desires for these goals are the source of much that is good in human life. Yet, as has long been known, these desires can be excessive. Worse, they can be badly educated regarding the nature of their object, sometimes with tragic result: we get what we ask for only to discover that it is very far from what we really wanted. Finally, they can be pursued in harmful ways and with improper means, often at the price of deforming the very goals being sought. To guard against such outcomes, we need to be alert in advance to the more likely risks and the more serious concerns. We begin with those that are more obvious and familiar.

II. FAMILIAR SOURCES OF CONCERN

The first concerns commonly expressed regarding any uses of biotechnology beyond therapy reflect, not surprisingly, the dominant values of modern America: health and safety, fairness and equality, and freedom. The following thumbnail sketches of the issues should suffice to open the questions—though of course not to settle them.

A. Health: Issues of Safety and Bodily Harm

In our health-conscious culture, the first reason people worry about any new biotechnical intervention, whatever its intended purpose, is safety. This will surely be true regarding "elective" uses of biotechnology that aim beyond therapy. Athletes who take steroids to boost their strength may later suffer premature heart disease. College students who snort Ritalin to increase their concentration may become addicted. Melancholics taking mood-brighteners to change their outlook may experience impotence or apathy. To generalize: no biological agent used for purposes of self-perfection or self-satisfaction is likely to be entirely safe. This is good medical common sense: anything powerful enough to enhance system A is likely to be powerful enough to harm system B (or even system A itself), the body being a highly complex yet integrated whole in which one intervenes partially only at one's peril. And it surely makes sense, ethically speaking, that one should not risk basic health pursuing a condition of "better than well."

Yet some of the interventions that might aim beyond therapy—for example, genetic enhancement of muscle strength, retardation of aging, or pharmacologic blunting of horrible memories or increasing self-esteem—may, indirectly, lead also to improvements in general health. More important, many good things in life are filled with risks, and free people—even if properly informed about the magnitude of those risks—may choose to run them if they care enough about what they might gain thereby. If the interventions are shown to be *highly* dangerous, many people will (later if not sooner) avoid them, and the Food and Drug Administration or tort liability will constrain many a legitimate would-be producer. But if, on the other hand, the interventions work well and are indeed highly desired, people may freely accept, in trade-off, even considerable risk of later bodily harm for the sake of significant current benefits. Besides, the bigger ethical issues in this area have little to do with safety; the most basic questions concern not the hazards associated with the techniques but the benefits and harms of using the perfected powers, assuming that they may be safely used.

B. Unfairness

An obvious objection to the use of enhancement technologies, especially by participants in competitive activities, is that they give those who use them an unfair advantage: blood doping or steroids in athletes, stimulants in students taking the SATs, and so on. This issue, briefly discussed in Chapter Three, has been well aired by the International Olympic Committee and the many other athletic organizations who continue to try to formulate rules that can be enforced, even as the athletes and their pharmacists continue to devise ways to violate those rules and escape detection. Yet as we saw, the fairness question can be turned on its head, and some people see in biotechnical intervention a way to compensate for the "unfairness" of *natural* inequalities—say, in size, strength, drive, or native talent. Still, even if everyone had equal access to genetic improvement of muscle strength or mind-enhancing drugs, or even if these gifts of technology would be used only to rectify the inequalities produced by the unequal gifts of nature, an additional disquiet would still perhaps remain: The disquiet of using such new powers in the first place or at all, even were they fairly distributed. Besides, as we have emphasized, not all activities of life are competitive, and the uses of biotechnologies for purposes beyond therapy are more worrisome on other grounds.*

C. Equality of Access

A related question concerns inequality of access to the benefits of biotechnology, a matter of great interest to many Members of this Council, though little discussed in the previous chapters. The issue of distributive justice is more important than the issue of unfairness in competitive activities, especially if there are systemic disparities between those who will and those who won't have access to the powers of biotechnical "improvement." Should these capabilities arrive, we may face severe aggravations of existing "unfairnesses" in the "game of life," especially if people who need certain agents to treat serious illness cannot get them while other people can enjoy them for less urgent or even dubious purposes. If, as is now often the case with expensive medical care, only the wealthy and privileged will be able to gain easy access to costly enhancing technologies, we

---

* For example: It mattered to the young woman we cited in Chapter Five that the young man said he loved her only because he was high on Ecstasy. It matters to all of us that the people we have dealings with are not psychotropically out of their right minds. In neither case is the issue one of unfair advantage.

might expect to see an ever-widening gap between "the best and the brightest" and the rest. The emergence of a biotechnologically improved "aristocracy"—augmenting the already cognitively stratified structure of American society—is indeed a worrisome possibility, and there is nothing in our current way of doing business that works against it. Indeed, unless something new intervenes, it would seem to be a natural outcome of mixing these elements of American society: our existing inequalities in wealth and status, the continued use of free markets to develop and obtain the new technologies, and our libertarian attitudes favoring unrestricted personal freedom for all choices in private life.

Yet the situation regarding rich and poor is more complex, especially if one considers actual benefits rather than equality or relative well-being. The advent of new technologies often brings great benefits to the less well off, if not at first, then after they come to be mass-produced and mass-marketed and the prices come down. (Consider, over the past half-century, the spread in the United States of refrigerators and radios, automobiles and washing machines, televisions and VCRs, cell phones and personal computers, and, in the domain of medicine, antibiotics, vaccines, and many expensive diagnostic and therapeutic procedures.) To be sure, the gap between the richest and the poorest may increase, but in absolute terms the poor may benefit more, when compared not to the rich but to where they were before. By many measures, the average American today enjoys a healthier, longer, safer, and more commodious life than did many a duke or prince but a few centuries back.

Nevertheless, worries about possible future bio-enhanced stratification should not be ignored. And they become more poignant in the present, to the extent that one regards spending money and energy on goals beyond therapy as a misallocation of limited resources in a world in which the basic health needs of millions go unaddressed. Yet although the setting of priorities for research and development is an important matter for public policy, it is not unique to the domain of "beyond therapy." It cannot be addressed, much less solved, in this area alone. Moreover, and yet again, the inequality of access does not remove our uneasiness over the thing itself. It is, to say the least, paradoxical, in discussions of the dehumanizing dangers of, say, future eugenic selection of better children, that people vigorously complain that the poor will be denied equal access to the danger: "The food is contaminated, but why are my portions so small?" Huxley's *Brave New World* runs on a deplorable and impermeably rigid class system, but few people would want to live in that world even if offered the chance to enjoy it as an alpha (the privileged caste). Even an elite can be dehumanized, can dehumanize itself. The questions about access and distributive justice are, no doubt, socially important. Yet the more fundamental ethical questions about taking biotechnology "beyond therapy" concern not equality of access, but the goodness or badness of the things being offered and the wisdom of pursuing our purposes by such means.

D. Liberty: Issues of Freedom and Coercion, Overt and Subtle

A concern for threats to freedom comes to the fore whenever biotechnical powers are exercised by some people upon other people. We encountered it in our discussion of "better children" (the choice of a child's sex or the drug-mediated alteration of his or her behavior; Chapter Two), as well as in the coerced use of anabolic steroids by the East German Olympic swimmers (Chapter Three). This problem will of course be worse in tyrannical regimes. But there are always dangers of despotism within families, as many parents already work their wills on their children with insufficient regard to a child's independence or long-term needs, jeopardizing even the "freedom to be a child." To the extent that even partial control over genotype—say, to take a relatively innocent example, musician parents selecting a child with genes for perfect pitch—would add to existing social instruments of parental control and its risks of despotic rule, this matter will need to be attended to.*

Leaving aside the special case of children, the risk of overt coercion does not loom large in a free society. On the contrary, many enthusiasts for using technology for personal enhancement are libertarian in outlook; they see here mainly the enlargement of human powers and possibilities and the multiplication of options for private choice, both of which they

---

* The danger of despotism of one generation over the next is, in fact, one of the arguments sometimes voiced against human cloning. See our report, *Human Cloning and Human Dignity: An Ethical Inquiry*, Washington, D.C.: Government Printing Office, 2002.

see as steps to greater human freedom. They look forward to growing opportunities for more people to earn more, learn more, see more, and do more, and to choose—perhaps several times in one lifetime—interesting new careers or avocations. And they look with suspicion at critics who they fear might want to limit their private freedom to develop and use new technologies for personal advancement or, indeed, for any purpose whatsoever. The coercion they fear comes not from advances in technology but from the state, acting to deny them their right to pursue happiness or self-improvement by the means they privately choose.

Yet no one can deny that people living in free societies, and even their most empowered citizens, already experience more subtle impingements on freedom and choice, operating, for example, through peer pressure. What is freely permitted and widely used may, under certain circumstances, become practically mandatory. If most children are receiving memory enhancement or stimulant drugs, failure to provide them for your child might be seen as a form of child neglect. If all the defensive linemen are on steroids, you risk mayhem if you go against them chemically pure. And, a point subtler still, some critics complain that, as with cosmetic surgery, Botox, and breast implants, many of the enhancement technologies of the future will very likely be used in slavish adherence to certain socially defined and merely fashionable notions of "excellence" or improvement, very likely shallow and conformist. If these fears are realized, such exercises of individual freedom, suitably multiplied, might compromise the freedom to be an individual.*

This special kind of reduction of freedom—let's call it the problem of conformity or homogenization—is of more than individual concern. In an era of mass culture, itself the by-product of previous advances in communication, manufacture, and marketing techniques, the exercise of uncoerced private choices may produce untoward consequences for soci-

---

* Freedom does not automatically increase with a growing range of options. On the contrary, if the options differ but little from one another (Nike rather than Adidas, Budweiser rather than Coors), and if the choosing agent expends growing energies on choices that contribute but little to his or her genuine well-being, enjoying one's greater number of options might represent a curtailment of a deeper and more genuine freedom.

ety as a whole. Trends in popular culture lead some critics to worry that the self-selected nontherapeutic uses of the new biotechnical powers, should they become widespread, will be put in the service of the most common human desires, moving us toward still greater homogenization of human society—perhaps raising the floor but also lowering the ceiling of human possibility, and reducing the likelihood of genuine freedom, individuality, and greatness. (This is an extension of Tocqueville's concern about the leveling effects of democracy, now possibly augmented by the technological power to make those effects ingrained and perhaps irreversible.)

Indeed, such constriction of individual possibility could be the most important society-wide concern, if we consider the aggregated effects of the likely individual choices for biotechnical "self-improvement," each of which might be defended or at least not objected to on a case-by-case basis (the problem of what the economists call "negative externalities"). For example, it might be difficult to object to a personal choice for a life-extending technology that would extend the user's life by three healthy decades or a mood-brightened way of life that would make the individual more cheerful and untroubled by the world around him. Yet as we have suggested more than once, the aggregated social effects of such choices, widely made, could lead to a Tragedy of the Commons, where benefits gained by individuals are outweighed by the harms that return to them from the social costs of allowing everyone to share the goodies. And, as Huxley strongly suggests in *Brave New World*, when biotechnical powers are readily available to satisfy short-term desires or to produce easy contentment, the character of human striving changes profoundly and the desire for human excellence fades. Should this come to pass, the best thing to be hoped for might be the preservation of pockets of difference (as on the remote islands in *Brave New World*) where the desire for high achievement has not been entirely submerged or eroded.*

---

* Which of the imaginable social consequences will in fact occur is, of course, an empirical question, though it is worthwhile to think about the alternatives in advance. Indeed, anticipatory reflection might play a role in helping to forestall some of the worst possible outcomes. We return to the relation of biotechnology to American society in the last section of this chapter.

III. ESSENTIAL SOURCES OF CONCERN

Our familiar worries about issues of safety, equality, and freedom, albeit very important, do not exhaust the sources of reasonable concern. When richly considered, they invite us to think about the deeper purposes for the sake of which we want to live safely, justly, and freely. And they enable us to recognize that even the safe, equally available, non-coerced and non-faddish uses of biomedical technologies to pursue happiness or self-improvement raise ethical and social questions, questions more directly connected with the essence of the activity itself: the use of technological means to intervene into the human body and mind, not to ameliorate their diseases but to change and improve their normal workings. Why, if at all, are we bothered by the voluntary *self*-administration of agents that would change our bodies or alter our minds? What is disquieting about our attempts to improve upon human nature, or even our own particular instance of it?

The subject being relatively novel, it is difficult to put this worry into words. We are in an area where initial revulsions are hard to translate into sound moral arguments. Many people are probably repelled by the idea of drugs that erase memories or that change personalities, or of interventions that enable seventy-year-olds to bear children or play professional sports, or, to engage in some wilder imaginings, of mechanical implants that would enable men to nurse infants or computer-brain hookups that would enable us to download the *Oxford English Dictionary*. But can our disquiet at such prospects withstand rational, anthropological, or ethical scrutiny? Taken one person at a time, with a properly prepared set of conditions and qualifications, it will be hard to say what is wrong with any biotechnical intervention that could improve our performances, give us (more) ageless bodies, or make it possible for us to have happier souls. Indeed, in many cases, we ought to be thankful for or pleased with the improvements our biotechnical ingenuity is making possible.

If there are essential reasons to be concerned about these activities and where they may lead us, we sense that it may have something to do with challenges to what is naturally human, what is humanly dignified, or to attitudes that show proper respect for what is naturally and dignifiedly human. As it happens, at least four such considerations have already been treated in one place or another in the previous chapters: appreciation of and respect for "the naturally given," threatened by hubris; the dignity of human activity, threatened by "unnatural" means; the preservation of identity, threatened by efforts at self-transformation; and full human flourishing, threatened by spurious or shallow substitutes.

A. Hubris or Humility: Respect for "the Given"

A common, man-on-the-street reaction to the prospects of biotechnological engineering beyond therapy is the complaint of "man playing God." If properly unpacked, this worry is in fact shared by people holding various theological beliefs and by people holding none at all. Sometimes the charge means the sheer prideful presumption of trying to alter what God has ordained or nature has produced, or what should, for whatever reason, not be fiddled with. Sometimes the charge means not so much usurping God-like powers, but doing so in the absence of God-like knowledge: the mere playing at being God, the hubris of acting with insufficient wisdom.

Over the past few decades, environmentalists, forcefully making the case for respecting Mother Nature, have urged upon us a "precautionary principle" regarding all our interventions into the natural world. Go slowly, they say, you can ruin everything. The point is certainly well taken in the present context. The human body and mind, highly complex and delicately balanced as a result of eons of gradual and exacting evolution, are almost certainly at risk from any ill-considered attempt at "improvement." There is not only the matter of unintended consequences, a concern even with interventions aimed at therapy. There is also the matter of uncertain goals and absent natural standards, once one proceeds "beyond therapy." When a physician intervenes therapeutically to correct some deficiency or deviation from a patient's natural wholeness, he acts as a servant to the goal of health and as an assistant to nature's own powers of self-healing, themselves wondrous products of evolutionary selection. But when a bioengineer intervenes for nontherapeutic ends, he stands not as nature's servant but as her aspiring master, guided by nothing but his own will and serving ends of his own devising. It is far from clear that our delicately integrated natural bodily powers will take kindly to such impositions, however desirable the sought-for change may seem to the intervener. And there is the further question of the unqualified goodness of the goals being sought, a matter to which we shall return.*

One revealing way to formulate the problem of hubris is what one of our Council Members has called the temptation to "hyper-agency," a Promethean aspiration to remake nature, including human nature, to serve our purposes and to satisfy our desires. This attitude is to be faulted not only because it can lead to bad, unintended consequences; more fundamentally, it also represents a false understanding of, and an improper disposition toward, the naturally given world. The root of the difficulty seems to be both cognitive and moral: the failure properly to appreciate and respect the "giftedness" of the world. Acknowledging the giftedness of life means recognizing that our talents and powers are not wholly our own doing, nor even fully ours, despite the efforts we expend to develop and to exercise them. It also means recognizing that not everything in the world is open to any use we may desire or devise. Such an appreciation of the giftedness of life would constrain the Promethean project and conduce to a much-needed humility. Although it is in part a religious sensibility, its resonance reaches beyond religion.[1]

Human beings have long manifested both wondering appreciation for nature's beauty and grandeur and reverent awe before nature's sublime and mysterious power. From the elegance of an orchid to the splendor of

---

* The question of the knowledge and goodness of goals is often the neglected topic when people use the language of "mastery," or "mastery and control of nature," to describe what we do when we use knowledge of how nature works to alter its character and workings. Mastery of the means of intervention without knowing the goodness of the goals of intervening is not, in fact, mastery at all. In the absence of such knowledge of ends, the goals of the "master" will be set rather by whatever it is that happens to guide or move his will—some impulse or whim or feeling or desire—in short, by some residuum of nature still working within the so-called master or controller. To paraphrase C. S. Lewis, what looks like man's mastery of nature turns out, in the absence of guiding knowledge, to be nature's mastery of man. (See his *The Abolition of Man*, New York: Macmillan, 1965, paperback edition, pp. 72-80.) There can, in truth, be no such thing as the *full* escape from the grip of our own nature. To pretend otherwise is indeed a form of hubristic and dangerous self-delusion. For reasons given in the text, therapeutic medicine, though it may use the same technologies, should not be regarded as "mastery of nature," but as service to nature, as we come to know, through medical science, how it might best be served.

the Grand Canyon, from the magnificence of embryological development to the miracle of sight or consciousness, the works of nature can still inspire in most human beings an attitude of respect, even in this age of technology. Nonetheless, the absence of a respectful attitude is today a problem in some—though by no means all—quarters of the biotechnical world. It is worrisome when people act toward, or even talk about, our bodies and minds—or human nature itself—as if they were mere raw material to be molded according to human will. It is worrisome when people speak as if they were wise enough to redesign human beings, improve the human brain, or reshape the human life cycle. In the face of such hubristic temptations, appreciating that the given world—including our natural powers to alter it—is not of our own making could induce a welcome attitude of modesty, restraint, and humility. Such a posture is surely recommended for anyone inclined to modify human beings or human nature for purposes beyond therapy.

Yet the respectful attitude toward the "given," while both necessary and desirable as a restraint, is not by itself sufficient as a guide. The "giftedness of nature" also includes smallpox and malaria, cancer and Alzheimer disease, decline and decay. Moreover, nature is not equally generous with her gifts, even to man, the most gifted of her creatures. Modesty born of gratitude for the world's "givenness" may enable us to recognize that not everything in the world is open to any use we may desire or devise, but it will not *by itself* teach us *which* things can be tinkered with and which should be left inviolate. Respect for the "giftedness" of things cannot tell us which gifts are to be accepted as is, which are to be improved through use or training, which are to be housebroken through self-command or medication, and which opposed like the plague.

To guide the proper use of biotechnical power, we need something in addition to a generalized appreciation for nature's gifts. We would need also a particular regard and respect for the special gift that is our own given nature. For only if there is a *human* "givenness," or a given humanness, that is also good and worth respecting, either as we find it or as it could be perfected *without ceasing to be itself,* will the "given" serve as a *positive* guide for choosing what to alter and what to leave alone. Only if there is something precious in our given human nature—beyond the fact of its giftedness—can what is given guide us in resisting efforts that would degrade it. When it comes to human biotechnical engineering beyond therapy, only if there is something inherently good or dignified about, say, natural procreation, the human life cycle (with its rhythm of rise and fall), and human erotic longing and striving; only if there is something inherently good or dignified about the ways in which we engage the world as spectators and appreciators, as teachers and learners, leaders and followers, agents and makers, lovers and friends, parents and children, citizens and worshippers, and as seekers of our own special excellence and flourishing in whatever arena to which we are called—only then can we begin to see why those aspects of our nature need to be defended against our deliberate redesign.

We must move, therefore, from the danger of hubris in the powerful designer to the danger of degradation in the designed, considering how any proposed improvements might impinge upon the nature of the one being improved. With the question of human nature and human dignity in mind, we move to questions of means and ends.

B. "Unnatural" Means: The Dignity of Human Activity

Until only yesterday, teaching and learning or practice and training exhausted the alternatives for acquiring human excellence, perfecting our natural gifts through our own efforts. But perhaps no longer: biotechnology may be able to do nature one better, even to the point of requiring less teaching, training, or practice to permit an improved nature to shine forth. As we noted earlier, the insertion of the growth-factor gene into the muscles of rats and mice bulks them up and keeps them strong and sound without the need for nearly as much exertion. Drugs to improve alertness (today) or memory and amiability (tomorrow) could greatly relieve the need for exertion to acquire these powers, leaving time and effort for better things. What, if anything, is disquieting about such means of gaining improvement?

The problem cannot be that they are "artificial," in the sense of having man-made origins. Beginning with the needle and the fig leaf, man has from the start been the animal that uses art to improve his lot by altering or adding to what nature alone provides.* Ordinary medicine makes extensive use of similar artificial means, from drugs to surgery to mechanical implants, in order to treat disease. If the use of artificial means is absolutely welcome in the activity of healing, it cannot be their unnaturalness alone that disquiets us when they are used to make people "better than well."

Still, in those areas of human life in which excellence has until now been achieved only by discipline and effort, the attainment of similar results by means of drugs, genetic engineering, or implanted devices looks to many people (including some Members of this Council) to be "cheating" or "cheap." Many people believe that each person should work hard for his achievements. Even if we prefer the grace of the natural athlete or the quickness of the natural mathematician—people whose performances deceptively appear to be effortless—we admire also those who overcome obstacles and struggle to try to achieve the excellence of the former. This matter of character—the merit of disciplined and dedicated striving—is surely pertinent. For character is not only the source of our deeds, but also their product. As we have already noted, healthy people whose disruptive behavior is "remedied" by pacifying drugs rather than by their own efforts are not learning self-control;** if anything, they may be learning to think it unnecessary. People who take pills to block out from memory the painful or hateful aspects of a new experience will not learn how to deal with suffering or sorrow. A drug that induces fearlessness does not produce courage.

Yet things are not so simple. Some biotechnical interventions may assist in the pursuit of excellence without in the least cheapening its attainment. And many of life's excellences have nothing to do with competition or overcoming adversity. Drugs to decrease drowsiness, increase alertness, sharpen memory, or reduce distraction may actually help people interested in their natural pursuits of learning or painting or performing

---

* By his very nature, man is the animal constantly looking for ways to better his life through artful means and devices; man is the animal with what Rousseau called "perfectibility."

** We have also noted that other people, suffering from certain neuro-psychiatric disorders, become capable of learning self-control only with the aid of medication addressed to their disorders.

their civic duty. Drugs to steady the hand of a neurosurgeon or to prevent sweaty palms in a concert pianist cannot be regarded as "cheating," for they are in no sense the source of the excellent activity or achievement. And, for people dealt a meager hand in the dispensing of nature's gifts, it should not be called cheating or cheap if biotechnology could assist them in becoming better equipped—whether in body or in mind.

Nevertheless, as we suggested at some length in Chapter Three, there remains a sense that the "naturalness" of means matters. It lies not in the fact that the assisting drugs and devices are artifacts, but in the danger of violating or deforming the nature of human agency and the dignity of the naturally human way of activity. In most of our ordinary efforts at self-improvement, whether by practice, training, or study, we sense the relation between our doings and the resulting improvement, between the means used and the end sought. There is an experiential and intelligible connection between means and ends; we can see how confronting fearful things might eventually enable us to cope with our fears. We can see how curbing our appetites produces self-command. Human education ordinarily proceeds by speech or symbolic deeds, whose meanings are at least in principle directly accessible to those upon whom they work.

In contrast, biotechnical interventions act directly on the human body and mind to bring about their effects on a passive subject, who plays little or no role at all. He can at best *feel* their effects *without understanding their meaning in human terms.* Thus, a drug that brightened our mood would alter us without our understanding how and why it did so— whereas a mood brightened as a fitting response to the arrival of a loved one or to an achievement in one's work is perfectly, because humanly, intelligible. And not only would this be true about our states of mind. All of our encounters with the world, both natural and interpersonal, would be mediated, filtered, and altered. Human experience under biological intervention becomes increasingly mediated by unintelligible forces and vehicles, separated from the human significance of the activities so altered. The relations between the knowing subject and his activities, and between his activities and their fulfillments and pleasures, are disrupted.

The importance of human effort in human achievement is here properly acknowledged: the point is less the exertions of good character against hardship, but the manifestation of an alert and self-experiencing agent making his deeds flow intentionally from his willing, knowing, and embodied soul. If human flourishing means not just the accumulation of external achievements and a full curriculum vitae but a lifelong being-at-work exercising one's *human* powers *well* and without great impediment, our genuine happiness requires that there be little gap, if any, between the dancer and the dance.*

C. Identity and Individuality

With biotechnical interventions that skip the realm of intelligible meaning, we cannot really own the transformations nor can we experience them as genuinely ours. And we will be at a loss to attest whether the resulting conditions and activities of our bodies and our minds are, in the fullest sense, our own as human. But our interest in identity is also more personal. For we do not live in a generic human way; we desire, act, flourish, and decline *as ourselves*, as individuals. To be human is to be someone, not any-one—with a given nature (male or female), given natural abilities (superior wit or musical talent), and—most important—a real history of attachments, memories, and experiences, acquired largely by living with others.

In myriad ways, new biotechnical powers promise (or threaten) to transform what it means to be an individual: giving increased control over our identity to others, as in the case of genetic screening or sex selection of offspring by parents; inducing psychic states divorced from real life and lived experience; blunting or numbing the memories we wish to escape; and achieving the results we could never achieve unaided, by acting as ourselves alone.

To be sure, in many cases, biomedical technology can restore or pre-serve a real identity that is slipping away: keeping our memory intact by

---

* This is not merely to suggest that there is a disturbance of human agency or freedom, or a dis-ruption of activities that will confound the assignment of personal responsibility or undermine the proper bestowal of praise and blame. To repeat: most of life's activities are non-competitive; most of the best of them—loving and working and savoring and learning—are self-fulfilling beyond the need for praise and blame or any other external reward. In these activities, there is at best no goal beyond the activity itself. It is the possibility of natural, unimpeded, for-itself human activity, that we are eager to preserve against dilution and distortion.

holding off the scourge of Alzheimer disease; restoring our capacity to love and work by holding at bay the demons of self-destroying depression. In other cases, the effect of biotechnology on identity is much more ambiguous. By taking psychotropic drugs to reduce anxiety or overcome melancholy, we may become the person we always wished to be—more cheerful, ambitious, relaxed, content. But we also become a different person in the eyes of others, and in many cases we become dependent on the continued use of psychotropic drugs to remain the new person we now are.

As the power to transform our native powers increases, both in magnitude and refinement, so does the possibility for "self-alienation"—for losing, confounding, or abandoning our identity. I may get better, stronger, and happier—but I know not how. I am no longer the agent of self-transformation, but a passive patient of transforming powers. Indeed, to the extent that an achievement is the result of some extraneous intervention, it is detachable from the agent whose achievement it purports to be. "Personal achievements" impersonally achieved are not truly the achievements of persons. That I can use a calculator to do my arithmetic does not make *me* a knower of arithmetic; if computer chips in my brain were to "download" a textbook of physics, would that make *me* a knower of physics? Admittedly, the relation between biological boosters and personal identity is much less clear: if I make myself more alert through Ritalin, or if drugs can make up for lack of sleep, I may be able to learn more using my unimpeded native powers while it is still unquestionably *I* who am doing the learning. And yet, to find out that an athlete took steroids before the race or that a test-taker (without medical disability) took Ritalin before the test is to lessen our regard for the achievement of the doer. It is to see not just an acting self, but a dependent self, one who is less himself for becoming so dependent.

In the deepest sense, to have an identity is to have limits: my body, not someone else's—even when the pains of aging might tempt me to become young again; my memories, not someone else's—even when the traumas of the past might tempt me to have someone else's memories; my achievements and potential, not someone else's—even when the desire for excellence might tempt me to "trade myself in" for a "better model." We seek to be happy—to achieve, perform, take pleasure in our experiences, and catch the admiring eye of a beloved. But we do not, at least self-consciously, seek such happiness at the cost of losing our real identity.

D. Partial Ends, Full Flourishing

Beyond the perils of achieving our desired goals in a "less-than-human way" or in ways "not fully our own," we must consider the meaning of the ends themselves: better children, superior performance, ageless bodies, and happy souls. Would their attainment in fact improve or perfect our lives as human beings? Are they—always or ever—reasonable and attainable goals?

Everything depends, as we have pointed out in each case, on how these goals are understood, on their specific and concrete content. Yet, that said, the first two human ends—better children and superior per-formance—do seem reasonable and attainable, sometimes if not always, to some degree if not totally. When asked what they wish for their chil-dren, most parents say: "We want them to be happy," or "We want them to live good lives"—in other words, to be better and to do better. The desire is a fitting one for any loving parent. The danger lies in misconceiv-ing what "better children" really means, and thus coming to pursue this worthy goal in a misguided way, or with a false idea of what makes for a good or happy child.

Likewise, the goal of superior performance—the desire to be better or do better in all that we do—is good and noble, a fitting human aspiration. We admire excellence whenever we encounter it, and we properly seek to excel in those areas of life, large and small, where we ourselves are engaged and at-work. But the danger here is that we will become better in some area of life by diminishing ourselves in others, or that we will achieve superior results only by compromising our humanity, or by corrupting those activities that are not supposed to be "performances" measured in terms of external standards of "better and worse."

In many cases, biotechnologies can surely help us cultivate what is best in ourselves and in our children, providing new tools for realizing good ends, wisely pursued. But it is also possible that the new technological means may deform the ends themselves. In pursuit of better children, biotechnical powers risk making us "tyrants"; in pursuit of superior performance, they risk making us "artifacts." In both cases, the problem is not the ends themselves but our misguided idea of their attainment or our false way of seeking to attain them. And in both cases, there is the ubiquitous problem that "good" or "superior" will be reconceived to fit the sorts of goals that the technological interventions can help us attain. We may come to believe that genetic predisposition or brain chemistry holds the key to helping our children develop and improve, or that stimulant drugs or bulkier muscles hold the key to excellent human activity. If we are equipped with hammers, we will see only those things that can be improved by pounding.

The goals of ageless bodies and happy souls—and especially the ways biotechnology might shape our pursuit of these ends—are perhaps more complicated.[2] The case for ageless bodies seems at first glance to look pretty good. The prevention of decay, decline, and disability, the avoidance of blindness, deafness, and debility, the elimination of feebleness, frailty, and fatigue, all seem to be conducive to living fully as a human being at the top of one's powers—of having, as they say, a "good quality of life" from beginning to end. We have come to expect organ transplantation for our worn-out parts. We will surely welcome stem-cell-based therapies for regenerative medicine, reversing by replacement the damaged tissues of Parkinson disease, spinal cord injury, and many other degenerative disorders. It is hard to see any objection to obtaining a genetic enhancement of our muscles in our youth that would not only prevent the muscular feebleness of old age but would empower us to do any physical task with greater strength and facility throughout our lives. And, should aging research deliver on its promise of adding not only extra life to years but also extra years to life, who would refuse it?

But as we suggested in Chapter Four, there may in fact be many human goods that are inseparable from our aging bodies, from our living in time, and especially from the natural human life cycle by which each generation gives way to the one that follows it. Because this argument is so counterintuitive, we need to begin not with the individual choice for an ageless body, but with what the individual's life might look like in a world in which everyone made the same choice. We need to make the choice universal, and see the meaning of that choice in the mirror of its becoming the norm.

What if everybody lived life to the hilt, even as they approached an ever-receding age of death in a body that looked and functioned—let's not be too greedy—like that of a thirty-year-old? Would it be good if each and all of us lived like light bulbs, burning as brightly from beginning to end, then popping off without warning, leaving those around us suddenly in the dark? Or is it perhaps better that there be a shape to life, everything in its due season, the shape also written, as it were, into the wrinkles of our bodies that live it—provided, of course, that we do not suffer years of painful or degraded old age and that we do not lose our wits? What would the relations between the generations be like if there never came a point at which a son surpassed his father in strength or vigor? What incentive would there be for the old to make way for the young, if the old slowed down little and had no reason to think of retiring—if Michael could play basketball until he were not forty but eighty? Might not even a moderate prolongation of life-span with vigor lead to a prolongation in the young of functional immaturity—of the sort that has arguably already accompanied the great increase in average life expectancy experienced in the past century?*

Going against both common intuition and native human desire, some commentators have argued that living with full awareness and acceptance of our finitude may be the condition of many of the best things in human life: engagement, seriousness, a taste for beauty, the possibility of virtue, the ties born of procreation, the quest for meaning.[3] This might be true not just for immortality—an unlikely achievement, likely to produce only false expectations—but even for more modest prolongations of the maximum lifespan, especially in good health, that would permit us to live as if there were always tomorrow. The pursuit of perfect bodies and further life-extension might deflect us from realizing more fully the aspirations to which our lives naturally point, from living well rather than merely staying alive. A concern with one's own improving agelessness might finally be incompatible with accept-

---

* The gift of added years of expected future life is surely a great blessing for the young. But is the correlative perception of a seemingly limitless future an equal blessing? How preciously do people regard each day of life when its limits are out of sight?

ing the need for procreation and human renewal. And far from bringing contentment, it might make us increasingly anxious over our health or dominated by the fear of death. Assume, merely for the sake of the argument, that even a few of these social consequences would follow from a world of much greater longevity and vigor: What would we then say about the simple goodness of seeking an ageless body?

What about the pursuit of happy souls, and especially of the sort that we might better attain with pharmacological assistance? Painful and shameful memories are disturbing; guilty consciences trouble sleep; low self-esteem, melancholy, and world-weariness besmirch the waking hours. Why not memory-blockers for the former, mood-brighteners for the latter, and a good euphoriant—without risks of hangovers or cirrhosis—when celebratory occasions fail to be jolly? For let us be clear: If it is imbalances of neurotransmitters that are largely responsible for our state of soul, would it not be sheer priggishness to refuse the help of pharmacology for our happiness, when we accept it guiltlessly to correct for an absence of insulin or thyroid hormone?

And yet, as we suggested in Chapter Five, there seems to be something misguided about the pursuit of utter and unbroken psychic tranquility or the attempt to eliminate all shame, guilt, and painful memories. Traumatic memories, shame, and guilt, are, it is true, psychic pains. In extreme doses, they can be crippling. Yet, short of the extreme, they can also be helpful and fitting. They are appropriate responses to horror, disgraceful conduct, injustice, and sin, and, as such, help teach us to avoid them or fight against them in the future. Witnessing a murder should be remembered as horrible; doing a beastly deed should trouble one's soul. Righteous indignation at injustice depends on being able to feel injustice's sting. And to deprive oneself of one's memory—including and especially its truthfulness of feeling—is to deprive oneself of one's own life and identity.

These feeling states of soul, though perhaps accompaniments of human flourishing, are not its essence. Ersatz pleasure or feelings of self-esteem are not the real McCoy. They are at most shadows divorced from the underlying human activities that are the essence of flourishing. Most people want both to feel good and to feel good about themselves, but only as a result of being good and doing good.

At the same time, there appears to be a connection between the possibility of feeling deep unhappiness and the prospects for achieving genuine happiness. If one cannot grieve, one has not truly loved. To be capable of aspiration, one must know and feel lack. As Wallace Stevens put it: Not to have is the beginning of desire. In short, if human fulfillment depends on our being creatures of need and finitude and therewith of longings and attachment, there may be a double-barreled error in the pursuit of ageless bodies and factitiously happy souls: far from bringing us what we really need, pursuing these partial goods could deprive us of the urge and energy to seek a richer and more genuine flourishing.

Looking into the future at goals pursuable with the aid of new biotechnologies enables us to turn a reflective glance at our own version of the human condition and the prospects now available to us (in principle) for a flourishing human life. For us today, assuming that we are blessed with good health and a sound mind, a flourishing human life is not a life lived with an ageless body or an untroubled soul, but rather a life lived in rhythmed time, mindful of time's limits, appreciative of each season and filled first of all with those intimate human relations that are ours only because we are born, age, replace ourselves, decline, and die—and know it. It is a life of aspiration, made possible by and born of experienced lack, of the disproportion between the transcendent longings of the soul and the limited capacities of our bodies and minds. It is a life that stretches towards some fulfillment to which our natural human soul has been oriented, and, unless we extirpate the source, will always be oriented. It is a life not of better genes and enhancing chemicals but of love and friendship, song and dance, speech and deed, working and learning, revering and worshipping.

If this is true, then the pursuit of an ageless body may prove finally to be a distraction and a deformation. And the pursuit of an untroubled and self-satisfied soul may prove to be deadly to desire, if finitude recognized spurs aspiration and fine aspiration acted upon *is itself* the core of happiness. Not the agelessness of the body, nor the contentment of the soul, nor even the list of external achievements and accomplishments of life, but the engaged and energetic being-at-work of what nature uniquely gave to us is what we need to treasure and defend. All other "perfections" may turn out to be at best but passing illusions, at worst a Faustian bargain that could cost us our full and flourishing humanity.

Summing up these "essential sources of concern," we might succinctly formulate them as follows:

> In wanting to become more than we are, and in sometimes acting as if we were already superhuman or divine, we risk despising what we are and neglecting what we have.

> In wanting to improve our bodies and our minds using new tools to enhance their performance, we risk making our bodies and minds little different from our tools, in the process also compromising the distinctly human character of our agency and activity.

> In seeking by these means to be better than we are or to like ourselves better than we do, we risk "turning into someone else," confounding the identity we have acquired through natural gift cultivated by genuinely lived experiences, alone and with others.

> In seeking brighter outlooks, reliable contentment, and dependable feelings of self-esteem in ways that bypass their usual natural sources, we risk flattening our souls, lowering our aspirations, and weakening our loves and attachments.

> By lowering our sights and accepting the sorts of satisfactions that biotechnology may readily produce for us, we risk turning a blind eye to the objects of our natural loves and longings, the pursuit of which might be the truer road to a more genuine happiness.

To avoid such outcomes, our native human desires need to be educated against both excess and error. We need, as individuals and as a society, to find these boundaries and to learn how to preserve and defend them. To do so in an age of biotechnology, we need to ponder and answer questions like the following:

When does parental desire for better children constrict their freedom or undermine their long-term chances for self-command and genuine excellence?

When does the quest for self-improvement make the "self" smaller or meaner?

When does a preoccupation with youthful bodies or longer life jeopardize the prospects for living *well*?

When does the quest for contentment or self-esteem lead us away from the activities and attachments that prove to be essential to these goals when they are properly understood?

Answers to these questions are not easily given in the abstract or in advance. Boundaries are hard to define in the absence of better knowledge of the actual hazards. Such knowledge will be obtainable only in time and only as a result of lived experience. But centrally important in shaping the possible future outcomes will be the cultural attitudes and social practices that shape desires, govern expectations, and influence the choices people make, now and in the future. This means reflecting more specifically on how biotechnology beyond therapy might affect and be affected by American society.

IV. BIOTECHNOLOGY AND AMERICAN SOCIETY

In free societies such as our own, choices about using biotechnologies are not made by central planners looking to realize some dream of a more perfect future society. They are made largely by private individuals looking to realize their personal dream of a better life, for themselves and for their children. The choices that they make will, of course, be constrained by boundaries set by law and by the limits of their own resources. More subtly, they will be influenced by the social norms, cultural ideals, and institutional practices of their communities—as these norms, ideals, and practices are themselves reciprocally shaped by the aggregated results of countless private choices. No account of our subject would be complete without a brief look at these larger social implications.

Looking over the horizon, what sort of society might we be getting in the coming age of biotechnology? What sort of society are we, in fact, bringing into being, knowingly or unknowingly, by our private choices? And how might our existing American norms, ideals, and practices frame and color the "big picture" whose outlines are only now becoming visible?

On the optimistic view, the emerging picture is one of unmitigated progress and improvement, yielding a society in which more and more people are able to realize the American dream of liberty, prosperity, and justice for all. Projecting that the present century will continue the remarkable achievements of the one just ended, it is easy to imagine a society whose citizens are healthier, longer-lived, livelier, freer, more competent, better educated, more productive, better accomplished, and happier than they have ever been in any society now known, including our own. Many more human beings—now biologically better equipped, aided by performance-enhancers, and more liberated from the constraints of nature and fortune—might someday live on a much higher human plane than has hitherto been possible save for very few people. This rosy picture of the future, encouraged by our past successes, cannot be lightly gainsaid.

Yet, as we have suggested throughout this report, there are reasons to expect more mixed or even unattractive outcomes. For example, there are risks—small in today's United States—of a sex-unbalanced society, the result of unrestrained free choice in selecting the sex of children; or of a change-resisting gerontocracy, with the "elders" still young in body but old and tired in outlook. And there are still uglier possibilities: an increasingly stratified and inegalitarian society, now with purchased biological enhancements, with enlarged gaps between the over-privileged few and the under-privileged many; a society of narcissists focused on personal satisfaction and self-regard, with little concern for the next generation or the common good; a society of social conformists but with shallow attachments, given over to cosmetic fashions and trivial pursuits; or a society of fiercely competitive individuals, caught up in an ever-spiraling struggle to get ahead, using the latest biotechnical assistance both to perform better and to deal with the added psychic stress.

Lacking prophetic powers, we will not hazard any guesses as to which of these prospects is more likely to be our future. Up until now, such visionary work has been best left to the imaginative gifts of science fiction writers, who, more than everyone else, have thought seriously aboutwhere biotechnology may be taking us, for better and for worse. From now on, however, we will do well to pay attention to this matter, devising the sorts of social indicators and empirical research that could teach us which way the social and cultural winds are blowing.

But if we can only dimly perceive our possible or likely futures, we can clearly recognize some features of contemporary American life that will, almost certainly, exercise great influence over the future that is likely to emerge. Among them we would identify the importance of commerce, the practice of medicine, and the ruling ideals and ethos of the American polity. They are already playing major roles in determining which of the many possible social futures our grandchildren and great-grandchildren will inherit.

A. Commerce, Regulation, and the Manufacture of Desire

Whether one likes it or not, progress in biology and biotechnology is now intimately bound up with industry and commerce. Although the federal government is still the major sponsor of biomedical research, more and more scientists work in partnership with industry. And the emergence of a vigorous biotech industry, growing rapidly even before it has delivered very much of its great promise, is a sign of things to come. Whatever one finally thinks about the relative virtues and vices of contemporary capitalism, it is a fact that progress in science and technology owes much to free enterprise. The possibility of gain adds the fuel of interest to the fire of genius, and even as the profits accrue only to some, the benefits are, at least in principle, available to all. And the competition to succeed provides enormous incentives to innovation, growth, and progress. We have every reason to expect exponential increases in biotechnologies and, therefore, in their potential uses in all aspects of human life.

Two aspects of the marriage between biotechnology and free-market commerce pose challenges to our ability to keep control of how those powers will be used. First, scientists and entrepreneurs, for perfectly understandable reasons, want no interference with research or development. Freedom to experiment is essential to discovery; freedom to invent and to market is essential to technological advance. Distrustful of governmental regulation and leery of public scrutiny of their activities, biologists and technologists are especially inclined to resist legal limitations that might be imposed on their activities based on ethical considerations. Like those who would prefer to "go slow," they vigorously make their interests felt in the deliberations of government. Yet in the long run, as members of American society, they have as much to gain or lose as anyone else from the kind of society that their own efforts are helping to create. What sort of society it will be will depend in part on whether industry and the broader public will collaborate in finding ways to monitor and regulate the uses of biotechnology beyond therapy.

Entrepreneurs not only resist governmental limitation of their work or restrictions on the uses to which their products may be put. They also promote public demand. The success of enterprise often turns on anticipating and stimulating consumer demand, sometimes even on creating it where none exists. Suitably stimulated, the demand of consumers for easier means to better-behaved children, more youthful or beautiful or potent bodies, keener or more focused minds, and steadier or more cheerful moods is potentially enormous. If the existing cosmetic industry may be taken as a model, the sky may be the limit for a truly effective "cosmetic pharmacology" that would deliver stronger muscles, better memories, brighter moods, and peace of mind. The direct-to-consumer advertising of pharmaceutical and other companies—for mood-brighteners, fatigue lesseners, youth preservatives, and behavior modifiers—is a harbinger of things to come. Today it is Ritalin, Botox, Rogaine, Viagra, and Prozac; could tomorrow be "Memorase," "Popeye's Potion," "Eroticor," "Self-love," or "Soma"? Desires can be manufactured almost as effectively as pills, especially if the pills work more or less as promised to satisfy the newly stimulated desires. By providing quick solutions for short-term problems or prompt fulfillment of easily satisfied desires, the character of human longing itself could be altered, with large aspirations for long-term flourishing giving way before the immediate gratification of smaller desires. What to do about this is far from clear; but its importance should not be underestimated.

B. Medicine, Medicalization, and a Stance "Beyond Therapy"

Wherever they may be invented and manufactured, most new biotechnologies, including those serving goals beyond therapy, will probably enter ordinary use through the offices of the medical profession. Should this occur, the pursuit of happiness and self-perfection would become part of the doctor's business, joining many other aspects of human life that formerly had little to do with doctors and hospitals: childbirth, infertility, sexual mores and practices, aspects of criminal behavior, alcoholism, abnormal behavior, anxiety, stress, dementia, old age, death, grief, and mourning—all these have over the past century been at least partially medicalized, and often with good reasons and welcome results.* The causes of medicalization are many, among them, the power of modern biological explanation and technique; the growth in medical knowledge and competence; the expanding domain of psychiatry, the "doctoring of the psyche"; increased success using medical interventions; and rising patient expectations of cure, relief, and salvation coming from health care professionals. It is also driven by deep cultural and intellectual currents, for example, to see more and more things in life not as natural givens to be coped with but as objects rightly subject to our mastery and control; to have compassion for victims, even when the victims are victimized by

---

* "Medicalization," a term coined by sociologists, means in the first instance a way of thinking and conceiving human phenomena in medical terms, which then guides ways of acting and organizing social institutions. More fully, it is the tendency to *conceive* an activity, phenomenon, condition, behavior, etc., as a disease or disorder or as an affliction that should be regarded as a disease or disorder: (1) people *suffer* it (the essence of patient-hood) or it befalls them; they are *victims* of it, hence not responsible for it; (2) the causes are *physical* or *somatic*, not "mental" or "spiritual" or "psychic"; (3) it requires (needs) and demands (has a claim to) *treatment*, aimed at *cure* or at least relief and abatement of symptoms; (4) at the hands of persons trained in the healing arts and licensed as *healers*; and (5) this conception of the condition will be supported by the society, which will also support efforts at treatment out of its interest in the *health* (as opposed to the morals or the education) of its people. The term is used—both in the literature and by us here— as neutral description, without any implied judgment. We have discussed medicalization of mental life briefly in Chapter Five.

their own foolish conduct; to see the human person not in spiritual or moral terms, but as a highly complex and successful product of blind evolutionary forces (which still perturb him through no fault of his own); and—very important—the acceptance of "health" as the one readily recognized and utterly uncontroversial human good (in contrast, say, with virtue, morality, or wisdom). With the decline in the cultural authority of religious institutions, and with the shrinking of other communal systems of help and support for people in difficulty, physicians often find themselves simply "neighbor to the problem." Rightly extending a helping hand, they often conceive and treat the problems they encounter in a purely medical fashion.

As new biotechnologies appear, with novel uses beyond therapy, the tendency toward medicalization will almost certainly be strengthened, both as a matter of practice and as a matter of thought. Physicians are the gatekeepers of biomedical technologies. They are judges of proper use. They are aware of dangerous side effects. They prescribe and dispense as they see fit. The medical profession is clothed in venerable ethical dress; in the United States there are also professional standards of good practice that offer guidance and principles of reimbursement that set limits on free professional and patient choices. Nevertheless, the practice of medicine is highly decentralized, and each physician has enormous discretion in dealing with patients, able to adapt general practices to the special needs and circumstances of each individual. All this is comforting and reassuring, more so than if the new biotechnical powers were wielded by an upstart group of technicians lacking these professional assets and virtues.

But there are difficulties when medical practice moves beyond therapy. Where the goal is restoring health, the doctor's discretion is guided by an agreed-upon and recognizable target. But a physician prescribing for goals beyond therapy is in uncharted waters. Although fully armed with the means, he has no special expertise regarding the end—neither what it is nor whether it is desirable. To the extent that the patient is transformed from a sick person needing healing into a consumer of technical services, medicine will be transformed from a profession into a trade and the doctor-patient relationship into a species of contract, ungoverned by any deep ethical norms. Should this occur, the medical profession and the health care system will be called upon to practice retail sanity regarding the technologies and wholesale madness regarding the ends, the costs, and the possible consequences of their use. The health-care system in the United States already constitutes roughly one-sixth of the gross national product. What might it become in the coming age beyond therapy?

There is yet a second and perhaps more fundamental danger in the growth of medicalization, a danger of thinking and outlook whose consequences could well be profound. The therapeutic intention at the heart of medicine—the goal of making whole that which is broken or disabled—runs the risk of looking increasingly upon the entire human condition in this way and, as a result, of regarding biotechnological measures as the royal road to improving our lot in life. Two opposing dangers need to be avoided. On the one hand, there is the risk of viewing everything in human life—not only human frailties, disappointments, and death itself, but also human relationships, pride and shame, love and sorrow, and all self-discontent—under the lens of disease and disability. Such a tendency would encourage everywhere the idea of human life as "victimhood" in need of rescue; it would discourage everywhere the idea that human beings are responsible agents and, at their best, noble creatures aspiring to and capable of genuine excellence and flourishing. On the other hand, there is the risk of attacking human limitation altogether, seeking to produce a more-than-human being, one not only without illnesses, but also without foibles, fatigue, failures, or foolishness.[*]

Seen against these problematic temptations, the remedy for the dangers lurking in the drift toward greater medicalization and "beyond therapy" is, paradoxically, to be found in rethinking the very idea of "beyond therapy." It is to be found in adopting a standpoint toward human life that is, in another sense of the term, radically *beyond* therapy. It does not start with medicine to discover the terrain that lies beyond the goals of medicine. It looks beyond the therapeutic view of life altogether. It rejects and goes beyond the "therapy versus enhancement" distinction for a reason deeper than those we gave at the outset of this report (see Chapter One): for medicine, sickness, and healing are not the natural or best lens

---

[*] Or without birthmarks, the superficial sign of being marked from birth as finite and frail. See Nathaniel Hawthorne, "The Birth-mark."

through which to look upon the whole of human life. Health, though a primary human good, is not the only—or even the supreme—human good.

Going "beyond therapy" in this sense means returning to an account of the human being seen not in material or mechanistic or medical terms but in psychic and moral and spiritual ones. It is to see the human being as a creature "in-between," neither god nor beast, neither dumb body nor disembodied soul, but as a puzzling, upward-pointing unity of psyche and soma whose precise limitations are the source of its—our—loftiest aspirations, whose weaknesses are the source of its—our—keenest attachments, and whose natural gifts may be, if we do not squander or destroy them, exactly what we need to flourish and perfect ourselves—*as human beings.* Readers, we hope, will recognize that this entire report has been written from this more-than-therapeutic perspective and with this richly humanistic intent.

C. Biotechnology and American Ideals

The significance of these two prominent features of American life—the power of free markets and the prestige of medicine—points us also toward a greater understanding of the implications of our new biotechnical powers for our American ideals. In a certain sense, as a people committed to life, liberty, and the pursuit of happiness, we may tend to be especially drawn to the promise of biotechnology. Some of the techniques we have discussed offer the prospect of longer and livelier life, of expanded liberty made possible by improved abilities and powers, and of a more successful and fulfilling pursuit of happiness. Medicine thrives in a culture that values life; science and enterprise thrive in a society that values freedom; technology flourishes in a nation eager to make life more prosperous and comfortable.

And yet, these very ideals also offer reasons to moderate the desires that drive us toward greater biotechnological prowess, and to look upon new possibilities through the lens of a rich yet temperate understanding of the human condition. Even as they encourage progress, the American principles may serve to moderate a dangerous utopianism. Our devotion to life is understood in light of the human dedication to *the good life,* and so calls for reflection on our most basic priorities, and on just what it is that gives life its significance. Our aspiration to liberty is grounded in some sense that we men and women are the beings deserving of liberty, and capable of using it well. It reminds us, also, that our actions always run the risk of curtailing the freedom of others, including especially that of future generations—to whom we owe the same liberty passed down to us. And our nation's declared commitment to the pursuit of happiness— understood in light of our devotion to life, and our dedication to meaningful liberty—invites us to consider the nature (and also the limits) of happiness, and to wonder what sort of happiness a people so devoted and dedicated might rightly pursue.

But these American ideals, and the character of the nation they have helped to shape, moderate not only our hopes but also our fears. The reservations we have raised in this report are the worries of a free and decent people—concerned for its character and its goodness and its soul. Had we looked only at the perils of the technologies that seem to lie in our future, and had we sought to imagine the worst, it would not have been difficult to raise up specters of terrifying and inhuman violations, or of an unprecedented despotism of man over man, with powerful new technologies serving as the whips of new slave-masters. The recent history of the human race offers no dearth of sources for such nightmarish visions. But that is not what we perceive when we peer over the horizon, because our society, dedicated as it is to life and liberty and happiness, is always alert to repel such excesses.

Rather, the concerns we have raised here emerge from a sense that tremendous new powers to serve certain familiar and often well-intentioned desires may blind us to the larger meaning of our ideals, and may narrow our sense of what it is to live, to be free, and to seek after happiness. If, by informing and moderating our desires and by grasping the limits of our new powers, we can keep in mind the meaning of our founding ideals, then we just might find the means to savor some fruits of the age of biotechnology, without succumbing to its most dangerous temptations.

To do so, we must first understand just what is at stake, and we must begin to imagine what the age of biotechnology might bring, and what human life in that age could look like. In these pages, we have sought to begin that vital project, in the hope that these first steps might spark and inform a public debate, so that however the nation proceeds, it will do so with its eyes wide open.

ENDNOTES

[1] This discussion depends heavily on a paper by Michael J. Sandel, "What's Wrong with Enhancement," prepared for the President's Council on Bioethics, Washington, D.C., December 12, 2002. Copy available at the Council's website, www.bioethics.gov.

[2] The discussion that follows depends heavily on a paper by Leon R. Kass, "Beyond Therapy: Biotechnology and the Pursuit of Human Improvement," prepared for the President's Council on Bioethics, Washington, D.C., January 16, 2003. Copy available at the Council's website at www.bioethics.gov.

[3] See, for example, Jonas, H., "The Blessings and Burdens of Mortality," *Hastings Center Report*, January/February 1992; Kass, L., "*L'Chaim* and Its Limits: Why Not Immortality," in *Life, Liberty, and the Defense of Dignity: The Challenge for Bioethics*, San Francisco: Encounter Books, 2002.

BIBLIOGRAPHY

Abraham, C. "Gene Pioneer Urges Human Perfection." *Toronto Globe and Mail,* 26 October 2002.

American College Health Association. *National College Health Assessment: Reference Group Executive Summary Spring 2002.* Baltimore: American College Health Association, 2002.

American Psychiatric Association. *Diagnostic and Statistical Manual of Mental Disorders.* Fourth Edition. Text Revision ["DSM-IV-TR"]. Washington, D.C.: American Psychiatric Association, 2000.

American Society for Reproductive Medicine (Ethics Committee). "Preconception Gender Selection for Nonmedical Reasons." *Fertility and Sterility* 75: 5, 2001.

American Society for Reproductive Medicine (Ethics Committee). "Sex Selection and Preimplantation Genetic Diagnosis." *Fertility and Sterility* 72: 4, 1999.

Angold, A., et al. "Stimulant treatment for children: A community perspective." *Journal of the American Academy of Child and Adolescent Psychiatry* 39: 975-984, 2000.

Aristotle. *Nicomachean Ethics.*

Aristotle. *Rhetoric.* trans. L. Cooper, Englewood Cliffs, N.J.: Prentice-Hall, 1960.

Asakura, A., et al. "Muscle satellite cells are multipotential stem cells that exhibit myogenic, osteogenic, and adipogenic differentiation." *Differentiation* 68(4-5): 245-253, 2001.

Austad, S. "Adding Years to Life: Current Knowledge and Future Prospects." Presentation at the President's Council on Bioethics, Washington, D.C. (www.bioethics.gov), 12 December 2002.

Austen, Jane. *Mansfield Park*, 1814.

Baard, E. "The Guilt-Free Soldier." *Village Voice*, 28 January 2003.

Barbaresi, W., et al. "How common is attention-deficit/hyperactivity disorder? Incidence in a population-based birth cohort in Rochester, Minnesota." *Archives of Pediatric and Adolescent Medicine* 156: 217-224, 2002.

Barondes, S. *Better Than Prozac: The Future of Psychiatric Drugs.* Oxford: Oxford University Press, 2003.

Barton-Davis, E., et al. "Viral mediated expression of insulin-like growth factor I blocks the aging-related loss of skeletal muscle function." *Proceedings of the National Academy of Sciences* 95(26): 15603-15607, 1998.

Benetos, A., et al. "Telomere length as an indicator of biological aging: The gender effect and relation with pulse pressure and pulse wave velocity." *Hypertension* 37(2): 381-385, 2001.

Biederman, J., et al. "Pharmacotherapy of Attention-Deficit Hyperactivity Disorder Reduces Risk for Substance Use Disorder." *Pediatrics* 104: e20, 1999.

Blackburn, E. "Telomere states and cell fates." *Nature* 408(6808): 53-56, 2000.

Borges, J. "Funes the Memorious" in *Ficciones,* ed. John Sturrock, 1942 [English translation, Grove Press, 1962; reprinted by Knopf/Everyman, 1993].

Bradley, C. "The Behavior of Children Receiving Benzedrine." *American Journal of Psychiatry* 94: 577-585, 1937.

Braude, P., et al. "Preimplantation Genetic Diagnosis." *Nature Review Genetics* 3(12): 941-953, December 2002. (See also erratum, *Nature Review Genetics* 4(2): 157, February 2003.)

Braun, S. *The Science of Happiness: Unlocking the Mysteries of Mood.* New York: John Wiley & Sons, 2000.

Brown, W. "A method for estimating the number of motor units in thenar muscles and the changes in motor unit count with aging." *Journal of Neurology, Neurosurgery, and Psychology* 35: 845-852, 1972.

Cahill, L., et al. "Beta-Adrenergic activation and memory for emotional events." *Nature* 371: 702-704, 1994.

Castellanos F., et al. "Anatomic brain abnormalities in monozygotic twins discordant for attention-deficit hyperactivity disorder." *American Journal of Psychiatry* 160(9): 1693-1696, 2003.

Castellanos, F., et al. "Neuroscience of Attention-Deficit/Hyperactivity Disorder: The Search for Endophenotypes." *Nature Reviews Neuroscience* 3: 617-628, 2002.

Cawthon, R., et al. "Association between telomere length in blood and mortality in people aged 60 years or older." *Lancet* 361(9355): 393-395, 2003.

Chan, A., et al. "Foreign DNA transmission by ICSI: injection of spermatozoa bound with exogenous DNA results in embryonic GFP expression and live rhesus monkey births." *Molecular Human Reproduction* 6(1): 26-33, 2000.

Cohen, E. "Our Psychotropic Memory." SEED, no. 8, Fall 2003.

Collins, F. "Genetic Enhancements: Current and Future Prospects." Presentation at the President's Council on Bioethics, Washington, D.C. (www.bioethics.gov), 13 December 2002.

Coyle, J. "Psychotropic drug use in very young children." *Journal of the American Medical Association*, 283(8): 1059–1060, 2000.

Cuttler, L., et al., "Short stature and growth hormone therapy: a national study of physician recommendation patterns." *Journal of the American Medical Association* 276: 531-537, 1996.

Davis, D. *Genetic Dilemmas: Reproductive Technology, Parental Choices, and Children's Futures.* New York: Routledge, 2001.

DeGrandre, R. *Ritalin Nation: Rapid-Fire Culture and the Transformation of Human Consciousness.* New York: Norton, 1999.

Descartes, R. *Discourse on the Method of Conducting One's Reason Well and Seeking Truth in the Sciences,* 1637.

Descartes, R. *The Passions of the Soul,* 1649.

Diller, L. "Prescription Stimulant Use in American Children: Ethical Issues." Presentation at the President's Council on Bioethics, Washington, D.C. (www.bioethics.gov), 12 December 2002.

Diller, L. *Running on Ritalin: A Physician Reflects on Children, Society and Performance on a Pill.* New York: Bantam Books, 1998.

Dillin, A., et al. "Rates of behavior and aging specified by mitochondrial function during development." *Science* 298(5602): 2398-2401, 2002.

Dillin, A., et al., "Timing requirements for insulin/IGF-1 signaling in C. elegans." Science 298(5594): 830-834, 2002.

Dunlop, S., et al. "Pattern Analysis Shows Beneficial Effect of Fluoxetine Treatment in Mild Depression." *Psychopharmacology Bulletin* 26: 173-180, 1990.

Eberstadt, N. "Choosing the Sex of Children: Demographics." Presentation at the President's Council on Bioethics, Washington, D.C. (www.bioethics.gov), 17 October 2002.

Eberstadt, M. "Why Ritalin Rules." *Policy Review* 94, April/May 1999.

Elliott, C. *Better Than Well: American Medicine Meets the American Dream.* New York: Norton, 2003.

Enge, M. "Ad Seeks Donor Eggs for $100,000, Possible New High." *Chicago Tribune,* 10 February 2000.

Eriksson, M., et al. "Recurrent de novo point mutations in lamin A cause Hutchinson-Gilford progeria syndrome." *Nature* 423: 293-298, 2003.

Fletcher, J. "Ethics and Amniocentesis for Fetal Sex Identification." *Hastings Center Report,* 10(1): 16, 1980.

Fried, S. "Addicted to Antidepressants? The Controversy Over a Pill Millions of Us Are Taking." *Glamour*, April 2003.

Fukuyama, F. *Our Posthuman Future: Consequences of the Biotechnology Revolution.* New York: Farrar, Straus and Giroux, 2002.

Gates, D. "The Case of Dr. Strangedrug." *Newsweek*, 19 June 1993.

German National Ethics Council. *Genetic diagnosis before and during pregnancy: opinion.* Berlin: Nationaler Ethikrat, 2003.

Glader, P. "From the Maker of Effexor: Campus Forums on Depression." *Wall Street Journal*, 10 October 2002, p. B1.

Gladwell, M. "The Sporting Scene: Drugstore Athlete." *New Yorker*, 10 September 2001.

Glass, B. "Science: Endless Horizons or Golden Age?" *Science*, 171: 23-29, 1971.

Goodman, E. "Matter Over Mind?" *Washington Post*, 16 November 2002.

Hancock, L. "Mother's Little Helper." *Newsweek*, 18 March 1996.

Hardin, G. "The Tragedy of the Commons." *Science* 162: 1243-1248, 1968.

Hawthorne, N. "The Birth-mark," in *Nathaniel Hawthorne, Tales and Sketches*, ed. R. Pearce. New York: Library of America, 1982. (Originally published in *Twice-Told Tales*, 1843.)

Healy, D. *The Antidepressant Era.* Cambridge, MA: Harvard, 1997.

Homer, *The Odyssey*.

Hübner, K., et al. "Derivation of oocytes from mouse embryonic stem cells." *Science* 300(5620): 1251-1256, 2003.

Huxley, A. *Brave New World*, Norwalk, CT: Easton Press, 1978. (First published 1932.)

Hyman, S. "Pediatric Psychopharmacology." Presentation at the President's Council on Bioethics, Washington, D.C. (www.bioethics.gov), 6 March 2003.

Jonas, H. "The Burden and Blessing of Mortality." *Hastings Center Report* 22(1): 24-40, January/February 1992.

Juengst, E. "What does *enhancement* mean?" in E. Parens, ed., *Enhancing Human Traits: Ethical and Social Implications.* Washington, D.C.: Georgetown University Press, 1998, pp. 29-47.

Kass, L. "Beyond Therapy: Biotechnology and the Pursuit of Human Improvement." Paper prepared for the President's Council on Bioethics, Washington, D.C. (www.bioethics.gov), 16 January 2003.

Kass, L. "*L'Chaim* and Its Limits: Why Not Immortality" in *Life, Liberty, and the Defense of Dignity: The Challenge for Bioethics.* San Francisco, CA: Encounter Books, 2002.

Kessler, R., et al. "Posttraumatic Stress Disorder in the National Comorbidity Survey." *Archives of General Psychiatry* 52(12): 1048-1060, 1995.

Klam, M. "Experiencing Ecstasy." *New York Times Magazine*, 21 January 2001.

Klerman, G., et al. "Increasing rates of depression." *Journal of the American Medical Association* 261(15): 2229-2235, 1989.

Knutson, B., et al. "Selective Alteration of Personality and Social Behavior by Serotonergic Intervention." *American Journal of Psychiatry* 155: 373-379, 1998.

Kramer, P. "Happiness and Sadness: Depression and the Pharmacological Elevation of Mood." Presentation at the President's Council on Bioethics, Washington, D.C. (www.bioethics.gov), 12 September 2002.

Kramer, P. *Listening to Prozac.* Second edition. New York: Penguin, 1997.

Kramer, P. "The Valorization of Sadness: Alienation and the Melancholic Temperament." *Hastings Center Report* 30(2): 13-18, 2000.

Kulka, R., et al. *Trauma and the Vietnam War Generation: Report of Findings from the National Vietnam Veterans Readjustment Study.* New York: Brunner/Mazel, 1990.

Lane, M., et al. "The Serious Search for an Anti-Aging Pill." *Scientific American* 287(2): 36-41, 2002.

Langer, G. "Use of Anti-Depressants Is a Long-Term Practice." Abcnews.go.com. 10 April 2003.

Langreth, R. "Viagra for the Brain." *Forbes,* 4 February 2002.

Lewis, C. S. *The Abolition of Man.* New York: Macmillan, 1965.

LeDoux, J. "Emotion, Memory, and the Brain." *Scientific American* 270, 32-39, 1994.

Liotti, M., et al. "Differential Limbic-Cortical Correlates of Sadness and Anxiety in Healthy Subjects: Implications for Affective Disorders." *Biological Psychiatry* 48: 30-42, 2000.

Locke, J. *Essay Concerning Human Understanding.* 1690.

Luria, A. *The Mind of a Mnemonist: A little book about a vast memory,* trans. L. Solotaroff. New York: Basic Books, 1968.

Mandavilli, A. "Fertility's new frontier takes shape in a test tube." *Nature Medicine* 9(8): 1095, 2003.

Marshall, E. "Gene Therapy a Suspect in Leukemia-like Disease." *Science* 298: 34, 2002.

Marshall, E. "Second Child in French Trial Is Found to Have Leukemia." *Science* 299: 320, 2003.

McGaugh, J. "Emotional Activation, Neuromodulatory Systems and Memory" in D. Schacter, et al., eds., *Memory Distortion: How Minds, Brains, and Societies Reconstruct the Past.* Cambridge, MA: Harvard University Press, 1995, pp. 255-273.

McGaugh, J. "Enhancing Cognitive Performance." *Southern California Law Review* 65(1): 383-395, 1991.

McGaugh, J. "Memory consolidation and the amygdala: a system perspective." *Trends in Neuroscience* 25(9): 456-461, 2002.

McGaugh, J. "Remembering and Forgetting: Physiological and Pharmacological Aspects." Presentation at the President's Council on Bioethics, Washington, D.C. (www.bioethics.gov), 17 October 2002.

McGaugh, J. "Significance and Remembrance: The Role of Neuromodulatory Systems." *Psychological Science* 1: 15-25, 1990.

McHugh, P., et al. *The Perspectives of Psychiatry.* Baltimore: Johns Hopkins, 1998.

Meilaender, G. "Why Remember?" *First Things* No. 135: 20-24, August/September 2003.

Montaigne, M. "That to Philosophize Is to Learn to Die" in *The Complete Essays of Michel Montaigne,* trans. D. Frame. Stanford, CA: Stanford University Press, 1965.

Murphy, C., et al. "Genes that act downstream of DAF-16 to influence the lifespan of Caenorhabditis elegans." *Nature* 424: 277-283, 2003.

Musaro, A., et al. "Localized Igf-1 transgene expression sustains enlargement and regeneration in senescent skeletal muscle." *Nature Genetics* 27: 195-200, 2001.

National Human Genome Research Institute. "News Release: Researchers Identify Gene for Premature Aging." Washington, D.C.: National Institutes of Health (www.genome.gov), 16 April 2003.

National Institute of Mental Health. *Medication.* Washington, D.C.: NIH Publication No. 02-3929, 2002.

National Institute of Mental Health. *The Numbers Count: Mental Disorders in America.* Washington, D.C.: NIH Publication No. 01-4584, 2003.

National Research Council/National Academy of Sciences, Committee on Life Sciences and Social Policy. *Assessing Biomedical Technologies: An Inquiry into the Nature of the Process.* Washington, D.C.: National Academy of Sciences, 1975.

National Science Foundation. *Converging Technologies for Improving Human Performance: Nanotechnology, Biotechnology, Information Technology and Cognitive Science.* Arlington, VA: National Science Foundation, 2003.

Nestler, E., et al. "Neurobiology of Depression." *Neuron* 34: 13-25, 2002.

Olshansky, S., et al. "No Truth to the Fountain of Youth." *Scientific American*, June 2002, pp. 92-95.

Owino, V., et al. "Age-related loss of skeletal muscle function and the ability to express the autocrine form of insulin-like growth factor-1 (MGF) in response to mechanical overload." *FEBS Letters* 505: 259-263, 2001.

Parens, E., ed. *Enhancing Human Traits: Ethical and Social Implications.* Washington, D.C.: Georgetown University Press, 1998.

Pinker, S. *The Blank Slate: The Modern Denial of Human Nature.* New York: Viking, 2002.

Pinker, S. "Human Nature and Its Future." Presentation at the President's Council on Bioethics, Washington, D.C. (www.bioethics.gov), 6 March 2003.

Pitman, R., et al. "Pilot Study of Secondary Prevention of Posttraumatic Stress Disorder with Propranolol." *Biological Psychiatry* 51: 189-192, 2002.

Plato. "Symposium," trans. S. Benardete, in *The Dialogues of Plato.* New York: Bantam Books, 1986.

Powledge, T., and J. Fletcher. "A Report from the Genetics Research Group of Hastings Center Institute of Society, Ethics, and Life Sciences." *New England Journal of Medicine* 300(4): 168-172, 1979.

President's Commission for the Study of Ethical Problems in Medicine and Biomedical and Behavioral Research. *Screening and Counseling for Genetic Conditions: A Report on the Ethical, Social, and Legal Implications of Genetic Screening, Counseling, and Education Programs.* Washington, D.C.: Government Printing Office, 1983.

President's Council on Bioethics. *Human Cloning and Human Dignity: An Ethical Inquiry.* Washington, D.C.: Government Printing Office, 2002. *Human Cloning and Human Dignity: The Report of the President's Council on Bioethics.* New York: PublicAffairs, 2002.

Qu-Peterson, Z., et al. "Identification of a novel population of muscle stem cells in mice: potential for muscle regeneration." *Journal of Cell Biology* 157(5): 851-864, 2002.

Ramsey, J., et al. "Dietary restriction and aging in rhesus monkeys: the University of Wisconsin study." *Experimental Gerontology* 35(9-10):1131-1149, 2000.

Rapoport, J., et al. "Dextroamphetamine: its cognitive and behavioral effects in normal and hyperactive boys and normal men." *Archives of General Psychiatry* 37: 933-943, 1980.

Riddle, M., et al. "Pediatric Psychopharmacology." *Journal of Child Psychology and Psychiatry* 42(1): 73-90, 2001.

Rose, S. "'Smart drugs': do they work, are they ethical, will they be legal?" *Nature Reviews Neuroscience* 3: 975-979, 2002.

Rosenberg, I. "Summary Comments." *American Journal of Clinical Nutrition* 50: 1231-1233, 1989.

Rosenberg, L. "Brainsick: A Physician's Journey to the Brink." *Cerebrum* 4: 43-60, 2002.

Roubenoff, R., et al. "Sarcopenia: Current concepts." *The Journals of Gerontology, Biological and Medical Sciences,* Series A, 55A, M716-M724, 2000.

Rousseau, J.-J. "Discourse on the Origin and Foundations of Inequality (Second Discourse)," trans. R. and J. Masters, in *The First and Second Discourses,* ed. R. Masters. New York: St. Martin's Press, 1964.

Rudman, D., et al. "Effects of human growth hormone in men over sixty years old." *New England Journal of Medicine* 323: 1-5, 1990.

St. Augustine. *The Confessions of St. Augustine,* trans. J. Pilkington. Norwalk, CT: Easton Press, 1979.

Sandel, M. "What's Wrong with Enhancement." Paper prepared for the President's Council on Bioethics, Washington, D.C. (www.bioethics.gov), 12 December 2002.

Santarelli, L., et al. "Requirement of Hippocampal Neurogenesis for the Behavioral Effects of Antidepressants." *Science* 301: 805-809, 2003.

Sapolsky, R. "Will We Still Be Sad Fifty Years from Now?" in J. Brockman, ed. *The Next Fifty Years: Science in the First Half of the Twenty-First Century.* New York: Vintage, 2002.

Schacter, D. "Remembering and Forgetting: Physiological and Pharmacological Aspects." Presentation at the President's Council on Bioethics, Washington, D.C. (www.bioethics.gov), 17 October 2002.

Schacter, D. *The Seven Sins of Memory: How the Mind Forgets and Remembers.* New York: Houghton Mifflin, 2001.

Schatten, G., "Assisted Reproductive Technologies in the Genomics Era." Presentation at the President's Council on Bioethics, Washington, D.C. (www.bioethics.gov), 13 December 2002.

Science Magazine. "Random Samples." *Science* 290(5500): 2249, 22 December 2000.

Shakespeare, W. *King Henry the Fourth, Part 2.*

Shakespeare, W. *A Midsummer Night's Dream.*

Sheline, Y., et al. "Hippocampal atrophy in recurrent major depression." *Proceedings of the National Academy of Sciences* 93: 3908-3913, 1996.

Silver, L. *Remaking Eden.* New York: Avon Books, Inc., 1998.

Simpson, J., et al. "Sex Selection" in C. De Jonge and C. Barratt, eds., *Assisted Reproductive Technologies: Current Accomplishments and New Horizons.* Cambridge, U.K.: Cambridge University Press, 2002, pp. 384-396.

Sinsheimer, R., "The Prospect of Designed Genetic Change." *Engineering and Science Magazine,* California Institute of Technology, April 1969.

Slater, L. "Prozac Mother and Child." *New York Times Magazine,* 17 October 1999, pp. 15-17.

Smalley, S., et al. "Genetic linkage of attention-deficit hyperactivity disorder on chromosome 16p13, in a region implicated in autism." *American Journal of Human Genetics* 71: 959-963, 2002.

Stock, G. *Redesigning Humans: Our Inevitable Genetic Future.* New York: Houghton Mifflin, 2002.

Sweeney, H. L. "Genetic Enhancement of Muscle." Presentation at the President's Council on Bioethics, Washington, D.C. (www.bioethics.gov), 13 September 2002.

Swift, J. *Gulliver's Travels*, 1726.

Tsien, J., et al. "Genetic enhancement of learning and memory in mice." *Nature* 401: 63-69, 2 September 1999.

Tzankoff, S., et al. "Effect of Muscle Mass on Age-Related BMR Changes." *Journal of Applied Physiology* 43: 1001-1006, 1977.

United States Drug Enforcement Administration. *Methylphenidate-/amphetamine yearly production quotas.* Washington, D.C.: Department of Justice, 2000.

Vitiello, B. "Psychopharmacology for young children: Clinical needs and research opportunities." *Pediatrics* 108(4): 983-989, 2001.

Vitiello, B. "Stimulant Treatment for Children: A Community Perspective: Commentary." *Journal of the American Academy of Child and Adolescent Psychiatry* 39: 992-994, 2000.

Vonnegut, K. "Harrison Bergeron" in *Welcome to the Monkey House.* New York: Delacorte, 1968.

Wade, N. "Of Smart Mice and an Even Smarter Man." *New York Times,* 7 September 1999.

Wadman, M. "So You Want a Girl?" *Fortune,* 9 February 2001.

Weber, M. "Effects of growth hormone on skeletal muscle." *Hormone Research* 58(3): 43-48, 2002.

Weindruch, R., et al. *The Retardation of Aging and Disease by Dietary Restriction.* Springfield, Ill.: Charles Thomas Publishers, 1998.

Wheeler, T. "Miracle Molecule, 50 Years On." *Baltimore Sun,* 4 February 2003, p. 8A.

Wilson, J. Q. *The Marriage Problem: How Our Culture Has Weakened Families.* New York: HarperCollins, 2002.

Wolterstorff, N. *Lament for a Son.* Grand Rapids, MI: Eerdman's, 1987.

Yesavage, J., et al. "Donepezil and flight simulator performance: effects on retention of complex skills." *Neurology* 59: 123-125, 9 July 2002.

Zammit, P., et al. "The skeletal muscle satellite cell: stem cell or son of stem cell?" *Differentiation* 68(4-5): 193-204, 2001.

Zito, J., et al. "Psychotropic Practice Patterns for Youth: A 10-Year Perspective." *Archives of Pediatric and Adolescent Medicine* 157: 17-25, 2003.

Zito, J., et al. "Trends in the prescribing of psychotropic medications to preschoolers." *Journal of the American Medical Association* 283: 1025-1030, 2000.

COUNCIL STAFF AND CONSULTANTS

ISBN 0-16-073099-6

9 780160 730993

90000